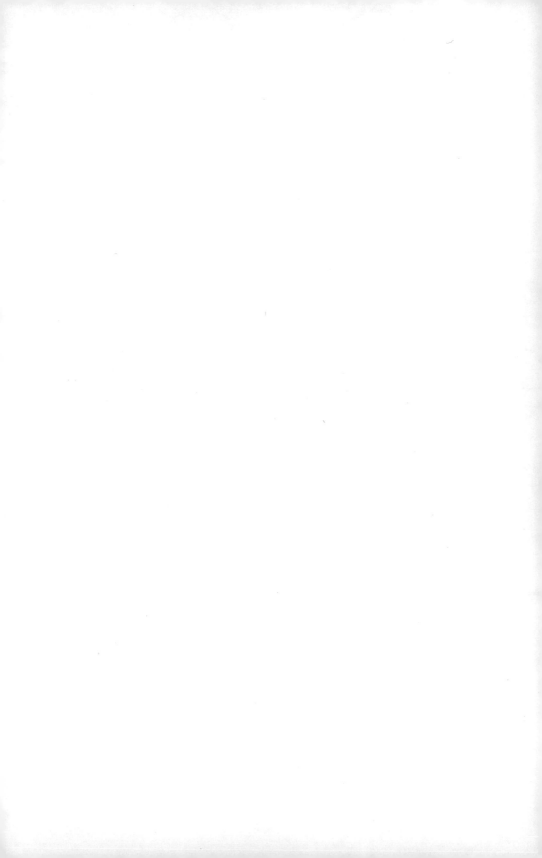

Evaluation of Dysphagia in Adults

FOR CLINICIANS BY CLINICIANS

Deanie Vogel and Michael P. Cannito, Series Editors

This book, *Evaluation of Dysphagia in Adults: Expanding the Diagnostic Options,* is the 11th book in the For Clinicians by Clinicians series of texts on the diagnosis and clinical management of speech, language, and voice disorders. Each text provides a contemporary perspective on one major disorder or clinical area and is designed for use in clinical methodology courses and continuing education programs. Authors have been selected who represent a broad spectrum of clinical interests and theoretical positions and who hold the common belief that their viewpoints, experiences, and successes should be shared in order to provide a forum for clinicians by clinicians.

The idea for this series came from Dr. Harris Winitz, who served as editor of the series until 1997. During Winitz's tenure as series editor, many important titles were added to the series, including the following volumes: *Treating Language Disorders, Treating Articulation Disorders, Case Studies in Aphasia Rehabilitation, Treating Cerebral Palsy, Alaryngeal Speech Rehabilitation, Treating Disordered Speech Motor Control, Cleft Palate,* and *Language Intervention: Beyond the Primary Grades.*

The last three additions to the series, *Aging and Communication, Alaryngeal Speech Rehabilitation,* and this book, have been guided by the new series co-editors, Deanie Vogel and Michael P. Cannito. Their intent is to continue the rich tradition of this important series that was established many years ago by Dr. Winitz.

Evaluation of Dysphagia in Adults

Expanding the Diagnostic Options

For Clinicians by Clinicians

Edited by

Russell H. Mills

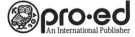

8700 Shoal Creek Boulevard
Austin, Texas 78757-6897
800/897-3202   Fax 800/397-7633
Order online at http://www.proedinc.com

BS

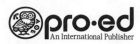

© 2000 by PRO-ED, Inc.
8700 Shoal Creek Boulevard
Austin, Texas 78757-6897
800/897-3202   Fax 800/397-7633
Order online at http://www.proedinc.com

Library of Congress Cataloging-in-Publication Data

Evaluation of dysphagia in adults : expanding the diagnostic options / edited by Russell
H. Mills.
     p.   cm.—(For clinicians by clinicians)
    Includes bibliographical references and index.
    ISBN 0-89079-836-2 (alk. paper)
    1. Deglutition disorders—Diagnosis.   I. Mills, Russell H.   II. Series.
RC815.2.C58   2000
616.3'1—dc21   99-039484

This book is designed in Eras and Palatino.

Production Director: Alan Grimes
Production Coordinator: Dolly Fisk Jackson
Managing Editor: Chris Olson
Art Director: Thomas Barkley
Designer: Jason Crosier
Print Buyer: Alicia Woods
Preproduction Coordinator: Chris Anne Worsham
Staff Copyeditor: Martin Wilson
Project Editor: Debra Berman
Publishing Assistant: John Means Cooper

Printed in the United States of America

1 2 3 4 5 6 7 8 9 10   04 03 02 01 00

4/18/02

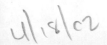

Dedication

This book is dedicated to family and friends, to
Earl who showed me that wisdom is not classroom taught;
Virginia who demonstrated that persistence is truly essential;
Gordon who always provided a benchmark for excellence;
Milt and Dot for giving me a long-term loan of their only daughter;
Dorothy Fosness who wouldn't let the slowest kid in the class give up;
Jennifer whose world flies on wings of compassion;
Joshua whose zest for the joy of life is a reminder of how we should be;
Zachary who reveals to me the beauty of words, both spoken and written;
Molly who without hesitation ventures forth to shape her unique world;
and Janet who has steadfastly endured it all, for her lifelong love and
friendship.

Dedication

Evaluation of Dysphagia in Adults: Expanding the Diagnostic Options is dedicated to Dr. JoAnne Robbins in recognition of her contributions to dysphagia management. While the advancement of this emerging subspecialty is based on the input of a large number of investigators and clinicians, a select few have provided a continuous stream of seminal work that has fundamentally influenced the way we practice. Dr. Robbins is a member of that very august group.

Dr. Robbins serves as the associate director for research of the Geriatric Research, Education and Clinical Center (GRECC) at the William S. Middleton Veterans Affairs Medical Center and as associate professor of the Department of Medicine at the University of Wisconsin. She is director of the combined VA/University of Wisconsin Swallowing Research Laboratory and has served as president of the Dysphagia Research Society. Her investigations have increased clinicians' understanding of the effect of age and age-related disease processes on swallowing, the impact of dysphagia on quality of life, and the short- and long-term effects of the interventions applied. The enduring quality of Dr. Robbins's research is reflected in the fact that her investigations have received continuous funding from the National Institutes of Health since 1983. It is a quality that has changed and will continue to fundamentally change the landscape in dysphagia management.

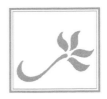

Contents

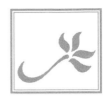

Contributors

Roperto Chua, RRT
Instructor
School of Respiratory Therapy
New York University
New York, NY

Karen J. Dikeman, MA, CCC-SLP
Co-Director
Department of Speech Pathology
New York Hospital Medical Center of
    Queens and Silvercrest Extended
    Care Facility
New York, NY

Jo Edwards, EdD
Adams Chair of Healthcare Excellence
Department of Nursing
Middle Tennessee State University
Murfreesboro, TN

Sue Fleming, PhD
Part-time Faculty
Communication Disorders and
    Sciences
Wayne State University
Detroit, MI

Michael E. Groher, PhD
Clinical Professor
Department of Communicative
    Disorders
University of Florida Health Sciences
    Center
Gainesville, FL

Dianne Hawkins, BS, RT
Consultant Radiology Technician
P.O. Box 345
Smithville, TN 37166

John C. Hudson, DDS, MPH
Chief, Dental Service, Retired
Alvin C. York Veterans Affairs Medical
    Center
Murfreesboro, TN

Marta S. Kazandjian, MA, CCC-SLP
Co-Director
Department of Speech Pathology
New York Hospital Medical Center of
    Queens and Silvercrest Extended
    Care Facility
New York, NY

Bryan Kobylik, MSN
Infection Control Nurse
Alvin C. York Veterans Affairs Medical
    Center
Murfreesboro, TN

Susan E. Langmore, PhD
Chief, Audiology and Speech
    Pathology Service
Veterans Affairs Medical Center
Ann Arbor, MI

Russell H. Mills, PhD
Chief, Audiology and Speech
    Pathology Service
Alvin C. York Veterans Affairs Medical
    Center
Murfreesboro, TN

Virginia Zachary, RD
Clinical Dietitian
Nutrition and Food Services
Alvin C. York Veterans Affairs Medical
    Center
Murfreesboro, TN

Pamela Zenner, MA
Chief, Restorative Services
Veterans Affairs Medical Center
St. Cloud, MN

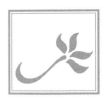

Preface

Although the history of the management of oropharyngeal dysphagia is short, the body of knowledge has increased substantially in the 17 years since Jeri Logemann's (1983) landmark textbook appeared. Some practitioners now find that dysphagia management has become their subspecialty of care, the focal point of their practice. How does it happen that an interest area appears, develops, and matures? Is the developmental process that dysphagia management is undergoing anything more than a random accumulation of clinical observations and assorted research findings? A retrospective view of the much lengthier development of the field of medicine provides some interesting insights, particularly in regard to the importance of diagnostic technologies and methods employed.

Although it is difficult to pinpoint a beginning for medicine, a code for physicians created by Hammurabi, the king of Babylon (1700 B.C.), and the Ebers Papyrus (1500 B.C.) were two landmark documents. The Hammurabi Code outlined what early physicians could treat and established acceptable charges for their services. The Ebers Papyrus was an early document that listed a number of remedies that were appropriate for the common human ailments that physicians encountered. As physicians practiced their profession over the next 3,000 years, a serious limitation persisted. In ancient practice diagnoses were based on patients' perceived symptoms and the degree to which physicians could observe them. Due to the lack of diagnostic techniques, there was little understanding of the causes that produced symptoms. Consequently, symptoms were treated as if they were causal entities. Fever was seen as a disease to be treated rather than as a symptom of an underlying cause. Thus, a physician of that time would be likely to prescribe similar treatments for coughs that had different etiological bases, such as diphtheria, the common cold, and tuberculosis.

Physicians continued to operate with severely limited vision until the dawning of the 18th century. During the 18th and 19th centuries, a flood of technologies emerged that extended physicians' senses to detect abnormalities within the living human organism. For the first time physicians were able to move beyond a description of symptoms to identify the causes of malady. In 1714 Daniel Gabriel Fahrenheit invented the mercury thermometer. Later Carl Wunderlich began to use it as a diagnostic tool and, for the first time, established fever as a symptom and not a disease. In Austria in 1761 Leopold Auenbrugger von Auenbrugg discovered that the presence of fluid in the chest could be detected by gently tapping on the chest wall. Fifty-five years later in France, Rene T. H. Laennec developed the stethoscope and introduced the practice of auscultation. Their developments allowed assessments of pulmonary and cardiac function not possible before. Other diagnostic developments that impacted medical practice in the 1800s included the microscope, ophthalmoscope, spirometer, laryngoscope, and, at the conclusion of the century, Röntgen's X-ray.

The impact that these instruments and technologies had on the practice of medicine was profound. The art and the science of the diagnosis became paramount to practice. Establishing causal relationships became the precursor to treatment. With the developing awareness of the importance of the diagnosis, there was also the realization that a diagnostic error could often have more serious consequences than an error of treatment. Physicians came to appreciate that the most certain route to untoward events was through the treatment of symptoms without developing an understanding the underlying causes.

A distinct parallel can be seen in the evolution of dysphagia management. When performing the dysphagia evaluation, the clinician can detect some of the symptoms of dysphagia even without instrumentation. If the patient coughs on the per oral (PO) intake of thin liquids, the clinician can infer aspiration and treat the symptom. However, the clinical examination can be problematic because, although it reveals symptoms, it may not illuminate the cause. Detection of coughing on PO intake cannot tell the clinician whether it is due to direct aspiration, is a result of penetration, or may be associated with pharyngeal stasis, gastroesophageal reflux, or something else. Also, the absence of a cough in association with aspiration is a common phenomenon and the source for false negative errors when instrumentation is not used. Evaluating dysphagia without the instrumentation needed to determine its causes forces the clinician to operate in a mode not unlike that used by physicians a thousand years ago.

From the preceding discussion the importance of instrumental evaluation to the understanding of dysphagia should be quite clear. Because the field of dysphagia management is evolving at the end of the 20th century, clinicians are advantaged in that a variety of important evaluative technologies have already been invented and perfected. Even though technologies such as X-ray, fluoroscopy, fiberoptics, laboratory assessment, scintigraphy, and others were not developed with the evaluation of swallowing in mind, with procedural focusing they can provide valuable diagnostic information regarding swallowing. Like theologian Mark Toulouse (1997), I am not a proponent of progressive history. Older is not automatically wiser. Things are not automatically better today than they were yesterday. The value of these technologies can be realized only if they are applied with thought and reason. Each has its strengths and limitations that must be appreciated and applied according to the needs of the patient and diagnostic questions that are posed.

Competent diagnostic practice requires knowledge that is, like the Mississippi River, both broad and deep. A broad base of knowledge implies that the dysphagia clinician must be capable of using a variety of diagnostic techniques, choosing the technology that is most appropriate to the diagnostic questions posed and to the patient being studied. Further, the clinician must have an in-depth knowledge of the diagnostic procedures he or she offers. This means that the clinician must offer more than a rote following of a standard protocol. With an in-depth knowledge of a diagnostic technique, the clinician can mold the examination to match the needs of the patient, making appropriate "on-the-fly" changes during the examination in response to the patient's performance. This level of familiarity will allow the underlying causes of the dysphagia symptoms to be revealed and appropriate management recommendations to be proposed.

In graduate-level courses and postgraduate workshops, clinicians are familiarized with the basic diagnostic concepts and tools. Most of this training addresses history taking, the clinical examination, and performing the videofluoroscopic swallowing study (VFSS). While the information that is provided is often sufficient to begin practice, practicing dysphagia clinicians often find themselves in need of more depth of knowledge regarding these central topics. This text provides that in-depth treatment of core diagnostic technologies. Based on extensive clinical experience, Michael Groher (Chapter 1) provides an insightful discussion of the collection and interpretation of case history information as a central part of the dysphagia evaluation. While the clinical examination continues as a core element in the dysphagia evaluation, it has been criticized for its limitations. Pamela Zenner (Chapter 2) discusses the use of an enhanced clinical dysphagia examination that couples the use of meal observation and auscultation as key elements. Russell H. Mills (Chapter 4) discusses the control of study variables to increase the precision of the VFSS procedures that are performed.

The second focus of the text is to familiarize the practicing dysphagia clinician with an array of topics that are important to practice, but usually not fully addressed in core curriculums. Susan Langmore (Chapter 5) provides a clinical orientation into the use of the Fiberoptic Endoscopic Evaluation of Swallowing (FEES). Sue Fleming (Chapter 9) outlines the benefits of scintigraphy, an important technique that can quantify the degree of aspiration that takes place with PO intake. Dysphagic patients who have significant pulmonary problems deserve special consideration and are discussed by Karen Dikeman, Marta Kazandjian, and Roperto Chua (Chapter 8). Virginia Zachary and Russell H. Mills devote a chapter (Chapter 6) to the use and interpretation of laboratory data that allow the clinician to begin to assess the impact of dysphagia on the organism. Finally, the reader is provided with important information about radiology concepts (Jo Edwards and Diane Hawkins in Chapter 3), the dental aspects of swallowing (John Hudson and Russell H. Mills in Chapter 7), and the considerations for infectious disease in dysphagia management (Russell H. Mills and Bryan Kobylik in Chapter 10). With the breadth and depth of information contained within the pages of this text, the practicing dysphagia clinician will be better prepared to evaluate dysphagia and provide appropriate management recommendations for his or her patients.

References

Logemann, J. (1983). *Evaluation and treatment of swallowing disorders.* Austin, TX: PRO-ED.

Toulouse, M. G. (1997). *Joined in discipleship: The shaping of contemporary disciples identity.* St. Louis: Chalice Press.

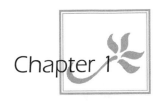

Chapter 1

The Case History

Michael E. Groher

Groher explains how a thorough case history taken from the patient with dysphagia should guide both diagnostic and treatment approaches. He develops a framework of investigation that affords the clinician a maximum amount of data prior to the physical or instrumental swallowing examination.

1. *List the important components in the history of a person who complains of a swallowing disorder.*

2. *Support the listing of the components by briefly commenting on the importance of each in setting the stage for the physical or instrumental swallowing examination.*

3. *Discuss potential differences in obtaining a case history from a patient who complains of solid food dysphagia and one who complains of dysphagia for liquids. Explain how complaints of both solid and liquid dysphagia could develop.*

꙳ ꙳ ꙳

The starting point of the evaluation of the patient with suspected dysphagia should be the case history. Further clinical and instrumental evaluations will be guided by meticulous attention to the details of the patient's complaint and prior medical history related to that complaint.

Students entering the health care arena learn about the importance of the medical history: how it can provide factual data about their patients, how it is integrated into the process of differential diagnosis, and how it might guide the treatments that are provided. In the reality of clinical practice, detailed medical histories are not always available, forcing the examiner to ask the patient or family to provide the necessary details. Details that are missing, incomplete, or unclear may be verified in discussions with the patient or family. Ideally, the examiner will gather data based on the presenting complaint. For the patient with extremity weakness, the examiner may spend more time reviewing neurologic data. For the patient with fainting spells, the examiner may be more interested in past histories related to cardiac function. Similarly, for the patient with a swallowing disorder, the history should be specific enough to fully describe the complaint but broad enough not to overlook an unsuspected etiology.

A thorough medical history can help guide subsequent physical and instrumental evaluations. For instance, patients with past histories of repeated aspiration pneumonias who do not have a recognizable etiology to support this diagnosis may require more extensive instrumental evaluation than the patient who presents with multiple episodes of aspiration with documented radiographic results that support the etiology of the aspiration. Similarly, if a patient's medical history has documented solid food dysphagia and postprandial regurgitation, it may be more appropriate to refer the patient to a gastroenterologist before subjecting the patient to an extensive physical evaluation and expensive instrumental studies that focus on the mouth or pharynx.

Because a majority of patients with neurogenic dysphagia may have accompanying disorders of cognition, the clinician may have difficulty completing a physical evaluation or instrumental study because the patient may be unable to cooperate. In this circumstance, the clinician might have to rely solely on the medical history. If the patient is eating, the clinician should focus the examination on informal observations of the eating circumstance.

Assembling the pieces of the medical history that might relate to dysphagia can be difficult for a number of reasons. First, the time and duration of onset may be difficult to establish. Patients with dysphagia often compensate for their problem for long periods of time before seeking medical attention (Buchholtz, 1987). Patients, therefore, are not always clear about symptom progression and the exact nature of their complaint. Second, the medical record may not document the problem as dysphagia, but use descriptions of other disorders or behaviors that suggest dysphagia, such as "the patient no longer can chew meat," "the patient chokes on his liquids," or "the patient has a past history of recurrent pneumonia." Third, because dysphagia is a symptom of many medical disorders, the inexperienced examiner is easily frustrated by not knowing which ones might help explain the patient's current problem.

The Medical History for Dysphagia

Figure 1.1 is an example of a form that examiners can use to assemble the medical and social history of a patient with the complaint of dysphagia. Some components of the form are clarified in the following text.

Sources of Information

Information relevant to the patient's medical history can come from a number of sources. These usually include the written medical record, observations from other health care professionals, and observations from the patient and family.

The Medical Record. Because dysphagia can be slowly progressive, intermittent, and potentially unrelated to other medical problems, it is necessary to review not only the recent medical history but also information that may be as old as 20 years. For instance, a patient who had radiation therapy to the neck 15 years ago could be suffering from the late effects of radiation fibrosis that now have restricted laryngeal movement. Or the patient with a past history of fundoplication of the lower esophageal sphincter as a child now might be experiencing dysphagia related to that procedure. Obvious attention should be spent on recent progress notes that mention symptoms of dysphagia or related symptoms such as anorexia, weight loss, dehydration, or undernutrition. Specific areas of concern in reviewing the medical record are discussed in the following text.

The Nursing Staff. Not all information, even in cases of obvious dysphagia, is fully documented in the medical record. Nurses who provide feeding assistance to patients with dysphagia are frequently excellent sources of information, particularly when the patient is not

Medical History Form for Dysphagia

Patient's Name _____   **Sources of information**

Age _____   Gender _____   ☐ Patient _____

I.D. # _____   ☐ Family _____

Ethnic Origin _____   ☐ Recent medical _____

Chief complaint (Ascertain by food   ☐ Past medical _____
type, volume, frequency, functional
impact) _____   ☐ Other provider _____

_____

_____

1. Congenital Family Illnesses _____

2. Neurologic Disease

   ☐ Stroke _____

   ☐ Progressive disease _____

   ☐ Traumatic injury _____

   ☐ Other CNS disorders _____

   ☐ Medication(s) taken for _____

3. Psychiatric Disease

   ☐ Medication(s) taken for _____

   ☐ Movement disturbance _____

4. Surgical Procedures

   ☐ Myotomy _____

   ☐ Alimentary tract resections _____

   ☐ Fundoplication _____

   ☐ Thyroidectomy _____

   ☐ Cervical/thoracic spine procedures _____

   Cancer-related:

   ☐ Irradiation _____

Figure 1.1. Medical History Form for Dysphagia.

☐ Chemotherapy _____

5. Systemic/Metabolic Disorders

☐ Medications taken _____

☐ Nutrition/hydration status _____

☐ Current weight _____

☐ Ideal body weight _____

☐ Laboratory values related to nutrition _____

☐ Infections _____

☐ Toxins _____

☐ Diabetes _____

6. Respiratory Impairment

☐ Obstructive disease _____

☐ History of aspiration pneumonia _____

☐ Cardiopulmonary disease _____

7. Esophageal Disease

☐ Reflux/regurgitation _____

☐ Motility disorders _____

Prior treatment:

☐ Dilatation _____

☐ Surgery _____

☐ Medications _____

8. Prior Test Results

☐ Radiographic _____

☐ Manometric _____

☐ Scintigraphic _____

☐ Ultrasonic _____

9. Current Advance Directive Status _____

Figure 1.1. *Continued.*

communicative or when there is no family support. For instance, nurses can provide information that may establish useful trends in care, such as "The patient always seems to eat better at breakfast," or "She never chokes until after I put her to bed." Casual observations rarely are documented in the progress notes yet can be important pieces of information in diagnosis and subsequent treatment. The first example suggests that (a) patient fatigue may be an issue because breakfast is the first meal of the day or (b) food items at that meal are more suited to the patient. In the second example, postprandial regurgitation or reflux may be more apparent because the patient is in a supine position. Both situations provide clues to the problem and should be pursued in the formal evaluation.

The Family. The family's description of the relative's swallowing disorder is particularly useful when the patient is unable to communicate. Even when the patient is a good communicator, confirmation of dates, times, and events may be beneficial. Because patients may tend to minimize the impact of the disorder, a family member's perspective, either of support or denial, often helps to provide a broader range of information. Of particular interest are the actions the family member has taken to minimize the disorder, such as altering methods of food preparation. Also important is the assessment of the impact of dysphagia on the family members' lives. This may be evidenced by an inability of patients to eat comfortably with their relatives.

Historical Elements

Because the etiologies for dysphagia are varied and often complex, the clinician needs to review many facets of the medical history that otherwise might be ignored. Those historical elements that are most relevant to the patient with suspected dysphagia are discussed below.

Age, Gender, Heredity, and Ethnic Background. Age alone is not readily correlated with dysphagia, although it has been an independent predictor of aspiration pneumonia in hospitalized patients with neurogenic disease (Mullan, Roubenoff, & Roubenoff, 1992). In a group of patients over the age of 80 who had no dysphagic symptoms, Kaatze (1991) found that 30% aspirated thin fluids. In a group of 56 older patients without dysphagic complaints, only 9 had normal radiographic evaluations of swallow (Ekberg & Feinberg, 1991). Dysphagia is more frequent in older age groups, not perhaps because of age alone but rather because those disorders that precipitate dysphagia are found more frequently in an aged population. Studies of the effects of age on the swallow mechanism suggest physiologic decompensation as early as 45 years (Robbins, Hamilton, Lof, & Kempster, 1992). The appearance of progressive neurologic disease may be suspected by age: multiple sclerosis (MS) in the 20s, motor neuron disease (amyotrophic lateral sclerosis) in the 40s, and Parkinsonism in the later years (Merritt, 1967). Some disorders, such as systemic lupus erythematosus, may be associated with child-bearing years (Andreoli, Carpenter, Plum, & Smith, 1990).

A person's gender may provide insight into some disorders that precipitate dysphagia. Some rheumatic disorders (connective tissue disease) may have a predilection for impacting the swallowing chain. For instance, when systemic lupus erythematosus is associated with polymyositis or dematomyositis, the ratio of females to males affected is 9:1 (Andreoli et al., 1990). Duchenne's type of progressive muscular dystrophy occurs almost exclusively in males (Merritt, 1967).

Some medical records may provide details about the medical histories of a patient's relatives. Some diseases of the nervous system are inherited or have a high familial occurrence and can be associated with dysphagia as a consequence. Some of these diagnoses include Alzheimer's disease, Pick's disease, cerebral palsy, Huntington's chorea, Friedreich's ataxia, and olivocerebellar atrophy (Merritt, 1967).

Although rare, some disease processes that precipitate oropharyngeal dysphagia are found in specific ethnic groups. Found almost exclusively in Jews, familial dysautonomia affects all levels of the central and peripheral nervous system, often resulting in dysphagia. Oculopharyngeal dystrophy, a rare disease found in French Canadians, involves exclusively the muscles of the eyes and the pharynx (Bradley, Daroff, Fenichel, & Marsden, 1991).

Neurologic Disease. The greatest number of patients with dysphagia have accompanying neurologic disease, in either the central or autonomic nervous system. The striated muscles of the head and neck that are under central nervous system control and the smooth muscle of the distal esophagus that is partially controlled by autonomic regulation may be affected. Both are prone to impairment from neurogenic causative factors. A general listing of neurogenic etiologies that precipitate dysphagia is presented in Table 1.1. Some progressive neurologic diseases such as Parkinson's disease and amyotrophic lateral sclerosis typically produce severe dysphagic symptoms in the terminal stages. Although stroke remains the primary etiology for dysphagia, less common causative factors such as Wilson's disease or progressive supranuclear palsy may need to be explored. Patients with traumatic brain injury may lose the necessary motor and cognitive controls needed to complete a normal

Table 1.1
Neuromuscular Disorders Causing Oropharyngeal Dysphagia

Central Nervous System (CNS)

Cerebral vascular accident (brainstem or pseudobulbar palsy)

Parkinson's disease

Wilson's disease

Multiple sclerosis

Amyotrophic lateral sclerosis

Brainstem tumors

Tabes dorsalis

Miscellaneous congenital and degenerative disorders of the CNS

Peripheral Nervous System

Bulbar poliomyelitis

Peripheral neuropathies (diphtheria, botulism, rabies, diabetes mellitus)

Motor End Plate

Myasthenia gravis

Muscle

Muscular dystrophies

Metabolic myopathy (thyrotoxicosis, myxedema, steroid myopathy)

Dermatomyositis

Amyloidosis

Systemic lupus erythematosis

Note. From "Evaluation of Dysphagia: A Careful History Is Crucial," by D. O. Castell and M. W. Donner, 1987, *Dysphagia, 2,* pp. 65–71. Copyright 1987 by Springer-Verlag. Reprinted with permission.

swallow. Despite the fact that a stated neurogenic diagnosis may usually be associated with dysphagia involving the nervous system, the clinician should remain unbiased because the current presentation may have additional, undiagnosed causative factors. A stated history of neurologic disease without good supporting documentation may signal the need for neurologic reevaluation, especially if the physical examination supports neurologic impairment as the source for dysphagia.

Patients with generalized cognitive impairment, such as those with Alzheimer's disease or encephalopathy, may lose the necessary cortical controls to participate in feeding. Frequent accompaniments of these disorders include not recognizing the importance of food, forgetting how to transport food, forgetting to initiate chewing, overmastication, inattentiveness at mealtime, and general disinterest in participating in the pleasures of eating.

Psychiatric Disease. Although psychiatric disorders are not usually viewed as primary etiologic diagnoses for dysphagia, the side effects of their treatment may be linked to dysphagia. Particularly problematic are the xerostomic side effects of the phenothiazine and antidepressant drug groups. Antipsychotropic drugs also have been implicated as the source for tardive dyskinesia. These rapid, uncontrolled movements of the oral peripheral structures may interfere with the normal propulsion and preparation of a food bolus. Combined with severe xerostomia, some patients with chronic psychiatric illness will evidence oral stage dysphagia that may significantly reduce total intake. Often, complaints of dysphagia from patients with known psychiatric illness are not given serious consideration; however, when they are coupled with significant weight loss, pulmonary infiltrates, or a marked change in food ingestion patterns, they should receive a thorough dysphagia evaluation.

Surgery. Surgical procedures that have resulted in the removal or loss of peripheral nervous innervation to any part of the alimentary tract should be noted. Surgery of the cardiopulmonary system (cardiac bypass surgery), the vascular system (endarterectomy), or the neck (thyroidectomy) may precipitate swallowing impairment because of the potential to impair the 10th cranial nerve. The results of surgery to reduce a Zenker's diverticulum in the hypopharynx also should be noted. Any surgery that involved the relaxation (myotomy) of either the upper or lower esophageal sphincters is important to the understanding of the etiology of the present complaint and the potential need for reevaluation. Other surgery such as cervical laminectomy may be the causative factor for oropharygeal swallowing disorders (Martin, Neary, & Diamant, 1997). When the surgery involves removal of cancerous structures, the side effects of radiation and chemotherapy may further decompensate the swallow response. Knowledge of cancer metastasis rates, and to which structures they are most likely to migrate, could be important information in understanding the current problem. The late effects of radiation therapy that result in tissue fibrosis, xerostomia, and neurologic injury are well known (Dreizen, Daly, Drane, & Brown, 1977). Complications of surgical procedures such as edema and bleeding may delay efforts in swallowing. More serious complications that require prolonged tracheostomy and ventilator support also interfere with swallow rehabilitation. Tracheostomy predisposes patients to events of aspiration by reducing the larynx's ability to raise and protect the airway. Additionally, tracheostomy serves as a barrier to the clearance of accumulated pulmonary secretions. Patients who continue to have voice disorders following a period of intubation with accompanying oropharygeal dysphagia will require direct visualization of the laryngopharyngeal complex.

Systemic/Metabolic Disorders. The clinician should thoroughly review medications because of the possibility that their side effects may be contributing to dysphagic symptoms. Those that produce xerostomia are particularly problematic because the initiation of a swallow response is severely impaired without adequate moisture in the oral cavity. A list of drugs that result in xerostomia as a side effect is presented by category and name in Table 1.2. Sudden-onset dysphagia accompanied by a recent change in medication should be pursued in the diagnostic evaluation. Medications such as alprazolam (Xanax) that produce sedative effects with a subsequent change in mental alertness should be noted, as well as those that might depress appetite. Other medications, such as potassium chloride and quinidine, may become lodged in the esophagus if not given with sufficient amounts of water, resulting in inflammation and the development of strictures (Ravich, 1997).

The clinician should look for a history of undernutrition and dehydration, either in the progress notes or in the laboratory results. Laboratory values that frequently are used to measure nutritional status and hydration include albumin, prealbumin, total lymphocyte count,

Table 1.2
Drugs Capable of Causing Xerostomia

Classification	Example
Anticholinergics	Atropine, Scopolamine, Propantheline
Antihypertensives	Guanethidine (Ismelin), Clonidine (Catapres)
Antihistamines	Diphenhydramine (Benedryl), Chlorpheniramine (Chlor-Trimeton)
Antipsychotics	Chlorpromazine (Thorazine), Promazine (Sparine), Thioridazine (Mellaril)
Anorectics	Amphetamines, Diethylpropion
Narcotics	Meridine (Demerol), Morphine
Anticonvulsants	Carbamazepine (Tegretol), Lithium Carbonate (Lithane)
Antiparkinsonian	Benztropine (Cogentin), Trihexyphenidyl (Artane)
Antineoplastics	Busulfan (Myleran), Procarbazine HCL
Antispasmodics	Dicyclomine HCL (Bentyl)
Sympathomimetics	Ephedrine
Antidepressants	Tricyclic (Doxepin, Amytriptyline), MAO inhibitors (Isocarboxazid, Pheneizine)
Antianxiety agents	Meprobamate (Miltown), Benzodiazepines (Valium, Librium, Serax, Ativan), Hydroxyzine (Atarax)
Muscle relaxants	Orphenadrine (Norflex), Cyclobenzaprine (Flexeril)
Diuretics	Hydrochlorothiazide (HydroDiuril)
Antiemetics	Metoclopramide (Reglan)

total protein, transferrin, serum sodium, and hemoglobin. Patients who are severely undernourished and dehydrated may need to receive adequate amounts of intake before they are able to cooperate either with a physical evaluation of swallowing or in treatment efforts. Patients who complain of dysphagia with significant weight loss require careful and serious attention. Consultation with the dietitian in these instances is warranted (see Chapter 6 of this text).

Histories of bacterial, viral, or fungal infections should be noted as possible causative factors. Candidiasis in the mouth, pharynx, or esophagus secondary to chronic disease or long-term use of antibiotics could be severe enough to create sufficient pain that interrupts the normal swallow sequence. Other infectious processes such as neurosyphilis, tuberculosis, herpes, AIDS, and Guillain-Barre syndrome affect the nervous controls for swallow. Knowledge of their course and treatment is useful in planning diagnostic tests and in subsequent treatment.

Histories of toxins that might decompensate the central nervous system and swallow include botulism (muscle weakness), metallic and lead poisoning (polyneuritis and ataxia), manganese and mercury exposure (chorea), and alcohol (Andreoli et al., 1990). Chronic alcoholism may lead to vitamin B deficiencies, precipitating pseudobulbar deficits and disorders of esophageal motility (Buchholtz, 1995).

Persons with histories of diabetes may be liable to peripheral nerve involvement (Cranial Nerves V and VII), esophageal dysmotility (Andreoli et al., 1990), and changes in mental status. Dietary options and treatment stimuli may be necessarily limited due to poor sugar tolerance.

Respiratory Disease. Because of the unique relationship between respiration and deglutition, persons with primary respiratory disease may be at risk for dysphagia. Therefore, persons with histories of asthma, congestive obstructive pulmonary disease, and other obstructive lung diseases may be liable to an increase in pulmonary symptoms related to their dysphagia, or may need to have their disease stabilized as a precursor to dysphagia therapy. Patients with histories of aspiration pneumonia are more likely to develop similar symptoms, dictating a conservative approach when resuming oral ingestion. Chapter 8 in this text includes an in-depth discussion of pulmonary function and dysphagia.

Esophageal Disease. The medical record may indicate that the patient has a history of esophageal-related disorders. Because primary esophageal disease may have secondary effects on both oral and pharyngeal stages of the swallowing response (Jones, Ravich, Donner, Kramer, & Hendrix, 1985), histories of esophageal disorders should not be overlooked and should be pursued with the patient or family. Patients with histories of esophageal obstruction treated with dilatation may have recurring problems, since most will require repeat dilatation for successful management (Ravich, 1997). Histories of motility disorders that were treated with medications are noteworthy. Motility disorders may have secondary effects on pharyngeal function or may require continued intervention with drugs if the patient previously discontinued their use. Although not correlated with dysphagia, patients with hiatal hernia may have associated disorders, such as gastroesophageal reflux disease (GERD) (Ravich, 1997). If the patient has been treated in the past for GERD, the type of treatment and the response to that treatment should be noted. Problems with gastrointestinal bleeding may preclude attempts at oral ingestion until the bleeding is controlled. An algorithm for assessing the patient with suspected esophageal-related dysphagia is presented in Figure 1.2.

Radiologic Study Results. The results of prior radiographic evaluations may be important either in uncovering a relevant swallowing disorder that was investigated in the past or as support to continue further evaluation. They also may eliminate the need to repeat tests that already have been performed. The results of any brain imaging studies, such as magnetic resonance imaging (MRI) or computerized axial tomography (CAT), may be useful in establishing a neurologic etiology for the dysphagia. Records of reports of upper gastrointestinal investigations, including barium swallow studies, may indicate previous concern that led to investigation of the esophagus and lower gastrointestinal tract. Prior reports from videofluorographic studies would suggest the need to image the upper (mouth, pharynx, and cervical esophagus) alimentary tract. Prior CAT scans of any structures of the alimentary system suggest possible concern for an anatomical abnormality. Manometric studies of the esophagus suggest that there was a need to rule out a motility disorder, or to measure the pressures within the upper or lower esophageal segments to evaluate a patient's candidacy for a surgical myotomy. Endoscopy of the upper airway or of the esophagus might be consistent with a need to rule out structural lesions in the pharynx, larynx, or esophagus.

Advance Directive Status. Knowledge of a patient's advance directive status can be very useful in planning diagnostic approaches and in establishing treatment options. For instance, if a patient with severe dysphagia has requested in writing not to be fed enterally, then the diagnostic tests would focus entirely on discovering methods to make ingestion as safe as possible. Some patients with dysphagia may refuse instrumental investigations because they no longer appreciate or trust

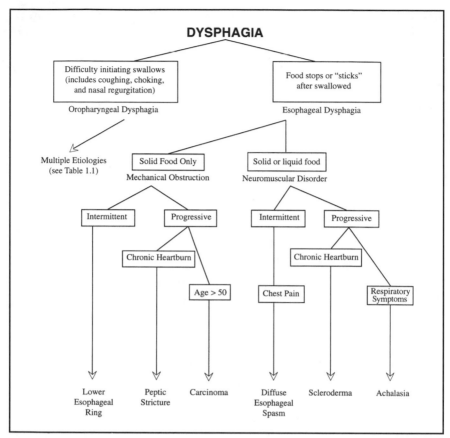

Figure 1.2. Diagnostic algorithm for the assessment of patients with dysphagia. *Note.* From "Evaluation of Dysphagia: A Careful History Is Crucial," by D. O. Castell and M. W. Donner, 1987, *Dysphagia, 2,* p. 67. Copyright 1987 by Springer-Verlag. Reprinted with permission.

their value. In this circumstance the dysphagia evaluation would be limited to the completion of a history and physical. If an advance directive statement pertinent to tube feeding has not been initiated, a wider range of diagnostic and treatment options may be available.

Patient and Family Reports

After reviewing the medical history, the clinician will resolve ambiguity, ask for the patient's impression of the problem, and ask questions that may provide additional information on key issues that may be crucial to the diagnosis. For instance, the examiner may want to know if the patient had experienced dysphagia following cardiac surgery, even though this was not documented in the medical record. Or the clinician might be interested in focusing on how the patient's dysphagia has changed his or her daily routine, an issue that frequently is overlooked in the medical record.

Information from the medical record that requires clarification usually includes specific documentation of the approximate onset of the swallowing disorder or how long the patient estimates that it has been a problem. Other issues that should be explored during this initial exchange of information include nondocumented visits to a specialist related to dysphagia or treatment for seemingly unrelated problems by the family physician. An example of the latter might be treatment for a prolonged cough that was diagnosed as bronchitis, but might be more related to episodes of GERD associated with chronic pulmonary irritation.

History Verification

The medical history review, as it relates specifically to dysphagia, is often incomplete or lacks information in sufficient detail. Particularly absent is a timeline of events indicating when the first dysphagic symptoms appeared, how the symptoms progressed, and when tests or studies to explain those symptoms were completed. Whether dysphagic symptoms immediately followed the first stroke or appeared only after the second stroke may be difficult to discern from the medical record, and therefore requires patient verification. Explanation of how prior dysphagia complaints have been managed, particularly the patient's response to that management, often helps to guide the direction of the evaluation. For instance, if a patient verifies that she received therapy for GERD but that the symptoms were abated only temporarily, reevaluation may be appropriate. If a patient who is suffering from head and neck cancer has had a stable swallow for 3 years but now reports that it is worse, the clinician might pursue an evaluation for disease recurrence, an evaluation of the late effects of radiotherapy-related fibrosis, or an etiology not related to cancer. Any information from the past medical history that seems to relate directly to the current clinical presentation should be confirmed in the patient interview. Copies of evaluation and treatment reports from other medical centers should be sought and the information contained in them verified with the patient. Often the patient's complaint on direct questioning may differ from the brief history of complaint given by the referral source. For instance, the referral source may indicate that the patient is having trouble swallowing all food items, whereas the patient only admits to having difficulty swallowing some liquids.

Chief Complaint. The patient should be given the opportunity to explain what he or she thinks is the essence of the swallowing complaint. The onset of the swallowing complaint should be established. In general, a sudden or recent change in swallowing performance, especially with liquids, is associated with neurologic impairment, whereas slowly progressive changes of dysphagia for solid foods are typically associated with esophageal disease. In some cases the onset is associated with complications following a surgical procedure or a recent change in medications. If the patient does associate dysphagia with these events, then the examiner will strive to focus on specific details of the post-surgical course or on the potential negative effects of medications on the swallow mechanism. Questioning should focus on the patient's perception of how the disorder has affected his or her lifestyle, such as changes in meal preparation or the avoidance of specific food items. Any information relative to how the patient has compensated for the problem, either by special postures or utensils or by a slower eating rate, could be useful in both diagnosis and treatment. Sometimes the patient's complaint as stated in the medical history is not consistent with the current complaint. Such inconsistency may shed doubt on the patient's ability as a reporter or may indicate that the previous examiner did not fully appreciate the nature of the problem. If the problem was not fully appreciated, perhaps the patient did not have the appropriate diagnostic studies. For instance, the patient who continues to complain of constant choking episodes on liquids, who has undergone three barium swallow studies focusing on esophageal function, may not have had the appropriate test to delineate the problem. Frequent choking would be more consistent with pharyngeal rather than esophageal symptoms and would require a modified instead of a standard barium swallow study. After reading the medical summary, the examiner may have formed a diagnostic hypothesis that may be at odds with the patient's stated complaint. This inconsistency requires resolution and may guide the direction of the physical and instrumental examination.

Problem Localization. In 750 patients with a variety of swallowing complaints, Logemann (1983) found that the anatomic location of the disorder correlated with the patient's perception of its location. Such localization may help the clinician initially to focus on a single anatomic region more intensely. For instance, if a patient pointed to his mouth and felt that his swallowing problem was related to poor tongue mobility, more time might be spent in detailed examination of the oral cavity.

In a large series of patients with confirmed esophageal-related disorders, Edwards (1974) found that although most patients could localize their disease within the esophagus, a considerable number did not. Fifty patients correctly pointed to the lower esophageal sphincter when in fact there was a stricture at that level; however, five patients localized the same pathology to the mouth and six localized it to the neck. At best, symptom localization should not be the final guide in deciding where to begin the physical evaluation or where emphasis in evaluation should be placed. Rather the patient's report of localization should stand as one piece of information from the elicited history and should be placed in the context of other information, only some of which might support the patient's impression.

Specific Foods. Even though patients with oropharygeal impairments typically have more swallowing complaints for liquids than solids, this may not always guide the focus of the examination. For instance, those with pharyngeal swallowing disorders can have difficulty swallowing both liquids and solids because the pharynx is too weak to propel semisolids and solid food boluses. Similarly, patients with confirmed obstructive esophageal disorders who complain only of solid food dysphagia also may complain of difficulty with liquids if the obstruction severely narrows the esophageal lumen. Questions that explore food temperature can be useful diagnostically. Those patients who report avoidance of cold food items and pain localized to the chest may have an esophageal motility disorder (Miller, 1997). Those who localize their disorder to the mouth or pharynx and complain that cold items interfere with swallow may have myotonic dystrophy

(Miller, 1997). In this syndrome, cold temperatures stimulate muscle contraction, but interfere with relaxation, with resultant dysphagia. Patients who report avoidance of hot or spicy foods may have lesions in the alimentary tract that are irritated by the chemistry of the spice. If the ingestion of spicy foods is associated with chest pain and dysphagia, the patient may be suffering from GERD. Reported changes in smell or taste may be associated with gingivitis and poor oral hygiene (Miller, 1997), Parkinson's disease (Doty, Deems, & Stellar, 1988), and the early stages of traumatic brain injury (Griffith, 1976).

Regurgitation and Reflux. Patients should be questioned about their perception of the presence of heartburn, especially when experienced in conjunction with chest pain during or after eating, acid taste in the throat or mouth, solid food dysphagia with fullness (globus sensation) in the neck (Jones et al., 1985), halitosis, nocturnal wheezing, belching, persistent and unexplained cough (Ravich, 1997), pain in the mouth or throat when swallowing, and vocal hoarseness (Pearlman, Steigmann, & Teter, 1988). GERD is the retropulsion of stomach acid, sometimes mixed with food, that reenters the esophagus, pharynx, or oral cavity. Regurgitation is the retropulsion of food that has not entered the stomach, and should be associated with disorders of esophageal function (Ravich, 1997). Patients who deny symptoms of reflux or regurgitation during the day should be questioned about nocturnal symptoms because the elimination of gravity effects while lying down may precipitate retropulsive disorders. Even patients who deny symptoms of reflux may have GERD as the etiology for their dysphagia (Ravich, 1997). The severity of GERD may be estimated by asking the patient about the frequency of episodes. The patient should be questioned about both over-the-counter and prescriptive medications that have been taken to control episodes of reflux. In particular, the patient's success in controlling reflux and compliance in taking prescriptions should be explored.

Neurologic Status. The patient should be questioned about the presence of any changes in motor performance in the arms or legs or muscles of articulation, including episodes of weakness or fatigue, incoordination, or loss of sensation. Although these symptoms may be associated with a wide array of nervous system diseases, they could provide the evidence required for the examiner to consult a neurologist.

The clinician should ask questions particular to abnormal fatigability of the voice or swallowing muscles or increased respiratory effort during swallowing to rule out the possibility of muscular disease such as muscular dystrophy or myasthenia gravis. Reports of dyskinetic movements may be secondary to medications as in tardive dyskinesia, Parkinson's disease, and Huntington's chorea.

Vocal Changes. The clinician should ask the patient about changes in vocal quality that may be secondary to injury of the 10th cranial nerve or to local irritation as from GERD. If there is a history of tracheal intubation with vocal changes and dysphagia, the clinician will want to pursue direct visualization of the larynx. Vocal changes in the absence of GERD or alcohol or tobacco use might be associated with the first symptoms of neurologic disease and require consultation of the neurologist.

Respiration. Patients who complain of choking on food or fluids may experience episodes of prolonged apnea if the episodes are secondary to airway obstruction. An elicited history of obstruction that requires the Heimlich maneuver is an indicator of the severity of the disorder and a need for careful evaluation. An increase in the respiratory rate during or after eating may be evidence for airway protection dysfunction. The examiner should ask patients with primary respiratory disease if they have experienced an increase in respiratory rate associated with the effort needed to swallow. Rapid respiratory changes may prevent the airway from closing for the time it takes a bolus to safely clear the pharynx before an ensuing inhalation. When patients exhibit respiratory instability during swallow because of primary respiratory disease, medical management of the disease may take precedence over treatment for dysphagia.

Dental Complaints. The examiner should ask the patient about complaints related to teeth, gums, or dentures. Ill-fitting dentures may cause mucosal irritation that interferes with swallow, whereas infected teeth or gums may contribute to odynophagia (painful swallow). Infection accompanied by pain also may be secondary to recent dental surgery. Patients who have self-treated painful gums or teeth with over-the-counter topical anesthetics may be liable to transitory sensory changes that interfere with bolus preparation and delivery.

Case Examples

The process of constructing a medical history related to dysphagia, assembling the pieces of information into relevant patterns, and formulating a diagnostic plan from those problems is demonstrated in the following case examples.

Case Example 1

A 77-year-old Caucasian male has a history of solid food dysphagia. A Zenker's diverticulum was discovered 2 years ago. He received a cervical myotomy to reduce the diverticulum, but was left with a true vocal fold weakness. Six months following the myotomy, he had a gelfoam injection of the left true vocal fold that improved voice and swallow. Six months following the gelfoam injection, he came to the outpatient clinic complaining of swallowing difficulty for liquid, characterized by choking episodes at each meal.

Important Historical Elements. His initial complaint was for solid food dysphagia associated with a Zenker's diverticulum (hypopharyngeal pouch), but now complains of dysphagia for liquids. Therefore, the complaint may not be related to a recurrence of the diverticulum, although it is a possibility. The true vocal fold weakness following the myotomy probably was the result of damage to the 10th cranial (vagus) nerve, especially if the vocal fold weakness was on the same side as the surgical entrance into the neck. The patient had a gelfoam injection into the vocal fold with a reported positive impact on speech and swallow; however, he continues to choke on liquids. The dysphagia for liquids may represent 10th cranial nerve injury that could be responsible for any or all of the following: reduced airway protection at the vocal fold level, reduced pharyngeal contraction, or reduced laryngeal elevation with accompanying decrease in the opening of the pharyngo-esophageal segment.

Interview Focus Items. The following questions need to be confirmed: (1) Is the dysphagia purely for liquids (indicating a change in complaint)? (2) Did his swallow really improve following the myotomy? (His solid food dysphagia may have been the only improvement.)

(3) Has there been a history of stroke in the past 2 years? (He is in the age group for stroke and it could be a new etiology.) (4) Has his voice become worse? (Differentiate vocal closure problems from laryngeal elevation disorders.) (5) Has he experienced a negative social impact from choking on liquids? (6) Has he had any other medical problems, such as an aspiration pneumonia that may indicate an intolerance for aspirants? (7) Has there been a history of reflux disease (as an etiology for the Zenker's diverticulum)?

Direction of Evaluation. There is a need to establish the etiology for the choking episodes. Are the current choking episodes the result of an airway closure problem (aspiration during swallow) or pharyngo-esophageal segment dysfunction (aspiration postswallow)?

Is the current problem more related to the iatrogenic effects of the myotomy, to undiagnosed disease, or to the recurrence of the Zenker's diverticulum? The history suggests the possibility of poor airway closure combined with poor pharyngoesophageal segment mechanics. Airway closure mechanics are best evaluated by endoscopy, whereas pharyngoesophageal segment mechanics are best evaluated by video-fluoroscopy.

Case Example 2

A 69-year-old black female has a long history of Alzheimer's disease that is in the end stages. She suddenly has stopped eating. The dysphagia team is asked to determine whether she has dysphagia.

Important Historical Elements. Speculation arises as to whether the current complaint is related to a loss of the ability to appreciate eating as in end-stage Alzheimer's disease, dysphagia from an unknown source, or a medical problem such as constipation or a related gastrointestinal disorder that would precipitate disinterest in eating. The clinician should review the medical history for evidence of a pattern of behavior such as refusal to eat. It is necessary to determine whether such refusal might be related to poor fluid intake, producing constipation; urinary tract infections accompanied by a change in comfort or mental status; alterations of medications; a change in environment; or a change in the diet offered to the patient. Any of these can cause a patient to refuse to eat.

Interview Focus Items. Because the patient is unable to report any specifics related to dysphagia, the examiner must seek out her caregivers. Verification of the sudden onset is necessary because the onset may have been more progressive than reported. A more progressive onset might rule out a new, neurologic event. A change in diet level or social ambiance could be verified with the caregiver as a possible explanation of food refusal. Other changes in mental status that might correlate with the loss of the idea of eating could be verified, such as a recent failure to self-feed or assist in dressing activities. Documentation of the patient's fluid intake should be established, as well as changes in urinary output or fever that might be consistent with an infection or dehydration. Recent dietary changes should be noted, such as the recent change from a soft mechanical to a pureed diet. Such a change in diet may cause disinterest in feeding because of the lack of flavor and texture in a pureed meal. Laboratory panels such as an SMA-12 (Sequential Multiple Analyzer) and a complete blood count should be requested to determine the metabolic impact of the patient's refused intake.

Direction of Evaluation. The patient cannot cooperate with either a physical or an instrumental examination because of her Alzheimer's disease. Evaluation of swallowing competency will have to be made at the bedside with real food items. Because she refuses to eat, the test items selected should be favorite foods, usually sweets. If she refuses favorite items, then she may need consultation for placement of a feeding tube unless an advance directive (written instructions from the patient) indicates the contrary. Underlying medical etiologies for refusal, such as constipation and any systemic or metabolic disorder, need to be considered.

Case Example 3

A 45-year-old Caucasian male complains of solid food dysphagia localized to the throat. A barium swallow study was negative.

Important Historical Elements. Localizing solid food dysphagia to the neck may be unreliable. The source of the patient's dysphagia may be esophageal, even though barium swallow studies were normal. Such studies, if done only with thin barium, may not have detected an obstruction that would have been detected with a solid bolus. Another possible source of dysphagia for this patient might be GERD, not detected by standard barium swallow unless it was severe, but associated with fullness in the neck region with solid food dysphagia.

Interview Focus Items. The clinician needs to establish the severity of the disorder from the patient's perspective. Has he lost weight, changed dietary habits, or avoided eating situations? Patients who chew food excessively or avoid tough, fibrous solids like steak may have an obstruction. In this case there is a need to establish with the patient if the feeling of fullness is associated with choking episodes. If there is a denial of choking episodes (associated with airway and pharyngoesophageal segment disorders), the interview should focus on esophageal-related questions. For instance, has he ever had a procedure to detect or treatment for an esophageal disorder? Because GERD may produce esophageal symptoms, questions should be asked that are specific to heartburn and regurgitation. The patient should be asked whether he has ever been treated for symptoms of GERD, whether he takes over-the-counter antacids, and whether there have been any voice or respiration changes (possibly secondary to reflux disease). For completeness, the clinician should ask whether the patient has experienced any neurologic changes.

Direction of Evaluation. If the patient denies neurologic changes and is not choking on liquids, but confirms solid food dysphagia and frequent episodes of reflux, referral to the gastroenterologist, even in the presence of normal barium swallow studies, is warranted. If the gastroenterologist's opinion is negative, evaluation of the pharyngoesophageal segment with videofluoroscopy is warranted to rule out an isolated abnormality in pharyngoesophageal mechanics, or an obstruction such as a web or fibrosis that might be associated with irritation from GERD.

Summary

The medical case history specific to the patient with complaints of dysphagia provides the focus for the ensuing physical and instrumental evaluation. In patients who are unable to cooperate with formal evaluation, it serves as the sole source of information. A good history, taken with sufficient detail, can establish a diagnosis. Because oral, pharyngeal, and esophageal stages of swallow are interdependent, historical information pertinent to these stages should be gathered. Due to the potential for multifactorial dysphagic etiologies, the clinician must be able to judge the relative importance of each as a variable contributing to the patient's complaint. Most important are those etiologies of central and peripheral neurogenic origin, obstructive disease, respiratory impairment, and metabolic insufficiency secondary to undernutrition and dehydration. Finally, the clinician must assess the impact of the dysphagic complaint on the patient's general health and psychosocial status.

References

Andreoli, T., Carpenter, C. C. J., Plum, F., & Smith, L. H. (1990). *Essentials of medicine.* Philadelphia: Saunders.

Bradley, W. G., Daroff, R. B., Fenichel, G. M., & Marsden, D. C. (1991). *Neurology in clinical practice.* Stoneham, MA: Butterworth-Heinemann.

Buchholtz, D. (1987). Neurologic evaluation of dysphagia. *Dysphagia, 1,* 187–192.

Buchholtz, D. (1995). Oropharyngeal dysphagia due to iatrogenic neurological dysfunction. *Dysphagia, 10,* 248–254.

Castell, D. O., & Donner, M. W. (1987). Evaluation of dysphagia: A careful history is crucial. *Dysphagia, 2,* 65–71.

Doty, R. L., Deems, D. A., & Stellar, S. (1988). Olfactory dysfunction in parkinsonism: A general deficit unrelated to neurologic signs, disease stage, or disease duration. *Neurology, 38,* 1237–1244.

Dreizen, S., Daly, T. E., Drane, J. B., & Brown, L. (1977). Oral complications of cancer radiotherapy. *Postgraduate Medicine, 61,* 85–92.

Edwards, D. A. W. (1974). History and symptoms of esophageal disease of the esophagus. In G. VanTrappen & J. Hellemans (Eds.), *Diseases of the esophagus* (pp. 72–137). New York: Springer-Verlag.

Ekberg, O., & Feinberg, M. (1991). Altered swallowing function in elderly patients with dysphagia: Radiologic findings in 56 cases. *American Journal of Radiology, 156,* 1181–1184.

Griffith, I. P. (1976). Abnormalities of smell and taste. *The Practitioner, 211,* 907–913.

Jones, B., Ravich, W. J., Donner, M. W., Kramer, S. S., & Hendrix, T. (1985). Pharyngoesophageal interrelationships: Observations and working concepts. *Gastrointestinal Radiology, 10,* 225–233.

Kaatze, M. (1991, May). *Aspiration in the normal elderly.* Paper presented at the Australian Speech and Hearing Convention, Adelaide, Australia.

Logemann, J. A. (1983). *Evaluation and treatment of swallowing disorders.* Austin, TX: PRO-ED.

Martin, R. E., Neary, M. A., & Diamant, N. E. (1997). Dysphagia following anterior cervical spine surgery. *Dysphagia, 12,* 2–8.

Merritt, H. (1967). *A textbook of neurology.* Philadelphia: Lea & Febiger.

Miller, R. M. (1997). Clinical examination for dysphagia. In M. E. Groher (Ed.), *Dysphagia: Diagnosis and management* (pp. 169–190). Newton, MA: Butterworth-Heinemann.

Mullan, H., Roubenoff, R. A., & Roubenoff, R. (1992). Risk of pulmonary aspiration among patients receiving enteral nutrition support. *Journal of Parenteral and Enteral Nutrition, 16,* 160–164.

Pearlman, N. W., Steigmann, G. V., & Teter, A. (1988). Primary upper aerodigestive tract manifestations of gastroesophageal reflux. *American Journal of Gastroenterology, 83,* 22–25.

Ravich, W. (1997). Esophageal dysphagia. In M. E. Groher (Ed.), *Dysphagia: Diagnosis and management* (pp. 107–130). Newton, MA: Butterworth-Heinemann.

Robbins, J., Hamilton, J., Lof, G., & Kempster, G. (1992). Oropharyngeal swallowing in normal adults of different ages. *Gastroenterology, 103,* 823–829.

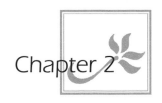

Chapter 2

The Clinical Examination for Dysphagia

Pamela Zenner

Zenner discusses the strengths and limitations of the clinical examination as it is often performed. She adds two components to the examination that strengthen it: meal observation and cervical auscultation.

1. *What are common environmental, cognitive-behaviorial, and physical factors that may contribute to a patient's swallowing or feeding disorders?*

2. *By use of auscultation it is possible to listen to the sounds of the swallow and of the sounds produced as air and liquids pass through the airway. Which of these proves most useful to the dysphagia clinician?*

3. *Describe how a dysphagia clinician can use a watch or a pulse oximeter to determine the impact of a swallowing disorder on the respiratory system.*

✻   ✻   ✻

Despite the failure of clinical examinations to consistently demonstrate validity at assessing the degree and characteristics of oropharyngeal dysphagia, the presence of aspiration, or diet textures for safe oral intake, clinicians continue to use and rely on their results as the first mode in the assessment of swallowing. This reliance on the clinical examination may occur for several reasons:

1. It incorporates more aspects of swallowing than only the mechanical movements of mouth, larynx, and pharynx.

2. It may provide information about the bigger picture of ingesting food to sustain nutrition and hydration.

3. It is more available as an assessment tool than other procedures that require expensive and elaborate equipment to complete.

4. It is not invasive, has no known health risks, and is much less burdensome to fragile patients who may find some techniques, or the act of moving to the examination room, intolerable.

Many of the components of the clinical examination may lack the validity that rigorous research could bring to bear. As such, the clinical examination may be more an art than a science, an art of extracting and integrating information into a congealable premise that allows the management of the swallowing problem within the context of the patient's daily life. This is a significant strength of the clinical examination. However, as a stand-alone evaluation, the clinical exam also has limitations. Therefore, clinicians should recognize both its strengths and limitations as it is employed. The three major components of the clinical examination include history taking, meal observation, and physical examination. The first of these, the case history, has been addressed by Groher in Chapter 1 of this text. In this chapter I deal with the observation of feeding during a meal and the clinical examination of the swallow.

Meal Observation

Although extra time is required, the clinician should observe a complete meal to evaluate the patient's ability to finish enough of the meal to sustain nutrition. As part of this observation, the clinician can assess the patient's ability to finish the meal unassisted and determine the time needed for the patient to complete the meal. An estimate of the amount of food and fluid intake should be noted and, unless unusual circumstances are present, this intake can be used as a good indication of the patient's typical intake during meals.

Too often, the clinician separates feeding from swallowing and omits an observation of the patient eating in the normal (or simulated normal) environment as a part of the comprehensive swallowing evaluation. Observing the patient in a natural eating situation provides an opportunity for the clinician to assess environmental and behavioral variables that contribute to the patient's success or failure with oral feeding. An observation of feeding not only helps the clinician reshape and revise the broad, preliminary assessment obtained as a result of history taking, but identifies variables that may be deleterious or beneficial to the patient in the natural feeding environment. The evaluation of feeding should include an examination of environmental factors, as well as the patient's cognitive and behavioral abilities, physical ability to self-feed, and ability to ingest an adequate amount of food and fluid.

Environmental Factors

During the meal observation, the clinician should first evaluate the atmosphere of the feeding environment, the feeding mates of the patient, and the manner in which the patient is seated during the meal. These environmental variables are often within the control of caregivers and, as such, can be manipulated to improve the patient's ability to function more successfully.

Atmosphere. The environment in which the patient regularly eats typically includes sights, sounds, and smells that should provide cues that meals are being prepared and eaten. In hospitals and skilled nursing facilities, an atmosphere that is conducive to eating is often absent, creating a significant problem. For many patients who eat in the isolation of their rooms, the external cues that provide the needed prompt that it is time to eat may be lacking. In some environments, the atmosphere can be deleterious to safe and satisfying eating because of foul smells, loud music and noise, or unpleasant and unappetizing surroundings. A desirable feeding environment provides appropriate sensory cues, such as dining tables covered with tablecloths, the sound of silverware hitting plates and cups, and the smell of food being prepared and served.

Feeding Mates. The people with whom the patient regularly eats are called feeding mates. Feeding mates who provide a pleasant meal experience and who provide necessary natural cues about appropriate feeding and social behaviors are a significant advantage over feeding mates who may have unpleasant medical or behavioral problems or who may be more cognitively impaired than the patient. Patients with milder degrees of dementing or psychiatric conditions often follow the lead of more cognitively intact feeding mates when they are unsure of appropriate feeding and social behaviors. Independence and function can often be improved for these patients by simply placing them at a table with more cognitively advanced feeding mates. Patients who eat alone in a bedroom as opposed to a dining room miss all of the social cues and pleasantries that are available to those who eat in a group setting. Intake can often be improved for these patients by arranging for them to take their meals in a dining room or other group setting.

Seating. How the patient is seated during the meal, including the kind of chair, the height of the table, and the distance of the chair from the table, is important for the clinician to note. Optimally, the patient is seated in a chair in such a way that hips are flexed at 90 degrees and feet are flat on the floor. The table should be of sufficient height to allow the chair to slide under it, but not so high that it interferes with self-feeding. The adequacy of seating functions not only as a variable for feeding but also as a positioning variable that may contribute to a patient's ability to protect the airway. I have observed some patients cough and choke during meals when they are semireclined in a geri-chair, whereas their clinical and radiographic examinations, completed in an upright position, did not identify significant aspiration risks.

Cognitive-Behavioral Factors

During the observation, the clinician should evaluate the patient's cognitive and behavioral abilities. Included in this observation are the patient's state of consciousness, the patient's overall mental status, the patient's response to food when it is presented, the amount of reinforcement the patient needs to eat, and the presence of behaviors that promote or interfere with safe eating.

Level of Consciousness. Level of consciousness refers to the patient's level of alertness and responsiveness to the environment (Berg, Franzen, & Wedding, 1987). Patients with altered states of consciousness or variable levels of alertness are especially vulnerable to aspiration if being fed by mouth (Huxley, Viroslav, Gary, & Pierce, 1978). It is wise for the clinician to rule out the side effects of medications for patients with altered consciousness, especially for elderly patients who are particularly susceptible to the sedating effects of medications. A clinical pharmacist is a valuable resource to consult when the clinician needs to assess the possible contribution of medications on the patient's impaired state of consciousness.

An assessment of alertness requires the clinician to observe the patient on multiple occasions or to seek information from those who care for the patient on a day-to-day basis. A patient who is alert can be active alert or passive alert. An active-alert patient is watchful and initiates actions, communication, or both, whereas a passive-alert patient is watchful but offers no resistance or emotional reaction. A patient who is semialert is awake but is slow to react to environmental stimuli, whereas a patient who is unresponsive does not react to stimulation. Depending on the patient's condition, the level of alertness may be stable or vary widely from active alert to unresponsive. The clinician should be cautious about generalizing what is observed on one occasion because a patient's state of consciousness can fluctuate considerably, especially if the patient's condition is unstable.

General Mental Status. Mental status refers to the patient's general cognitive condition. A general assessment of mental status can be structured or informal. Most clinicians can obtain an informal general assessment of the patient's mental status during the interview section of history taking, although more structured assessments such as the *Cognitive Performance Test* (Burns, Mortimer, & Merchak, 1994) can be used. The patient's mental status will help guide the clinician when recommendations that require the patient's self-monitoring are being contemplated. For example, a patient who is oriented and needs no cueing to self-feed or complete activities of daily living (ADLs) may be able to alter his or her feeding behavior in specific ways according to the clinician's instructions. On the other hand, a patient who is confused and requires cueing to self-feed or complete other ADLs will likely require verbal reminders, visual cues, or physical prompts to alter feeding behavior.

Of importance during an assessment of mental status are the presence of confusion and the degree of verbal, visual, or physical cueing that is required to obtain appropriate feeding responses. The patient who is oriented will likely be independent in feeding behavior, although some oriented patients require verbal cueing to remind them of appropriate adaptive behaviors. The patient with a mild level of confusion may respond well to verbal cueing, whereas patients with more advanced degrees of confusion may require visual cues in the form of pictures or modeling. Patients with severe confusion may require physical prompting to perform feeding behaviors or may be totally dependent on caregivers for feeding and other ADLs.

Response to Food. It is important to note the patient's response when presented with food at the beginning of the meal. Lack of interest in the visual presentation of food can result from many conditions, including depression, anorexia, confusion, and visual impairment (Albert & Moss, 1988). It is important to provide some cueing about the presence of the meal and the expected response before judging the cause of the absence of response. The presence of the clinician at the meal could alter the patient's normal response to food, especially if the patient is waiting for direction from the clinician before beginning to eat. In addition, the clinician should note inappropriate responses to the presentation of food as a possible clue to the underlying cause of the feeding and swallowing problem. The patient who inappropriately throws, mixes, or plays with food may have significant confusion, whereas the patient who looks away or pushes away food may have underlying depression or anorexia.

Amount of Reinforcement. The clinician should note the amount and type of reinforcement that the patient may need to continue and complete the meal. Patients who eat by themselves in their rooms may have dietary staff deliver and remove the meal tray without regard to their special physical or social needs. There are times when a small amount of encouragement from a staff member is all that is required to significantly improve a patient's intake. There are other occasions, however, during which the patient may need a considerable amount of encouragement to eat. Chronic staff shortages may be an important factor for patients who require considerable staff attention to reinforce and encourage their eating behavior and intake.

Feeding Behaviors. The clinician should be attuned to any unusual feeding behaviors that may interfere with safe oral intake. Patients who will not open their mouths to accept food pose special concern to the nursing staff who are charged with feeding patients. The clinician can generally expect one of two typical responses from nursing staff who are in this situation. One staff member may force the feeding upon the patient to ensure adequate intake, whereas another staff member may only offer, but will not force feeding upon the patient. Both responses place the patient at risk: risk of aspiration if force-fed and risk of dehydration and malnutrition if only offered food. Patients who eat rapidly stress the capacity of their swallowing ability and increase their risk for choking on food. Some patients with dementia or psychiatric conditions will present with this type of "behavioral dysphagia" (Leopold & Kagel, 1997).

Physical Factors

During the meal observation, the clinician should note physical factors such as feeding coordination and skill level. Included in this part of the observation are the patient's body alignment, head alignment, ability to eat finger foods, ability to use utensils, ability to cut food, ability to use a cup and glass, and physical efficiency with feeding. These factors provide the clinician with information about the patient's physical self-feeding skills and guidance when considering recommendations regarding feeding assistance. The clinician should consult an occupational therapist when assessing patients with complex physical disabilities that require specialized knowledge of positioning and adaptive feeding utensils. The rating scale developed by Drews (1983), adapted in Table 2.1, is a method through which the clinician can make simple assessments of posture and self-feeding ability.

The Physical Examination for Swallowing

The physical examination for swallowing provides the clinician with an opportunity to test and verify the preliminary assessment that has been made during the history and meal observation segments of the clinical examination. The physical examination is the low-tech test option that should precede any radiographic or invasive tests because

Table 2.1
Rating Posture and Self-Feeding Ability

Body and Head Alignment While Eating

1. Unsatisfactory 75% of the time or more (almost always).
2. Unsatisfactory 50% of the time (inconsistent).
3. Satisfactory with some assistance or adaptations, verbal or physical.
4. Consistently satisfactory, no adaptations 90% of the time.

Eating Finger Foods

1. No attempt to finger feed or use utensils.
2. Unskilled or awkward finger feeding.
3. Finger feeds most of the meal but is messy, no utensils used.
4. Satisfactorily eats a complete finger food meal.
5. Eats finger foods appropriately in combination with appropriate use of utensils.

Eating with a Spoon and Fork

1. No attempts to use a spoon or a fork.
2. Attempts to assist but attempts are awkward.
3. Brings food to mouth with frequent spills.
4. Scoops or spears and brings it to the mouth with some spillage; an adaptive utensil may be required.
5. Handles utensils appropriately and satisfactorily.

Cutting Food

1. Not applicable, food is blended or pureed.
2. Food is cut up for the patient, no attempt to cut food.
3. Able to cut food with a fork.
4. Unilateral hand use of knife or adapted utensil.
5. Bilateral hand use of fork and knife.

Using a Cup and Glass

1. No attempts to use a cup or glass.
2. Needs some assistance to prevent spills or to carry weight of cup/glass to mouth.
3. Independent with adapted cup or straw setup.
4. Independent use with one or two hands.

Efficiency of Feeding

1. Excessively messy eating, more than ¼ of food is spilled.
2. Messy eating pattern, about ¼ of food is spilled.
3. Some mess when eating, less than ¼ of food is spilled.
4. Neat feeding with minimal mess.

Note. Adapted from *Back to the Table: A Practical Approach to Long Term Care Dining Programs,* by J. Drews, 1983, Edina, MN: Saint Croix Therapy.

it may provide all the information the clinician needs to develop a treatment plan for the patient. Because the clinical examination does not allow the clinician to visualize the pharyngeal swallow, aspiration must be imperfectly inferred from the patient's reaction to the swallowing event. The presence of "silent aspiration" in a significant number of patients with dysphagia means that the detection of aspiration from overt symptomatology is imperfect. Likewise, the degree to which such an event can be understood without imaging the pharynx is also limited. The physical examination for swallowing involves two basic components: oral examination and test swallows.

Oral Examination

The oral examination completed during the clinical assessment of swallowing resembles the examination a clinician would complete during a speech evaluation because the musculature involved in both activities is essentially the same. Some components of the physical examination for swallowing receive relatively more weight given the specific requirements for bolus preparation, oral transit, and pharyngeal response. The physical examination at the bedside is considerably less instrumental than an examination completed in the clinic. Although instrumental examinations provide more measurement precision, there are relatively few normal adult values for muscle strength and coordination for swallowing. Four components of the oral examination should be completed regardless of the location: These are tests for motor speech performance, oral reflexes, and mobility and strength of the oral musculature, as well as a general inspection of the oral cavity.

Motor Speech Performance. It is important for the clinician to assess the integrity of the patient's voice, nasalence, and articulation because these three motor speech components have significant correlates to requirements for safe and efficient swallowing (see Table 2.2). While normal movements of the vocal cords and soft palate are needed for voice and nasalence, these movements also ensure tracheal and nasal airway protection. Likewise, the coordination and strength of tongue movement needed for articulation of speech are also required for adequate movement of the bolus within the mouth.

Voice. The primary function of the vocal cords is to protect the lower airway during swallowing, whereas their secondary function is

Table 2.2
Correlates of Speech and Swallowing

Structure	Speech	Swallowing
Vocal cords	Voice	Tracheal airway protection
Soft palate	Nasalence	Nasal airway protection
Tongue	Articulation	Bolus movement

the vibration of air to create sound for speech (Denk, Swoboda, & Steiner, 1998). Normal voice quality may not always correlate well with the vocal cords' ability to protect the airway during swallowing; however, alteration of voice quality is certainly a strong indicator that airway protection is compromised (Linden & Siebens, 1983). The clinician can complete a gross assessment of voice integrity during the interview section of history taking by simply listening to the patient's voice quality and noting any abnormalities that may require an instrumental examination. If voice disturbances are present, the clinician should be suspicious of impaired tracheal airway protection.

Nasalence. The primary functions of the soft palate are protection of the nasal airway and closure of the aerodynamic tract during swallowing. This closure allows the pharynx and esophagus to create strong negative pressures to facilitate rapid bolus transit through the pharynx and into the esophagus (Donner, Bosma, & Robertson, 1985). Nasalence that is normal may not always correlate well to the soft palate's ability to protect the nasal airway during swallowing; however, alteration of nasal quality, especially hypernasality, is a strong indicator that palatal function is disturbed. The clinician can complete a gross assessment of nasalence during the interview section of history taking by simply listening to the patient's voice quality and noting any abnormalities that may require an instrumental examination. Although the patient with hyponasality may have difficulty breathing while eating, the patient with hypernasalence will more likely present with disturbances of nasal airway protection during swallowing.

Articulation. Unlike the vocal cords and the soft palate whose function is airway protection, the tongue is responsible for bolus preparation and bolus transit through the mouth and pharynx. A patient with precise and well-paced speech demonstrates the ability to coordinate tongue movements normally. For patients who find it difficult to follow directions because of language or other cognitive disturbances, the precision and pace of their articulation during conversational speech may be the only manner in which a clinician can assess tongue mobility and strength. Abnormal articulation of speech provides strong evidence that a patient's tongue strength, range of motion, or coordination is also impaired for bolus preparation and transit. Patients with generalized slow and labored speech patterns do not have the agility of tongue movements needed for efficient mastication and bolus transit. Patients with imprecise /k, g/ sounds may have weakness of the tongue base and demonstrate weak tongue base retraction during the pharyngeal phase of swallowing. Patients with imprecise /ʃ, ʒ/ sounds may have weakness of the tongue blade and demonstrate weak tongue grooving that may also impair their ability to transport the bolus from the anterior to the posterior mouth during the oral transit phase of swallowing. It is wise for the clinician to ask the patient to repeat words with these sounds so that the clinician can focus on the sound production. Repetition of the word *shake* will closely mimic the tongue movements used during oral transit.

Oral Reflexes. Two types of oral reflexes that the clinician should be aware of and test are protective reflexes and primitive reflexes. The protective reflexes, which promote safe swallowing and protect the airway, are the swallow reflex, the gag reflex, the cough reflex, and the palatal reflex. Primitive reflexes are present at birth and are inhibited or suppressed as the brain matures during infancy. The reemergence of primitive reflexes indicates that the patient is likely to have bilateral or scattered cortical damage (Miller, 1984). These signs also signify to the clinician that the patient not only may have brain damage, but may be unable to voluntarily alter learned or habitual patterns while eating. This becomes important to the clinician when changes in habitual feeding and swallowing behaviors are contemplated as recommendations to improve feeding and swallowing performance. The primitive reflexes that are easy to test are the snout reflex, the sucking reflex, and the tonic bite reflex. Table 2.3 lists the protective and primitive oral reflexes that the clinician should assess during the clinical examination.

Swallow Reflex. The activation of the pharyngeal component of the swallow is mediated by what is called the swallow reflex. In fact, it is not a reflex in the traditional manner in which reflexes are defined

Table 2.3
Protective and Primitive Oral Reflexes

Protective Reflexes	Primitive Reflexes
Swallow	Snout
Gag	Sucking
Cough	Tonic bite
Palatal	

(Dodds, 1989). It is more precise to state that a pharyngeal response occurs as a result of a bolus stimulating the anterior faucial arches and posterior soft palate. During the physical examination, the clinician can test the swallow reflex in two ways: by asking the patient to dry swallow or by offering food or fluid during test swallows.

The swallow reflex cannot be directly observed during the clinical examination, although the clinician can use methods to enhance detection of the onset of the pharyngeal response. One method, often referred to as the four-finger method, involves placing four fingers along the patient's laryngeal sling and feeling the laryngeal sling elevate as the pharyngeal response occurs (Logemann, 1983). Another method involves placing a stethoscope along the lateral side of the neck and listening for the "clicks" that correspond to the opening and closing of the cricopharyngeus muscle during the pharyngeal response (Hamlet, Nelson, & Patterson, 1990).

Gag Reflex. The gag reflex is a protective response to foreign material entering the pharynx. The clinician can test the gag reflex with a blunt instrument, such as a laryngeal mirror or tongue blade. By briskly touching the posterior pharyngeal wall, a sharp pharyngeal wall constriction occurs that is often accompanied by retching.

Considerable controversy and misconception exist regarding how a clinician should interpret a weak or absent gag reflex. It is an error to assume that the absence of the gag reflex indicates the presence of a dysphagia. There are wide variations of normal responses to a gag stimulus and, by itself, a diminished or absent gag reflex means very little (Leder, 1997). The absence of a gag reflex can be interpreted as a diminished touch sensation at the posterior pharyngeal wall and, when combined with other abnormal findings, may indicate that the patient has an increased risk for aspiration and airway obstruction (Chusid, 1979).

Cough Reflex. The cough reflex is a pulmonary response to foreign material in the lower airway (Braman & Corrao, 1987). The point at which a cough occurs as a result of foreign material aspiration is an indication of the integrity of touch sensation within the larynx and lower airway. The only way a clinician can truly test the cough reflex is to wait for the patient to spontaneously cough after aspiration. Although it is important to be observant of such events, it is equally important to note the strength of the cough and the degree of voluntary control a patient has over this behavior. It is wise for the clinician to ask the patient to voluntarily cough to assess these variables.

Palatal Reflex. The palatal reflex is a velar response to a touch stimulus delivered on the soft palate. The clinician can test the palatal reflex by briskly touching the soft palate with a blunt instrument, such as a laryngeal mirror or tongue blade. The protective response is a sharp velar constriction and elevation, sometimes accompanied by retching as a result of gag reflex stimulation at that anterior position. The patient's response to a palatal stimulus is an indication of the integrity of touch sensation in the palatal region. Together with an assessment of the patient's speech nasalence, the clinician can estimate the patient's ability to protect the nasal airway during the swallow.

Snout Reflex. The snout reflex is a primitive reflex that is commonly elicited in infants, in patients who have sustained severe injury to the brain, or in those who have advanced dementing diseases (Haerer, 1992). Using a blunt instrument, such as a tongue blade or fingertip, the clinician taps either the upper or lower lip. An abnormal response is indicated by protrusion of the lips toward the instrument. Although an abnormal snout reflex does not have an exact correlate to a swallowing problem, it provides the clinician with an overall impression of the extent of the patient's brain damage and ability to alter voluntary behaviors.

Sucking Reflex. The sucking reflex is a primitive oral reflex that is elicited by placing a blunt instrument, such as a laryngeal mirror or tongue blade, firmly along the center of the tongue. A primitive response is closure of the mouth and a pursing of the lips around the instrument. Like the positive snout reflex, an abnormal sucking reflex does not have an exact correlate to a swallowing problem. It will, however, provide the clinician with an overall impression of the extent of the patient's brain damage and ability to alter voluntary behaviors.

Tonic Bite Reflex. The tonic bite reflex is a primitive oral reflex that is elicited by tapping or touching the front teeth. The primitive response is evidenced by a significant increase of muscle tone, resulting in clamping of the teeth on the instrument, facial grimacing, and head extension. Obviously, it is wise to use a strong, blunt instrument such as a tongue blade to test for a tonic bite reflex to protect both the patient and the clinician from injury. To release a bite reflex, the clinician should not pull on the instrument or force open the patient's mouth. These actions will only strengthen the bite response. The clinician must continue to hold the instrument and attempt to normalize the patient's muscle tone by bringing the patient's head and trunk forward. When the clenching releases, the clinician can safely remove the instrument. Obviously, the presence of a tonic bite reflex has significant implications for oral feeding and oral hygiene, and presents a considerable challenge to all caregivers. Because the tonic bite reflex has such a deleterious impact on feeding and oral care, the integration of the reflex is often a high rehabilitation priority.

Mobility and Strength of Oral Musculature. Testing the range of motion and the strength of the lips and tongue is a relatively straightforward assessment. The clinician should ask the patient to close the lips, maintain closure against resistance, purse the lips, and stretch the lips to the side. Although the clinician may test tongue movements outside of the mouth, I prefer to assess tongue movements within the mouth because they more closely approximate actual tongue movements necessary for swallowing. The patient should be asked to push the tongue against the anterior maxillary ridge and against the inside of each cheek, and to maintain pressure against the inside of the cheek against resistance. For both lip and tongue movements, the clinician should note generalized weakness of the musculature and asymmetry of range of motion or strength. Impaired mobility and strength of the oral musculature have implications for the patient's ability to efficiently masticate solid material, contain the bolus, and transport the material through the mouth and pharynx.

Inspection of the Oral Cavity. As part of the clinical examination for the swallow, the clinician should complete a thorough visual inspection

OOPA

of the mouth. This inspection should include a general assessment of the presence, fit, and health of the teeth or dental appliances. Special note should be made of absent opposing molars and loose or broken dentures, which often contribute to problems with masticating solid material (see Chapter 7). The overall health and hygiene of the mucosa, tongue, and palate should be assessed, with special concern given to any open sores, bleeding, inflammation, or xerostomia.

Test Swallows. For the final section of the clinical examination, the patient completes test swallows using a variety of food textures. During test swallows, the clinician assesses four major aspects of swallowing: mastication, oral transit of the prepared bolus, phase transition from the oral to the pharyngeal phase of swallowing, and the ability of the patient to protect the airway. A clinician should have the patient complete test swallows only if, in the clinician's opinion, the patient has sufficient cognitive and physical ability to do so safely. If the clinician knows that the patient will aspirate on all food textures before attempting test swallows, there is no need to complete this section of the examination. Patients who will clearly aspirate during test swallows but who are receiving oral feedings can be tested with less liability to the clinician since the patients are likely to aspirate during each meal. Decision making is not always clear, however, so the clinician should begin with food textures that are not easily aspirated and do not pose a significant threat to airway occlusion.

There is some controversy about what to feed the patient during this section of the examination. Some clinicians have concerns that offering food could result in pulmonary complications for the patient if the material is aspirated. I feel that the best way to judge the patient's safety with eating food is to complete test swallows with the kinds of food that are or will be normally eaten. It is best, however, to avoid food with high acid content because these materials are more likely to damage lung tissue than other foods (Bordow, 1991). In addition, when offering solid food, it is best to use foods that will not easily obstruct the airway. I use individual jars of pureed baby food for the pureed texture because they are safe to store, reduce food waste, and are relatively inexpensive. Individually wrapped packages of salt-free saltines or graham crackers are a good solid food for the evaluation of mastication, and water is a relatively safe liquid to use for liquid swallows. Commercial thickener and ice are convenient to have on hand for testing alternative liquids when patients aspirate tepid water. A list of test materials is provided in Table 2.4.

The clinician must also decide in which order to offer food textures. I suggest that the clinician start with a thick, pureed texture such as applesauce or pudding, and proceed to textures that require chewing if the patient swallows the pureed texture well. The examination should end with thin liquids.

Mastication. The clinician already should have assessed four key variables necessary for safe mastication: tongue mobility and strength, adequacy of saliva production, cognitive status, and presence of opposing molars. Tongue mobility and strength, dental integrity, and salivary function were assessed as part of the oral examination. Cognitive status was assessed as part of the meal observation. Before the clinician actually tests the patient's ability to chew, therefore, the clinician has a relatively good idea about how the patient will perform. During mastication, the clinician should assess the patient's ability to perform rotary chewing and to quickly prepare a completely masticated bolus. Rotary chewing occurs as the tongue throws material onto the molars. The clinician will observe a rotary motion of the mandible as the result of the coordination of the tongue movement and the grinding action of the molars. The absence of the rotary chewing

Table 2.4

Materials Needed for the Administration of Test Swallows

Jar of pureed baby food
Individually wrapped saltine or graham cracker
Glass of water
Thickener for liquids
Ice for liquids
Barrier gloves for infection control
Pen light
00 laryngeal mirror
Tongue blade
Stethoscope
Pulse oximeter
Oral lubricant for treatment of xerostomia

motion can be the result of impaired tongue movement, lack of opposing molars, or both. The speed at which the patient prepares a masticated bolus varies depending on the material that is masticated and the patient's age. An objective measurement of the time it takes the patient to masticate solid material is less valuable than the subjective assessment made by the clinician who can take multiple variables into account. If the clinician is suspicious that xerostomia is the cause of mastication problems, it is wise for the clinician to give the patient an oral lubricant and reassess mastication performance. Oral lubricants can be purchased over the counter at local drugstores or obtained through the facility's pharmacy. These lubricants rarely have side effects or drug interactions, although the clinician should always follow the product instructions.

Oral Transit. The clinician must attend to three key variables necessary for normal oral transit: tongue mobility and strength, adequacy of saliva production, and integrity of sensation, especially along the lateral buccal sulci located between the cheek and teeth. The clinician should attend to both the speed with which the patient can collect and transport the bolus through the mouth and the degree to which oral residue remains in the oral cavity following the swallow. Slow oral transit is generally the result of impaired tongue strength, coordination, or both, although impaired salivary production also results in slower performance. Residual material is most likely to be located in either buccal sulcus, indicating unilateral loss of sensory or motor impairment, or generally scattered through the mouth, indicating generalized weakness or xerostomia. Pastes or dry food textures may present a significant challenge to some patients with oral phase dysphagia so it is wise for the clinician to assess the patient's performance with these foods before making judgments about the safety of textures that may be more challenging.

Phase Transition. The clinician needs to assess the timing of the pharyngeal phase of swallowing in relation to the end of oral transit. A delay in the initiation of the pharyngeal phase increases the patient's risk for aspiration. Assessment can be accomplished in one of two ways, as described previously in the Swallow Reflex section of this chapter. One method involves placing the fingers along the laryngeal sling and feeling the laryngeal sling elevate as the pharyngeal response occurs.

Another method involves placing a stethoscope along the lateral side of the neck and listening for the "clicks" that can be heard as the pharyngeal response is triggered. I prefer to use auscultation to detect the occurrence of the pharyngeal response, although many professionals advocate the four-finger method. Neither method has been shown to be as sensitive as invasive techniques, but the clinician will be able to detect significantly slow phase transitions as well as the absence of a pharyngeal response.

Airway Protection. Although the clinician cannot directly observe aspiration during the clinical examination, useful information regarding airway protection can be gathered by observing pulmonary responses and auscultating breath sounds. Abnormal pulmonary responses that suggest aspiration include coughing, congestion, or wet voice quality after the swallow. Abnormal breath sounds through auscultation include variable or disorganized respiratory patterning surrounding the swallow or the presence of adventitious breath sounds after the swallow. It is important to understand that false negative and false positive errors may result should the clinical examination be used as the sole method of evaluation. Not all patients who aspirate will exhibit overt pulmonary responses, and cervical auscultation has yet to be shown to be effective in detecting minor degrees of aspiration. Also, not every patient who coughs does so due to an aspiration event. Because of the demonstrated utility of cervical auscultation in the clinical evaluation of swallowing, it is described in the following section.

Auscultation and the Physical Examination of Swallowing

For some clinicians, the clinical examination includes auscultation of the swallow. Auscultation is a general term that describes several techniques using a variety of instruments, each yielding different acoustic information about the swallow. These instrumentation alternatives include an accelerometer, a sonograph with Doppler, a laryngeal microphone, and a stethoscope. Data from each of these alternatives can be recorded for a permanent record of examination results if the clinician wishes to evaluate the results at a later time or feels that liability warrants permanent documentation. Auscultation with an accelerometer transduces surface body movement to an acoustic signal; the sonograph with Doppler records fluid flow and can be used to record the volume and movement of the bolus; and the laryngeal microphone and stethoscope detect the actual sounds that occur during the swallow. The stethoscope is designed to narrow the spectral range of sound detection to enhance the clinician's ability to hear breath sounds.

Acoustic analyses of the pharyngeal phase of the swallow have focused on either the mechanical sounds of the swallow itself or on the respiratory pattern that surrounds the swallow. Although attempts have been made to correlate the mechanical clicks heard with an accelerometer with specific physiologic events during the swallow, the clicks are not, as yet, fully understood (Hamlet et al., 1990). The respiratory pattern associated with normal and abnormal swallowing, however, has been described in the literature for over 40 years (Odanaka, 1952) and has practical implications for the clinician completing the clinical examination. Enhancement of breath sounds enables the clinician to assess the patient's ability to protect the airway while swallowing.

Breath Sounds Associated with Respiration

Breath sounds associated with respiration are different when heard over various parts of the pulmonary system. Normal breath sounds are usually classified as tracheal, bronchial, bronchovesicular, and vesicular.

Tracheal Breath Sounds. Tracheal breath sounds are heard when the stethoscope is placed over the larynx. These sounds are relatively loud, high pitched, and hollow. The duration of inspiration-to-expiration is 1:1 so that the clinician hears both respiratory phases equally.

Bronchial Breath Sounds. Bronchial breath sounds are heard when the stethoscope is placed over the trachea. Like the tracheal breath sounds, these sounds are relatively loud, high pitched, and hollow. The inspiration-to-expiration ratio is 2:3 so that the clinician hears the expiratory phase somewhat longer than the inspiratory phase.

Bronchovesicular Breath Sounds. Bronchovesicular breath sounds are heard when the stethoscope is placed at the main stem bronchus. The breath sounds are soft, low pitched, and breezy. The inspiration-to-expiration ratio is 1:1 so that the clinician hears both the inspiratory and the expiratory phases equally.

Vesicular Breath Sounds. Vesicular breath sounds are heard when the stethoscope is placed along the peripheral lung fields on the chest or back. Like the bronchovesicular breath sounds, these sounds are soft, low pitched, and breezy. The inspiration-to-expiration ratio is 3:1 so inspiratory sounds are heard for a longer period of time than expiratory sounds.

Adventitious Breath Sounds. Adventitious breath sounds refer to abnormal sounds such as rales or wheezes that indicate constriction of or fluid in pulmonary passages. Adventitious breath sounds also refer to the occasion of normal breath sounds heard in an area where it is not normally heard. For example, hearing brochovesicular breath sounds along the peripheral lung fields would be considered adventitious.

Breath Sounds Associated with Normal Swallowing

Swallow breathing, much like speech breathing in a normal adult, is a consistent pattern that involves a short, deep inhalation with the act of swallowing occurring during the exhalation (Selley, Flack, & Brooks, 1989a). As food or drink is being brought to the lips, the adult interrupts the normal respiratory pattern to take a relatively deep inhalation. If a breath is needed while the bolus is being prepared during the oral phase of swallowing, the pattern is short and shallow. As the bolus is transported through the mouth and pharynx into the esophagus, breathing is suspended (an apneic pause). This apneic pause typically occurs at the beginning of the expiratory phase of the breath, although some adults take their apneic pause near the end of the expiratory phase (Martin, Logemann, Shaker, & Dodds, 1992). The apneic pause lasts for approximately .6 to .8 seconds in young adults, begins as the thyroid cartilage elevates, and ends before the larynx returns to rest. The apneic pause does not always correspond to vocal cord adduction. Following the swallow, the exhalation is completed and the breath sounds are clear without evidence of adventitious sounds. Respiratory phasing associated with normal swallowing does not vary with bolus size unless a straw is used. In this case it is not uncommon to observe inhalation following the swallow (Boiron, Rouleau, & Metman, 1997).

Normal swallowing in the elderly varies slightly from this description. The apneic pause is generally longer (about 1.0 seconds), and approximately 30% of elderly adults take an inhalation following the swallow (Shaker et al., 1992). The underlying reasons for this developmental phenomenon are not understood.

Breath Sounds Associated with Dysphagia

Evidence suggests that the respiratory pattern during the swallow is different for adults with dysphagia (Selley, Flack, & Brooks, 1989b). The respiratory pattern is more variable from one swallow to the next, the apneic pause is less consistent, and inspiration occurs more frequently after the swallow. I have noted several unusual respiratory patterns that occur with patients with dysphagia. Some patients fail to produce an apneic pause and continue their normal breathing patterns while swallowing, leaving the airway totally unprotected during the swallow. Others begin and sustain the apneic pause several seconds before the mechanical swallow occurs, which has led clinicians to theorize that the actual mechanical swallow occurs late in the pattern, evidence of delayed phase transition. Still other patients, especially those with significant pulmonary disease, accelerate their breathing pattern while eating and, when they become short of breath, inhale during the swallow. In addition, breath sounds following the swallow are often characterized by respiratory bubbling, throat clearing, and vocal stridor in adults with dysphagia, suggesting that material penetration or aspiration has occurred.

Practical Considerations

Auscultation with a stethoscope involves placing the flat diaphragm of the stethoscope against the lateral side of the neck near the larynx and listening for tracheal breath sounds. The diaphragm is designed to enhance the frequency range in which breath sounds occur and is better than the bell side of the stethoscope for this purpose. The clinician should adjust the placement of the diaphragm until tracheal breath sounds can be easily heard. Placing the diaphragm in a posterior position along the neck may result in hearing carotid artery sounds that may interfere with breath sound auscultation. With some patients, the clinician may need to position the diaphragm low on the neck or close to the patient's ear to hear breath sounds well. It is prudent to listen to normal breath sounds for a few seconds before asking the patient to receive and swallow food or drink so that the clinician is familiarized with the patient's particular sound, rate, and pattern of breathing.

Studies that compare the clinical examination without auscultation to videofluoroscopy suggest that the examination identified true aspirators about one half of the time (Splaingard, Hutchins, Sulton, & Chaudhuri, 1988). Including auscultation with the clinical examination increases the clinician's ability to detect aspiration. Studies that include auscultation in the clinical examination identify true aspirators and true nonaspirators at a much higher rate (84% and 71%, respectively) than in the clinical examination alone (Zenner, Losinski, & Mills, 1995). Although these results indicate that auscultation can add significantly to the clinical examination, auscultation has a variety of limitations including nomenclature difficulties, observer variability, and the requirement that dysphagia clinicians develop a "trained ear." Given these limitations, it is important that the clinician understand that even including cervical auscultation with the clinical examination may not supplant the need for an instrumental evaluation (see Chapters 4 and 5 of this text for discussions of the videofluoroscopic swallowing study and fiberoptic endoscopic evaluation of swallowing techniques). Despite its limitations, auscultation is an inexpensive, noninvasive technique that does not expose the patient to radiation, can be used repeatedly without physical risk to the patient, and can add significantly to the quality of the information derived through the total swallowing evaluation.

Special Techniques for Assessing Airway Protection

Clinicians require additional skill and knowledge to accomplish a clinical examination of swallowing with patients who are seriously ill. Patients who are acutely ill or who have severe, chronic pulmonary disease are fragile, decompensate much more quickly than their healthy peers, and do not tolerate even small amounts of aspiration. It is wise for the clinician to add measurements of cardiopulmonary response as part of the assessment of airway protection to obtain a clearer picture of the patient's aspiration risks while eating.

Measurement of cardiopulmonary responses can be completed with the use of a pulse oximeter and a stethoscope, both portable and easy to use at bedside. A pulse oximeter is a noninvasive device that measures the patient's pulse (in beats per minute) and degree of oxygen saturation (in percent) through a sensor that is commonly clipped to a finger. Although the device is easy to use, the clinician needs to obtain sufficient training to operate the oximeter and to interpret its readings. Prior to test swallows, the clinician should obtain a resting respiratory rate and a resting pulse. In addition, the clinician should obtain a measure of oxygen saturation in blood (i.e., the S_pO_2 level). These measurements should be taken at regular intervals throughout the meal observation or test swallows to assess the patient's ability to tolerate the cardiopulmonary work effort of feeding, chewing, and swallowing.

By incorporating measures and results from pulse oximetry and auscultation with overt signs of aspiration (wet voice and coughing behavior), the clinician can obtain a fairly clear picture of the patient's ability to protect the tracheal airway during swallowing. Auscultation can identify an abnormal respiratory pattern surrounding the swallow and the presence of adventitious breath sounds. Abnormal swallow breathing can be characterized by abnormality of the apneic pause, inhalation after the swallow, or inconsistencies in respiratory patterns from one swallow to the next. Adventitious breath sounds such as wetness and stridor can indicate the presence of misdirected material in the laryngeal or tracheal airway. Pulse oximetry and measurement of the respiratory rate can identify abnormal increases in work effort. Abnormal work effort can be characterized by increased respiratory rate, increased heart rate, and decreased S_pO_2. Together, these measurements not only detect aspiration during the examination but provide the clinician with information regarding the impact of the aspiration on the patient's system and about the patient's ability to protect the tracheal airway from future aspiration.

Respiratory Rate

Respiratory rate is taken by counting the number of exhalations that occur in a 15-second period and then multiplying that number by 4. The normal adult respiratory rate is between 8 and 12 breaths per minute (Murray, 1986). An increase of the respiratory rate indicates increased workload for the patient. A respiratory rate that exceeds 30 breaths per minute is significantly elevated and indicates to the clinician that oral intake is most likely unsafe for the patient because the patient will be unable to coordinate swallowing with the heavy demands of breathing.

Oxygen Saturation Taken by Pulse

An S_pO_2 is an indirect measurement of oxygen saturation in the arterial blood taken by placing a probe on the fingertip or other peripheral body part. It tells the clinician how much oxygen is being carried on the hemoglobin in the red blood cells. S_pO_2 is expressed in terms of percent saturation. The normal S_pO_2 level for a healthy adult is 95% to 100%. S_pO_2 levels that drop below 90% indicate abnormal oxygen desaturation. If this level occurs during eating, it indicates that the work effort is greater than the patient's ability to provide a sufficient amount of oxygen to accomplish the work requirements. In an attempt to compensate for the drop in oxygen reserves, the patient will likely increase respiratory rate, heart rate, or both.

Pulse Rate

The pulse oximeter also displays the patient's pulse as part of its digital readout. A normal resting pulse for a healthy adult is 60 to 80 beats per minute (bpm). An increase of 10 bpm or more from baseline or an elevation of pulse above 100 bpm during a meal observation or during test swallows indicates an abnormal increase in cardiopulmonary work effort.

Special Considerations for Patients with Tracheostomy

The clinician needs to have specialized knowledge and skills to assess and manage the feeding and swallowing issues that occur as a result of or in conjunction with tracheostomy. The tracheostomy is an artificial airway that surgically introduces access to the lower airway through the trachea below the level of the larynx. It is used when the patient is unable to safely or efficiently maintain ventilation through normal structural access (mouth and nose). There are three basic types of tracheostomy tubes: cuffless, cuffed, and foam tubes. The inflated cuff and foam types of tracheostomy tubes create a seal in the trachea, whereas the deflated cuff and cuffless forms provide an air leak to the upper airway. The three general types of patients on whom a tracheostomy may be performed are those with total laryngectomy, those on mechanical ventilation, and those without laryngectomy or mechanical ventilation.

Patients with Total Laryngectomy

Clinicians cannot auscultate the swallow breathing of patients with total laryngectomy because there is no transfer of air through the pharynx. Airway protection during swallowing is rarely an issue for these patients because the airway has been totally diverted, surgically disconnecting the communication between the upper and lower airways. These patients present with very low risk of aspiration unless a tracheoesophageal fistula has developed, which allows material in the esophagus to enter the lower airway through the common wall of the esophagus and trachea.

Patients on Mechanical Ventilation

In completing the clinical swallowing examination on patients who are dependent on mechanical ventilation, the clinician should seek the assistance of a respiratory therapist or a registered nurse who is competent with mechanical ventilators. It is important for the patient to be medically stable because it is very difficult for a clinician to make judgments about the safety of feeding for a patient whose status changes rapidly. If the patient is on a ventilator-weaning protocol, it may be advisable to wait until the weaning process has been completed before introducing oral feeding as an additional variable for the medical team to manage.

Because a cuffed tracheostomy tube has many deleterious effects on safe swallowing, the clinician is not advised to complete test swallows or to begin oral feeding with a patient who requires a sealed (or inflated) tracheostomy cuff to maintain respiration and ventilation. A sealed tracheostomy tube cuff anchors the larynx and prevents it from accomplishing its normal excursion to remove the airway from the path of the food (Nash, 1988). In addition, both sensation and motor responses within the larynx are disturbed by the absence of airflow pressure through the larynx, impairing the patient's ability to detect misdirected material and to clear the airway of aspirated material (Buck-walter & Sasaki, 1984; Sasaki, 1977). Adjustment of ventilator parameters and assessment of the patient's tolerance of a leak in (or partial deflation of) the tracheostomy tube cuff can only be made by specialists such as the respiratory therapist. Under no circumstances should the clinician attempt to make any ventilator or tracheostomy tube cuff adjustments on his or her own.

When the clinician completes a clinical swallowing examination with a ventilator-dependent patient who is tolerating a leak in the tracheostomy tube cuff, it is particularly important to monitor pulse, respiratory rate, and S_pO_2 to evaluate effects of the work effort of feeding and swallowing on the patient's cardiopulmonary system. In addition, a drop in blood pressure, changes in the patient's color, and subjective patient responses such as anxiety and shortness of breath should be closely monitored and respected. With a cuff leak, the clinician is able to listen for voice abnormalities that are common to this population, such as stridor, breathiness, wetness, or harshness, that indicate conditions of the vocal cords that will require attention before swallowing is attempted.

When the patient can safely tolerate a cuff leak and voice quality is normal, the clinician can safely proceed with test swallows. Although its validity has been questioned (Thompson-Henry & Braddock, 1995), I suggest that the clinician use vegetable food coloring to blue-dye all food offered as part of test swallows, which facilitates detection of aspiration. Auscultation with patients who are ventilator dependent is much more difficult than with other patients because the mechanical ventilator produces a considerable amount of ambient noise. The technique may not provide the clinician with sufficient information about airway protection. The advantage the clinician has, however, is that tracheal suctioning can be completed at any time during or after test swallows to assess the patient's ability to protect the airway from aspiration of food. At a minimum, the clinician should have the patient suctioned at the end of test swallows and within 15 minutes of completion of the clinical examination. Qualified medical personnel should suction the patient whenever he or she requests it or when the clinician suspects that airway protection has been compromised. It is advisable for the clinician who works with patients who have tracheostomies to obtain training in oral and tracheal suctioning so that the clinician is prepared to perform the procedure in an emergency.

Patients Without Mechanical Ventilation

In some ways the patient who has been weaned from mechanical ventilation but who still requires tracheostomy for respiration is more fragile for oral feedings than patients who remain on mechanical ventilation. The patient on mechanical ventilation can rely on the ventilator to provide support for the effort and requirements of breathing, especially when completing tasks that may require additional work effort. Patients who have been weaned from the ventilator are essentially on their own, with the exception of oxygen support that may be offered. It is particularly important for the clinician to employ all of the techniques mentioned for patients on mechanical ventilation with this patient group. In addition, it is important that the patient who is weaned from the ventilator have a closed aerodynamic tract during swallowing to permit the normal pressure changes. That is, the tracheostomy tube should be occluded with a one-way speaking valve, a capped outer canula, or a tracheostomy tube button during test swallows. These special tracheostomy tube devices should be used only with the assistance of a respiratory therapist since occlusion of the tracheostomy may place the patient in respiratory distress. For an in-depth discussion of pulmonary function considerations in dysphagia management, see Chapter 8 in this text.

Outcomes and Decision Making

Following the completion of the three components of the clinical examination of swallowing—that is, history taking, feeding observation, and physical examination—the clinician may understand the extent of and the bases for the feeding or swallowing disturbances that the patient presents. If, at the completion of the clinical examination, the clinician recognizes the symptomatology but not the underlying physiologic basis for the swallowing problem, then an instrumental evaluation of swallowing is required, such as the videofluoroscopic swallowing study (VFSS) or a Fiberoptic Endoscopic Evaluation of Swallowing. Most medical centers rely on the VFSS as the primary instrumental method for the evaluation of swallowing. Whether a patient is referred for such an examination should depend on the diagnostic questions that are posed. As Mills points out in Chapter 4, few diagnostic questions can be sufficiently answered based on the results of a single examination technology. This is true of both the VFSS and the clinical examination. The VFSS can provide a visualization of the anatomy and physiology of the pharyngeal swallow that the clinical examination cannot, whereas the clinical examination can establish an environmental relevance for the instrumental findings that the VFSS cannot accomplish alone. Most often the patient is best served when both types of information are provided.

In many medical centers the vast majority of patients who are referred for dysphagia evaluations go on to receive the VFSS. If it is determined that such a study is not needed, that decision should be based on clinical rather than administrative or economic issues. Fluoroscopy is not commonly available in nursing home environments. Transporting a resident to an area medical center for the completion of a VFSS can be an expensive undertaking. Dysphagia clinicians must be alert to situations in which other than clinical factors may be considered in determining whether a resident receives an instrumental dysphagia examination. Should a patient or resident be denied a needed instrumental dysphagia examination, it becomes the dysphagia clinician's responsibility to act as an advocate to ensure that needed services are provided.

Through the clinical examination, the clinician can assess the patient's ability to protect the airway during swallowing, to ingest sufficient amounts of food and fluid to maintain nutrition and hydration, to self-feed within the current feeding environment, and to benefit from therapeutic interventions. The clinician can also assess how vital the unknown information is to the plan of care, and what benefits can be expected from further examinations. The bases for oropharyngeal dysphagia are complex, and no simple algorithm will lead the clinician through the decision-making process. The following discussion is meant to assist the clinician with considerations that may guide clinical decisions.

Airway Protection

The first question that the clinician must answer is how well the patient can protect the airway. Whether the patient aspirated material during the clinical examination is certainly important but does not tell the whole story. A patient who does not aspirate during the examination can also be at significant risk for airway compromise. Throughout the clinical examination, the clinician has gathered information that provides evidence about the patient's ability to protect the airway. During the history taking portion of the examination, the following information will lead the clinician to suspect that airway protection ability may be compromised:

1. Advanced age resulting in slower motor response times

2. Structural alterations including orolaryngeal resection, tracheotomy, or both

3. Amyotrophic lateral sclerosis and other neurologic conditions that impair diaphragm function

4. Acute or chronic pulmonary conditions

5. Conditions that can result in loss of sensation to orolaryngeal structures

6. Impaired judgment, aberrant feeding behaviors, or both

7. Patient or caregiver complaints of coughing or choking

The following occurrences during the meal observation provide the clinician with further evidence that the patient may be having problems with airway protection:

8. Impaired state of consciousness and alertness

9. Dependent feeding

10. Coughing or choking during observation

Abnormal findings during the physical examination add significant evidence that airway protection is compromised. These abnormal findings are often texture specific. That is, the patient may be able to sufficiently protect the airway when eating pureed foods but not when drinking thin liquids. The following abnormal findings signal that the patient most likely has difficulty protecting the nasal or tracheal airways:

11. Abnormal voice quality and nasalence of speech

12. Loss of protective oral reflexes (gag, cough, swallow, palatal)

13. Delayed phase transition during test swallows

14. Coughing, congestion, or wet voice quality after the swallow

15. Variable or disorganized respiratory patterning surrounding the swallow

16. Presence of adventitious breath sounds after the swallow

17. Increased respiratory rate during feeding, especially if more than 30 breaths per minute

18. Decreased S_pO_2 during feeding, especially if it drops below 90%

19. Increased pulse rate during feeding, especially if more than 100 beats per minute

20. Intolerance of leak in cuffed tracheostomy tube

Nutrition and Hydration

The second question the clinician must answer is whether the patient can ingest sufficient amounts of food and fluid by mouth to maintain nutrition and hydration. Although the clinician can make some broad judgments about the patient's nutrition and hydration status and needs, it is always best to obtain the expert advice of a registered dietitian. Together, these two professionals can design a nutrition program that best meets the patient's individual needs.

Throughout the clinical examination, the clinician will have gathered information that provides evidence about the patient's ability to ingest sufficient nutrients and fluids. Additional information will be derived from history taking. The presence of any of the following elements will cause the clinician to suspect that the patient may be unable to sustain himself or herself via oral feeding:

1. Advanced age resulting in decreased hunger and thirst

2. Drug-induced anorexia

3. Inability to ingest 1,500 cubic centimeters of fluid and 1,500 calories per day (48-hour intake record)

4. Undesirable weight loss by history

5. Depressed serum protein measures

6. Elevated serum electrolytes

During the meal observation, the following behaviors provide the clinician with further evidence that the patient may have difficulty with maintaining nutrition and hydration:

7. Aversive or indifferent response to food

8. Unusual amount of reinforcement needed to sustain eating behavior

9. Refusal to open mouth or displays of interfering behaviors

10. Poor intake during meal observation

The physical examination provides information about the effort the patient must exert to ingest sufficient amounts of food and fluid. Evidence of the following occurrences suggest that the patient's effort may be considerable to ensure sufficient oral intake:

11. Decreased strength of oral musculature

12. Slow or inefficient mastication

13. Slow oral transit

14. Increased respiratory rate during feeding, especially if more than 30 breaths per minute

15. Decreased S_pO_2 during feeding, especially if it drops below 90%

16. Increased pulse rate during feeding, especially if more than 100 beats per minute

Self-Feeding and the Feeding Environment

The third question that the clinician can answer is whether the available social and physical supports will allow the patient to maintain independence with self-feeding. The clinician may wish to enlist the assistance of an occupational therapist for cases that appear to be unusually complex, especially if the patient presents with significant physical problems that interfere with self-feeding.

Throughout the history taking portion of the clinical examination, the clinician has gathered information that can identify self-feeding problems. The following list of factors can be obtained from the history:

1. Degenerative neurologic disease impairing visuomotor ability

2. Acute neurologic condition impairing one or both upper extremities

3. Dementing diseases impairing judgment and self-care abilities

4. Psychiatric conditions impairing judgment and self-care abilities

5. Medications that may cause confusion

6. Pulmonary conditions that reduce the level of tolerated work effort

During the meal observation, the clinician has a first-hand opportunity to watch the patient's self-feeding behaviors. The following is a list of conditions or behaviors that, if observed, may affect self-feeding problems:

7. Distracting atmosphere of feeding environment

8. Feeding mates with medical or social problems

9. Type of chair or seating during the meal

10. Distance from the table during the meal

11. Impaired or variable state of consciousness

12. Verbal, visual, or physical cueing required to complete tasks

13. Aversion to or disinterest in food when offered

14. Unsatisfactory body and head alignment

15. Difficulty using feeding utensils

16. Spilling of food

During the physical examination, the presence of primitive oral reflexes, such as rooting, suckle, and tonic bite, indicates to the clinician that the patient will likely have difficulty altering habitual patterns of behavior. The presence of these reflexes contributes to the patient's inability to adapt behavior to compensate for medical, physical, and social changes.

Treatment

The fourth question that the clinician is called upon to answer from the clinical examination is what kind of treatment, if any, is indicated for the patient. Although the exact physiologic components of the pharyngeal phase of swallowing are not known from the clinical examination, the clinician is able to ascertain the appropriateness of other aspects of impaired feeding and swallowing.

Although the history portion of the clinical examination does not involve direct observation of the patient, there are specific conditions that, when evident in the history, will lead the clinician to identify patients who will likely benefit from treatment. The following is a list of treatable conditions that can be identified through the history:

1. Tooth loss, disrepair, and loose dentures may require a dentist's attention.
2. Presence of a sealed cuffed tracheostomy tube suggests a trial with a cuff leak.
3. Surgical resection of the mouth, pharynx, or larynx leads to specific therapeutic alternatives that should be considered.
4. Acute neurologic conditions such as stroke or traumatic brain injury suggest specific therapeutic alternatives.
5. Medications that can cause xerostomia, changes in muscle tone, anorexia, thrush, or confusion could be changed.
6. Malnutrition and dehydration require a dietitian's attention.

The meal observation allows the clinician to identify many environmental factors that could be changed to improve the patient's success. The following is a list of conditions that can be altered or managed for the patient:

7. Atmosphere of feeding environment can be changed to reduce noise and increase natural clues that food is being served.

8. Feeding mates can be changed to improve social cues.

9. Seating during the meal can be changed to improve function.

10. Distance from the table during the meal can be changed.

11. Verbal, visual, or physical cueing to assist self-feeding can be provided.

12. Body and head alignment can be improved.

13. Adaptive feeding utensils can be provided.

14. Finger foods can be substituted for foods requiring utensils.

Findings from the physical examination will identify specific conditions that may be amenable to treatment, thereby improving the patient's swallowing ability. The following is a list of conditions that may respond to treatment:

15. Abnormal voice, nasalence, and articulation can be treated.

16. Impaired protective reflexes may respond to sensory stimulation.

17. Tongue and lip weakness can be treated.

18. Impaired oral hygiene can be corrected with regular care.

19. Impaired mastication may be treated with chewing exercises.

20. Slow oral transit may be treated with tongue exercises.

21. Inconsistent or abnormal swallow breathing may respond to sensory stimulation in much the same way that protective reflexes will.

Summary

The clinical examination of swallowing provides the clinician with a wealth of information about the variables that contribute to the patient's success or failure with oral feeding. Unlike technical procedures that focus on the mouth, pharynx, or larynx, the clinical examination provides the "big picture" context from which the clinician can gather a significant amount of information that assists in treating or managing the patient's dysphagia. It allows the clinician to address the patient in a holistic manner so that recommendations make sense in the patient's life. It is within this context that the results from instrumental assessments truly become meaningful. Without the big picture that is recognized when the clinical examination is performed, clinicians are prone to make unrealistic and likely ineffective recommendations. The only way to properly manage a patient's dysphagia is with the inclusion of the totality of information gathered during the clinical examination.

References

Albert, M. S., & Moss, M. B. (1988). *Geriatric neuropsychology.* New York: Guilford Press.

Berg, R., Franzen, M., & Wedding, D. (1987). *Screening for brain impairment: A manual for mental health practice.* New York: Spring.

Boiron, M., Rouleau, P., & Metman, E. H. (1997). Exploration of pharyngeal swallowing by audiosignal recording. *Dysphagia, 12,* 86–92.

Bordow, R. A. (1991). *Manual of clinical problems in pulmonary medicine.* Boston: Little, Brown.

Braman, S. S., & Corrao, W. M. (1987). Cough: Differential diagnosis and treatment. *Clinical Chest Medicine, 8,* 177.

Buckwalter, J. A., & Sasaki, C. T. (1984). Effect of tracheostomy on laryngeal function. *Otolaryngology Clinics of North America, 17*(1), 41–48.

Burns, T., Mortimer, J. A., & Merchak, P. (1994). Cognitive Performance Test: A new approach to functional assessment in Alzheimer's disease. *Journal of Geriatric Psychiatry and Neurology, 7,* 46–54.

Chusid, J. G. (1979). *Correlative neuroanatomy and functional neurology.* Los Altos, CA: Lange Medical Publications.

Denk, D. M., Swoboda, H., & Steiner, E. (1998). Physiology of the larynx. *Der Radiologe, 38,* 63–70.

Dodds, W. J. (1989). The physiology of swallowing. *Dysphagia, 3,* 171–178.

Donner, M. W., Bosma, J. F., & Robertson, D. L. (1985). Anatomy and physiology of the pharynx. *Gastrointestinal Radiology, 10,* 196–212.

Drews, J. (1983). *Back to the table: A practical approach to long term care dining programs.* Edina, MN: Saint Croix Therapy.

Haerer, A. F. (1992). *The neurologic examination.* New York: Lippincott.

Hamlet, S. L., Nelson, R., & Patterson, R. (1990). Interpreting the sounds of swallowing: Fluid flow through the cricopharyngeus. *Annals of Otology, Rhinology, and Laryngology, 99,* 749–757.

Huxley, E. J., Viroslav, J., Gary, W. R., & Pierce, A. K. (1978). Pharyngeal aspiration in normal adults and patients with depressed consciousness. *American Journal of Medicine, 64,* 565–568.

Leder, S. B. (1997). Videofluoroscopic evaluation of aspiration with visual examination of the gag reflex and velar movement. *Dysphagia, 12,* 21–23.

Leopold, N. A., & Kagel, M. C. (1997). Dysphagia—ingestion or deglutition? A proposed paradigm. *Dysphagia, 12,* 202–206.

Linden, P., & Siebens, A. (1983). Dysphagia: Predicting laryngeal penetration. *Archives of Physical Medicine and Rehabilitation, 64,* 281–284.

Logemann, J. (1983). *Evaluation and treatment of swallowing disorders.* Austin, TX: PRO-ED.

Martin, B. J. W., Logemann, J. A., Shaker, R., & Dodds, W. J. (1992). Coordination between respiration and swallowing: Respiratory phase relationships and temporal integration. *Journal of Applied Physiology, 72*(2), 714–723.

Miller, R. M. (1984). Evaluation of swallowing disorders. In M. E. Groher (Ed.), *Dysphagia diagnosis and management* (pp. 85–110). Stoneham, MA: Butterworth.

Murray, J. F. (1986). *The normal lung.* Philadelphia: Saunders.

Nash, M. (1988). Swallowing problems in the tracheostomized patient. *Otolaryngology Clinics of North America, 21*(4), 701–709.

Odanaka, T. (1952). Studies on the mechanism for the appearance of swallowing respiration. *Japan Journal of Physiology, 14,* 352–354.

Sasaki, C. T. (1977). The effect of tracheostomy on the laryngeal closure reflex. *Laryngoscope, 89*(9, Part 1), 1428–1433.

Selley, W. G., Flack, F. C., & Brooks, W. A. (1989a). Respiratory patterns associated with swallowing: Part 1. The normal adult pattern and changes with age. *Age & Aging, 18,* 168–173.

Selley, W. G., Flack, F. C., & Brooks, W. A. (1989b). Respiratory patterns associated with swallowing: Part 2: Neurologically impaired dysphagic patients. *Age & Aging, 18,* 173–176.

Shaker, R., Li, Q., Ren, J., Townsend, W. F., Dodds, W. J., Martin, B. J., Kern, M. K., & Rynders, A. (1992). Coordination of deglutition and phases of respiration: Effect of aging, tachypnea, bolus volume, and chronic obstructive pulmonary disease. *American Journal of Physiology,* G750–755.

Splaingard, M. L., Hutchins, B., Sulton, L., & Chaudhuri, G. (1988). Aspiration in rehabilitation patients: Videofluoroscopy versus bedside clinical assessment. *Archives of Physical Medicine and Rehabilitation, 69,* 637–640.

Thompson-Henry, S., & Braddock, B. (1995). The modified Evan's blue dye procedure fails to detect aspiration in the tracheotomized patient: Five case reports. *Dysphagia, 10,* 172–174.

Zenner, P. M., Losinski, D. S., & Mills, R. H. (1995). Using cervical auscultation in the clinical dysphagia examination in long-term care. *Dysphagia, 10,* 27–31.

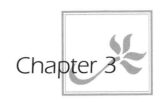

Chapter 3

Radiologic Concepts in the Management of Adult Dysphagia

Jo Edwards and Dianne Hawkins

Edwards and Hawkins explain the imaging process used in the diagnosis of speech and language disorders. They discuss the risks of radiation to the professional and the patient and give suggestions to minimize radiation exposure to both.

1. *Describe the imaging chain in fluoroscopy.*

2. *Describe the known effects of low-dose radiation.*

3. *Identify the ways in which speech–language pathologists can minimize the radiation received by themselves and patients during a videofluoroscopic swallowing study.*

✴   ✴   ✴

W hen speech–language pathologists provide videofluoroscopic examinations of swallowing for their patients, many are entering into a foreign environment. The scope of training provided to most of these clinicians does not afford them an understanding of the equipment and materials with which they will work. The purpose of this chapter is to familiarize clinicians who lack training in medical imaging with the information necessary to work safely and effectively in the radiology environment. This chapter describes the types of radiation commonly employed, the methods by which they are produced, and the radiation safety measures necessary to protect both the patient and the operator during radiologic procedures. Further, it discusses the construction and operation of radiographic and fluoroscopic equipment, as well as the types and uses of contrast media for studying the pharynx and esophagus.

Fundamental Radiation Concepts

Radiation Sources

All individuals are exposed daily to ionizing radiation. Most radiation exposure comes from background radiation, including the sun's ultraviolet rays and materials in the earth's surface such as uranium, radium, and thorium, to name a few. The amount of background radiation received by an individual also depends on where he or she lives. People living at high altitudes may receive twice as much background radiation as people living near sea level.

Since the harmful effects of excessive radiation exposure have been documented, human beings have been advised to limit their exposure to radiation. Aside from limiting exposure to the sun, it is difficult to control the amount of background radiation received. The best way of reducing radiation exposure is to limit the exposure to man-made radiation. According to the National Council on Radiation Protection (NCRP, 1987), 90% of all man-made radiation exposure comes from medical and dental radiologic procedures. Only 10% of man-made radiation exposure can be attributed to nuclear power plants, computer screens, and microwave ovens.

History of the X-ray

The man-made production of radiation was discovered on November 8, 1895, by Wilhelm Conrad Röntgen, a physicist working at the University of Wurtzburg, in Bavaria, Germany (Yochum, 1995). Working in his darkened laboratory one evening, Professor Röntgen applied an electrical charge to a cathode ray tube. Quite accidentally, he noticed that a piece of barium plantinocyanide lying on a workbench gave off a glow of light. When he moved the tube closer to the phosphor, the light became brighter. Because he did not know the nature of the ray he had discovered, he used x, the mathematical symbol for the unknown, to describe it. Although Thomas Edison and others also were experimenting with cathode ray tubes, Professor Röntgen was the first to publish his findings of this new X-ray. Beyond the discovery of X-ray, he also demonstrated, by use of his wife's hand, that the image could be captured on photographic film. The medical community quickly began to recognize the diagnostic potential of the discovery. Professor Röntgen received the first Nobel Prize in Physics in 1901.

Röntgen's "new light" soon found its way into hospitals. The discovery of X-ray by Röntgen and the isolation of radium by Madam Curie electrified the general public. Newspaper headlines touted radium as a substitute for gas and electricity and a positive cure for every disease. Due to the absence of laws governing its use, X-ray became available to the public in a variety of unusual forms. The public enjoyed glowing, radium-laced cocktails and soaked in radioactive hot springs. By the 1950s it was not uncommon to find fluoroscopy in the offices of family physicians and in shoe stores. With a growing awareness of the potential dangers, however, the Food and Drug Administration and other regulating bodies imposed limitations on the ownership and use of X-ray generating systems during that decade.

What Is X-ray?

X-ray is a form of electromagnetic radiation. Visible light, radio and television waves, and microwaves are also forms of electromagnetic radiation. The difference between X-ray and these other forms of electromagnetic rays lies in the wavelength of the radiation. Wavelength is described as the distance from peak to peak in a waveform. Radio and television waves and even visible light have long distances between peaks. Gamma rays are also electromagnetic radiation that is emitted from the nucleus of a radioisotope. X-rays are produced by electrical machines. The electromagnetic spectrum is demonstrated in Figure 3.1.

X-rays, used in both radiography and fluoroscopy, have very short wavelengths, which allow them to penetrate matter. In so doing X-rays are capable of causing damage to matter such as human tissue and organs. The damage produced by X-rays cannot be distinguished from tissue or organ damage produced in other ways.

How Is X-ray Produced?

Today as in Röntgen's time, X-rays are produced in a highly evacuated glass tube that contains a cathode (negative terminal) and an anode

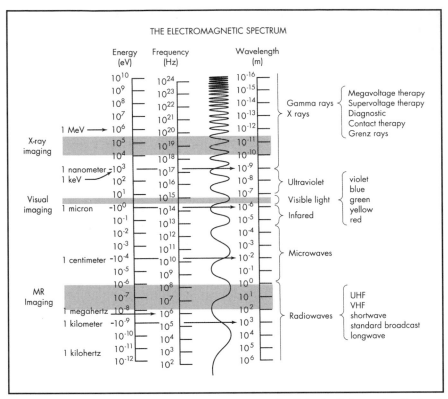

Figure 3.1. The electromagnetic spectrum. From *Radiologic Science for Technologists* (6th ed., p. 49), by S. C. Bushong, 1997, St. Louis: Mosby. Copyright 1997 by Mosby. Reprinted with permission.

(positive terminal) (see Figure 3.2). When an electrical current is applied to the cathode, an electron cloud is created. The amperage of the current determines the number of electrons produced and thus the *quantity* of X-ray photons that are ultimately produced. In the production of X-ray, only small amounts of amperage are needed, so small that they are measured in milliamperes (mA), or thousandths of an ampere. Once produced, the electrons are driven at a high speed to the positively charged anode. As they approach the anode, the electrons decelerate and form a packet of energy called a photon. It is the photon that can penetrate matter. The driving force in this process is the voltage (V) that is employed. In the production of X-rays, voltages are

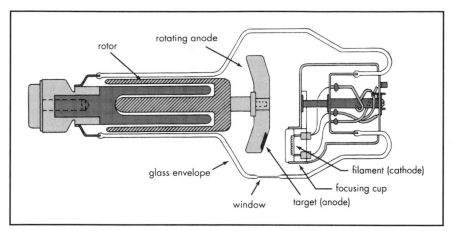

Figure 3.2. A schematic representation of an X-ray tube. From *Radiologic Science for Technologists* (6th ed., p. 110), by S. C. Bushong, 1997, St. Louis: Mosby. Copyright 1997 by Mosby. Reprinted with permission.

quite large and are measured in thousands of peak volts (kVp). The higher the kVp, the shorter the wavelength of the radiation produced. When the wavelength is decreased, X-rays can more easily penetrate tissue. The kVp determines the *quality* of the photons, or the energy level of the resulting photons. These two exposure factors—mA and kVp—affect the fluoroscopic image. As a general rule the kVp should be as high as possible consistent with adequate contrast, and the mA as low as possible consistent with adequate image brightness.

Photons have the ability to knock electrons out of their orbits, creating electrically charged ions. These ions have the ability to be absorbed by matter, scatter the electrons within the matter, or go completely through the matter without any interaction. There are three main types of X-ray photon interaction: photoelectric, Compton's, and pair production.

Photoelectric Interaction. The photoelectric effect occurs when a photon knocks an inner orbital electron out of its shell and in so doing transfers all of the photon's energy to it. This is the most common type of energy transfer in the diagnostic range of X-ray exposure and is responsible for radiographic contrast or the visible difference between the blacks and the whites in an X-ray image.

Compton's Interaction. Compton's interaction, named in honor of physicist Arthur H. Compton, occurs at slightly higher kilovoltage levels. It takes place when an incoming photon interacts with an orbital electron and gives only a portion of its energy to the orbital electron. This causes the electron to be knocked out of the orbit, which ionizes the atom. The remaining photon has less energy and changes directions, causing scatter. This is the type of energy that tends to fog or produce a graying effect on the X-ray image.

Pair Production. Pair production is a type of interaction that occurs at levels of energy much higher that those used in diagnostic X-ray. For this reason it is of little concern to the practicing clinician.

Radiation Measurement

As with all types of measurement, a quantifiable unit must be assigned to measure radiation exposure. In fact, several units are used depending on the nature of the measurement that is required. Thus, different units are used when discussing equipment testing as opposed to occupational exposure or absorbed dose levels. The terminology used has undergone transition in an attempt to produce a universal nomenclature. Although the older or traditional units are still used by some authors, preference should be given to the more recently accepted Standard International (SI) units. Traditional and corresponding SI units are provided in Table 3.1. Because of the relatively large size of most

Table 3.1

Abbreviation Table for Traditional
and International Radiation Units

Quantity Measured	Traditional Unit		SI unit	
	Name	Symbol	Name	Symbol
Exposure in air	röntgen	R	coulomb/kilogram	C/kg
Absorbed dose	rad	rad	gray	Gy
Dose equivalent	rem	rem	sievert	Sv

Note. SI = Standard International. Adapted from *Radiologic Science for Technologists* (6th ed., p. 14), by S. C. Bushong, 1997, St. Louis: Mosby. Copyright 1997 by Mosby. Reprinted with permission.

measurement units, the prefix *milli*, meaning ¹⁄₁,₀₀₀ of a unit, is frequently used to report measured radiation levels.

The ionizing radiation dose to humans is measured in rads or millirads (mrads) and is now called the gray (Gy). The rem or millirem (mrem) is the dose equivalent, and is now called the sievert. Thus, millirad, millirem, and millisievert (mSv) are often encountered.

Equipment Testing

The röntgen (R) or columb/kilogram (C/kg) is used as a unit of measurement primarily when testing radiologic equipment and measuring exposure in the air, such as leakage from the X-ray tube. These are the values reported as the equipment undergoes periodic calibration and safety testing.

Measurement of Absorbed Dose

Absorbed dose is defined as the amount of radiation imparted to matter per unit mass of irradiated material (Brill, 1982). The unit for absorbed dose, the rad or gray (Gy), is used in radiation therapy when a dose to a particular tumor must be given or in diagnostic X-ray when skin dose is measured. Measuring the skin dose in diagnostic X-ray is not done on a routine basis.

Measurement of Occupational Exposure

The rem or sievert (Sv) is the unit used to measure occupational exposure to personnel during radiographic procedures. It is referred to as dose equivalent because it takes into account the type of radiation the worker may be exposed to, including alpha, beta, and gamma radiation, as well as X-ray. In the diagnostic X-ray exposure range, it is generally considered that 1 R (C/kg) is equal to 1 rad (Gy) or to 1 rem (Sv).

Radiation Dose Limits

Occupational Dose Limits

Dose limits are assigned to occupationally exposed individuals by regulating agencies such as the NCRP (see Table 3.2). Dose limits are also assigned to student operators who are under the age of 18 years and who are exposed while in education and training programs. While working in environments that contain radiation, workers are required to wear a dosimeter that will monitor the amount of radiation received. The annual occupational whole body dose limit is 50 mSv. The lifetime occupational dosage is calculated as 10 mSv × age.

Patient Dose Limits

There is no limit to the amount of radiation exposure an individual can receive during needed medical procedures. If a medical procedure is necessary, it is assumed that the benefit outweighs the risk of any possible complication from radiation exposure. Table 3.2 also provides the dose limits assigned to the general public, approximately 1/10 the occupational exposure level.

Table 3.2
Occupational and Medical Radiation Dose Limits

Annual occupational exposure limit	
Whole body	50 mSv (5,000 mr)
Cumulative occupational exposure limit	
Whole body	10 mSv × age
Dose equivalent for tissues and organs	
1. Lens of the eye	150 mSv (15,000 mr)
2. All other organs (bone marrow, breast, lungs, gonads, etc.)	500 mSv (50,000 mr)
Annual public exposure	
Effective dose equivalent, infrequent exposure	5 mSv (500 mr)
Annual education/training exposure	
Effective dose equivalent	1 mSv (100 mr)
Embryo-fetus exposure during gestation	
Total dose equivalent	5 mSv (500 mr)

Note. See Table 3.1 for meanings of abbreviations. Adapted from *Radiologic Science for Technologists* (6th ed., p. 500), by S. C. Bushong, 1997, St. Louis: Mosby. Copyright 1997 by Mosby. Reprinted with permission.

Due to the young, immature, and rapidly dividing cells, the most dangerous time for a fetus to receive radiation is during the first trimester of the mother's pregnancy. Nonemergency radiologic procedures on the pregnant patient should be delayed until after delivery. If a procedure is deemed an emergency, it should be discussed with the radiologist to determine whether radiation exposure during the examination can in any way be reduced. Although most technologists do not receive more than the dose limits for the fetus (5 mSv or 500 mr) during a full year of occupational exposure, technologists and clinicians who are pregnant may wish to request a second badge for wearing under the lead apron at waist level during fluoroscopic procedures to measure the nonattenuated fetal dose. Aprons that allow room for growth during pregnancy are available.

Biological Effects of Radiation

Any amount of radiation exposure has the potential to produce negative effects on individuals. Radiation exposure has a linear, nonthreshold relationship in human tissue. This means that negative effects can occur at any dose and that the risk of negative effects increases with dose. For certain body organs a specific threshold exists at which negative effects may be seen.

Radiation exposure can produce negative somatic and genetic effects. Several are listed in Table 3.3. Somatic effects are those that directly affect the exposed individual, such as tissue reddening or burn immediately following exposure or abnormal cell development some time later. Genetic effects are those that affect the reproductive or germ cells, the evidence of which may appear in the subject's offspring. When considering reproductive health of the clinician and the patient, it is important to realize that genetic effects from radiation are considered to be nonthreshold.

Somatic Effects: Malignant Disease

One of the most serious potential effects of radiation exposure is the development of malignant disease. Exposure to high levels of radiation can produce cellular change and rapid growth commonly referred to as cancer. Studies have clearly shown that if the radiation dose is sufficient,

Table 3.3
Summary of Responses, Effects of Irradiation in Utero, and Protective Measures for the Pregnant Radiographer

Human Responses to Low-Level X-ray Exposure

Life-span shortening	10 days/rad
Cataracts	None below 200 rad
Leukemia	10 cases/10^6/rad
Cancer	100 cases/10^6/rad
Genetic effects	Doubling dose = 50 rad
Death from all causes	1:10,000/rad

Effects of Irradiation in Utero

0 to 14 days	Spontaneous abortion: 25% natural incidence; 0.1% increase/10 rad
2 to 8 weeks	Congenital abnormalities: 5% natural incidence; 1% increase/10 rad
Second to third trimester	Cell depletion: no effect at less than 50 rad: Latent malignancy: 4:10,000 natural incidence; 6:10,000/rad
0 to 9 months	Genetic effects: 10% natural incidence; 5×10^{-7} mutations/rad

Protective Measures for the Pregnant Radiographer

Two personal radiation monitors
Dose limit: 500 mrem every 9 months, 50 mrem every month

Note. See Table 3.1 for meanings of abbreviations. From *Radiologic Science for Technologists* (6th ed., p. 504), by S. C. Bushong, 1997, St. Louis: Mosby. Copyright 1997 by Mosby. Reprinted with permission.

a single exposure can elevate the risk for cancer development several years later. Also, no type of cancer is unique to radiation exposure; the incidence of all types of cancer can increase with exposure to radiation. Finally, it is known that certain body tissues (bone marrow, thyroid gland, breast, and gonads) are radiosensitive and that young children who have rapidly dividing cells are more radiosensitive than adults (Bushong, 1997).

Leukemia. The characteristics that define leukemia include an abnormal proliferation and incomplete maturation of leukocytes and lymphocytes (white blood cells). This disease may develop relatively early after radiation exposure. For this reason it has been well studied. Development of leukemia has been associated, for example, with radiation exposure in the form of fallout from nuclear testing (Johnson, 1984; Land, McKay, & Machado, 1984).

Thyroid Cancer. Research has established a clear relationship between exposure to external radiation and the development of thyroid cancer (Ron et al., 1995). Children in the 1930s and 40s were irradiated to the neck as a treatment for enlarged thymus glands. These children later developed a significant increase over the nonradiated matched controls in the development of thyroid tumors. More recently, a substantial increase in the incidence of thyroid cancer has been reported in Russia and the Ukraine as a consequence of the 1986 Chernobyl nuclear disaster (Williams, Pinchera, Karaoglou, & Chadwick, 1993).

Breast Cancer. Although early studies indicated that the risk associated with the radiation received during mammography did not outweigh the risk of receiving radiation, current technology has rendered mammography a successful screening tool for nonpalpable breast tumors and provides only small amounts of radiation. A longitudinal Canadian study tracked breast cancer development in women who received interventional irradiation for tuberculosis between 1930 and 1950. The results show a strong linear trend of increasing risk for breast cancer development with increasing radiation dose (Howe & McLaughlin, 1996). A study of 105,000 female radiology technologists spanning more than 50 years failed to show an increase in the development of breast cancer due to occupational exposure (Doody, Mandel, & Boice, 1995).

Somatic Effects: Nonmalignant Effects

In addition to the exposure-related development of metastatic lesions, radiation can also produce nonmalignant changes in the organism. Selected body systems show increased sensitivity to radiation.

Cataracts. The eye is sensitive to the effects of radiation. Radiation-induced cataracts were a complication associated with the early use of radiation, with increased frequency in the development of cataracts found among physicists and physicians working with radiation

(Bushong, 1997). The threshold dose for radiation-induced cataracts is considered to be approximately 200 rads for a single exposure with a 20-year latency period for their development (Singer, 1989). Modern fluoroscopy systems emit significantly less radiation so the risk to participating health care workers is much smaller.

Life Span Shortening. The somatic effect of a shortened life span has been more difficult to document. In the 1930s it was determined that as a group radiologists lived about 5 years less than their physician colleagues (Bushong, 1997). Recent large group studies completed by the American Registry of Radiologic Technologists did not show any significant life span shortening for radiologic technologists. This change is likely due to a variety of factors, including increased awareness of the importance of radiation safety, equipment improvements such as the development of image intensifiers, improved shielding materials, and procedural improvements.

Genetic Effects of Radiation Exposure

The effect of radiation on germ cells may result in genetic damage that may be passed on to future generations in the form of mutations. Genetic effects are considered to have a linear, nonthreshold, dose–response relationship. Thus, any dose is capable of producing a genetic change and the risk increases with dose.

Because most information relative to radiation genetics comes from animal studies, it is considered to be the weakest area of human radiobiology information. Still, it is generally agreed that, although radiation-induced mutations are very uncommon, any dose of radiation can potentially produce them. Whereas mutations similar to those that are radiation induced can also occur in the absence of radiation exposure, prevalence increased with radiation dose. The mutations that result are generally harmful to the developing organism and are usually recessive and more common in males than females.

Radiologic Equipment

Many types of diagnostic and fluoroscopic X-ray machines are in common use. Some are stationary, whereas others are mobile and capable of being moved from room to room. Stationary systems are installed in rooms with specific amounts of lead or lead-equivalent materials in the walls. Mobile equipment can be used in any room.

Stationary Equipment

The modern, general-purpose X-ray room contains a radiographic unit and sometimes a fluoroscopic unit with an electronic image intensifier and TV viewing system (see Figure 3.3). If the room has such a dual system, there are two X-ray tubes. One tube is attached to an overhead crane assembly for movement around the X-ray room and over the table. The other tube is located under the table and is used exclusively for fluoroscopy. As discussed elsewhere, recognition of the location of the radiation source will dictate certain radiation protection measures that are taken.

X-ray Tubes. The X-ray tube consists of a cathode (negative terminal) and an anode (positive terminal) within a highly evacuated glass envelope. The tube is immersed in oil and then placed within a lead housing.

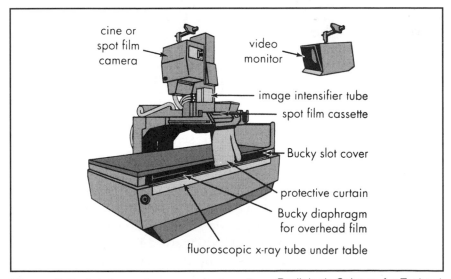

Figure 3.3. A stationary fluoroscopy system. From *Radiologic Science for Technologists* (6th ed., p. 322), by S. C. Bushong, 1997, St. Louis: Mosby. Copyright 1997 by Mosby. Reprinted with permission.

The beam can be focused through either a small or large focal spot perpendicular to the anode surface to which the electrons are focused. The smaller focal spot is chosen when detail on the radiograph is important. The larger focal spot is used for higher exposures necessary on large body parts. Because of the immense amounts of heat produced, manufacturers provide with each tube a rating chart that gives the maximum milliamperes, time, and kilovolts that are permissible, along with cooling requirements.

Fluoroscopy Equipment. The term *fluoroscopy* refers to the viewing of a fluoroscopic screen, which is a sheet of material that emits light (fluoresces) when exposed to X-ray. When performing a fluoroscopy study on a patient who is in the supine position, the under-table X-ray tube is in use with the fluoroscopic screen positioned above the patient. Thus, the radiation is generated from beneath the patient. The beam passes upward through the body and causes the screen to fluoresce or give off light. The fluoroscopy camera located above the patient detects emerging light caused by the photons. When the patient is in a seated position, the beam continues to be generated from beneath the table, but passes laterally through the patient's tissues to be detected by the camera. Fluoroscopy differs from radiography in that fluoroscopy is a dynamic study, meaning that fluoroscopic images are in motion, compared to radiographic images, which are static or still. The capability of fluoroscopy to record the full-motion swallow is the reason that it has become the "gold standard" in the evaluation of dysphagia.

Early fluoroscopy was performed with the radiologist looking directly into the fluoroscopic screen that dimly fluoresced in a totally darkened room. Today's modern equipment uses an image intensifier tube that is attached to the fluoroscopic screen. This tube converts the X-ray image at the input phosphor to an electron image at the photocathode that is bonded to the input phosphor. The electron image is focused through a series of electrostatic lenses toward the output phosphor. The resulting electrons that hit the output phosphor are 50 to 75 times brighter than before intensification. The image intensifier produces an image that can be readily viewed in full room lighting. The intensifier also produces a significant reduction in the radiation required to produce an acceptable image. A major advantage of image intensification is that the output image can be linked to a television camera by a lens system or a fiber-optic bundle, and the image displayed on a television monitor. Other advantages include the ability to control brightness and contrast electronically, the fact that multiple monitors can be used and placed away from the radiation source, electronic recording and playback capabilities, and digital manipulation of images. The major disadvantage of television monitoring is a loss of detail, with the television monitor being the weakest link in the video display chain.

Generators and Transformers. The function of a generator is to produce the power needed to create the radiation beam. Less than 1% of the total energy is actually converted to X-ray; the other 99% is given off as heat. Three types of generators are available for use today: single phase, three phase, and high frequency. Single-phase generators represent older technology and require almost twice the exposure to create an image equivalent to that of the newer types. Three-phase and high-frequency types used in fluoroscopes are the newest and have more efficient outputs. Transformers are used to step the voltage up or down to meet system needs. The step-up transformer is required to produce the kilovolts necessary to create X-ray.

Operating Consoles or Control Panels. The operating console is usually found in a shielded booth adjacent to the fluoroscopy suite. The control area will have a window close to the operating console and positioned so that the patient may be viewed when an X-ray exposure is made. The console is where selections are made for proper milliamperes, exposure time in seconds, kilovolts, and size of focal spot. Exposures for the under-table fluoroscopic tube are always made in the fluoroscopy room at the side of the table.

Examination Tables. The X-ray table can be either the stationary or tilting type. Tilting tables are necessary for fluoroscopy and for the proper completion of swallowing studies. The motorized tilting table can be placed in a vertical position (90 degrees), in a horizontal position (0 degrees), or any place in between. A variety of attachments, including the footplate, restraining straps, and foam wedges, allow additional positioning options for the patient who is studied while in a supine position. It is important for the dysphagia clinician to remember that the radiation source is typically located just below the table. When activated, the beam passes through the table top and the patient's tissue, and is received by the X-ray film or the fluoroscopy camera.

Automatic Exposure Control. X-ray systems are designed to take static films. The most common is the chest X-ray. Creating such a film is accomplished by loading a light-tight film cassette into the system, usually in the bucky tray that is located under the table. The bucky tray is loaded when static films are taken using the over-the-table camera. During the fluoroscopic swallowing study, static films can also be taken. These "spot films" are static and can be exposed through the overhead unit. On its underside, the fluoroscopy table contains a grid that is designed to absorb scattered radiation before it reaches the film and the automatic exposure control (AEC) detectors. For static images the AEC automatically stops exposure when a sufficient film density is reached; this includes images produced in the fluoroscopic spot-filming device. It is important that the right detectors are selected for the appropriate anatomy. With the pharynx and esophagus, only the center of what are usually three detectors should be used.

Mobile Fluoroscopy Equipment

Mobile fluoroscopy is performed by a fluoroscopic system that is portable and commonly referred to as a C-arm (see Figure 3.4). The C-arm can be easily transported to any location in a medical center or nursing home for on-site or off-site fluoroscopy studies. This technology is used extensively in operating rooms and surgical suites. The C-arm is battery operated, and is connected to a monitor for viewing and a VCR for recording the image. Whereas stationary units have viewing fields of up to 14 inches, the C-arm usually provides only a 6- or 9-inch field. These units often have digital imaging features that allow post-study image manipulation. The image analysis capability allows the examiner to enhance the image in a variety of ways that will aid in understanding the patient's swallowing problem. The same safety considerations appropriate for stationary fluoroscopy equipment need to be kept in mind when using the C-arm. As with stationary units, distance is still the best protection for the operator. If the C-arm unit is used outside the radiographic suite, all personnel should take the standard safety precautions. Personnel in adjacent rooms are not at significant risk, as the amount of radiation received 6 feet away

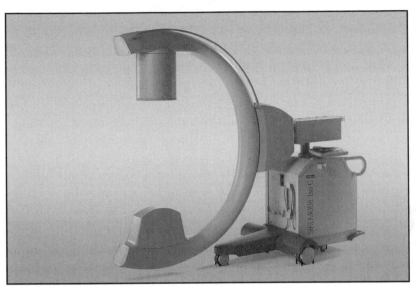

Figure 3.4. A C-arm (mobile) fluoroscopy system. Photo courtesy of Siemens Medical Systems, Inc.

from the unit is considered negligible. However, personnel should be apprised that a procedure using ionizing radiation is being performed within the adjacent room so that anyone concerned could take additional precautions.

Storage Systems for Imaging Data

Storage of Study Data: Videotape Recording. Although early image intensifiers represented a significant step forward, they allowed viewing by only one person at a time. Further, without video recording ability, there was no record of the transitory images upon which diagnoses were made. Today a video recording system can be coupled to the output phosphor of the image intensifier to allow viewing of the radiographic image by any number of observers in the fluoroscopy suite while the study is in progress.

A permanent video record of the swallowing study should be made and retained. Photo-spot films or cine may be used; however, it is easier to use a fluoroscopy system coupled with a videocassette recorder (VCR). The direct output of the fluoroscopy monitor can be cabled to the input of the VCR. Although a recorder in the standard VHS is acceptable, slightly improved recordings will result from the use of a Super-VHS system with S-VHS tapes. The VCR and fluoroscopy unit can be wired to each other in such a way that pressing the fluoroscope activation switch also engages the VCR in the record mode. The advantage is that only audio and video information that occurs during visualized swallows will be recorded on the tape, making for a more rapid review of swallow studies and conserving videotape. One significant limitation, however, is that there is a brief lag time between when the VCR is activated and when it begins recording. Consequently, unless a brief but consistent lead time is provided following swallows, the initial parts of swallows will be missed. Many dysphagia clinicians initiate the recorder at the beginning of the study and let it run uninterrupted until the end. This ensures that all swallows and between-swallow examiner comments are captured.

Storage of Study Data: Time and Date Recording. A signal from a time and date generator can be fed with the video signal to the recorder. As the fluoroscopy image is recorded, a timing channel is stamped, usually at the bottom or top of the screen. Timers used often have the ability to stamp each $\frac{1}{100}$ of a second. This exceeds the limits of the recording system that records at a rate of $\frac{1}{30}$ of a second. Still, when it comes to quantifying transit times, the channel is a necessity.

Storage of Study Data: Spot Films. In many studies, only select images are saved as "spot films." Although the fluoroscopic swallowing study is primarily a study of motion, at times the clinician may wish to record a static frame on film. Exposures with spot films require more patient dose, and the delay necessary before exposure can be made is undesirable. However, spot films do provide a familiar format for the radiologist and have high image quality should suspicious pathologies be identified and need further evaluation.

A photo-spot camera is similar to a movie camera except that it exposes only one frame when activated. It receives its image from the output phosphor of the image intensifier tube and therefore requires less patient exposure than the spot film. The older photo-spot camera uses film sizes of 70 and 105 millimeters (mm). As a general rule, the larger film format results in better image quality but greater patient dose. Even with 105-mm spot films, however, the patient dose is only approximately half of that with spot films. The photo-spot camera results in an adequate image quality without interruption of the fluoroscopic examination and has a rate of up to 12 images per second. The film is processed in the automatic processor used for conventional films.

Cine film, which is 16 mm and 35 mm in size, is smaller than photo-spot films, and is more commonly found in angiography suites. This film is especially useful in studies requiring rapid-sequencing filming, such as in swallowing studies. Cine film must be developed in a special cine processor prior to viewing. Cine and spot film systems are giving way to digital radiography, which has the advantage of digital enhancement such as contrast and density enhancement, magnification, subtraction, and real-time imaging. Dysphagia clinicians need to inform the radiographer which imaging system they intend to use, as appropriate cameras need to be loaded and attached prior to the procedure to avoid delays during the procedures.

NCRP Special Radiation Safety Considerations During Fluoroscopy

The NCRP (1989) provides specific safety guidelines to be followed when fluoroscopy is performed. These include the following:

1. Only persons whose presence is necessary shall be in the fluoroscopy room during the exposure. All persons shall be protected (provided with lead aprons, leaded gloves, and portable shields, as needed).

2. The hand of the fluoroscopist shall not be placed in the useful beam unless the patient attenuates the beam and a protective glove of at least 0.25 mm lead equivalent is worn. Shielding devices such as leaded screen drapes and tableside shields shall be provided to minimize scatter radiation reaching the operator.

3. Medical fluoroscopy should be performed only by or under the supervision of physicians properly trained in fluoroscopic procedures.

4. The operator should use the maximum source-to-skin distance (SSD), consistent with medical requirements of the
procedure. For fluoroscopic procedures, distances of less
than 30 cm (12 inches) *shall not* be used and distances of less
than 38 cm (15 inches) *should not* be used. The SSD must
be considered because the fluoroscopist has the ability to
move the fluoroscope very close to the patient. The source
means the target of the X-ray tube. The manufacturer will
design the unit so that it complies with the standards
regarding the distance from the source to the tabletop.

5. A cumulative timing device, activated by the fluoroscope
exposure switch, shall be provided. It shall indicate by
either audible or visual signal, or both, obvious to the user,
the passage of a predetermined period of irradiation not to
exceed 5 minutes. The signal should last at least 15 seconds
and require a manual reset.

Factors that Determine Exposure to Radiation

Three basic exposure factors are set on the radiographic equipment
before making an X-ray exposure: milliamperage (mA), exposure time
in seconds, and kilovoltage (kVp). These settings, made by the radiologic technologist (radiographer) or the radiologist, influence the quality of the visual image and determine, to a large degree, the amount of
radiation to which the patient is exposed.

Patient dose is not easily calculated, and needs to be measured
during the exposure to accurately represent the absorbed dose for any
procedure. Patient dose is, however, directly proportional to milliamperage second (mAs), or mA × time, if all other factors such as
distance from the patient to the source and kilovoltage are kept constant. During normal image-intensified fluoroscopy, low milliamperage
(< 5 mA) is used, resulting in a relatively low exposure rate for patient
and personnel. During spot and cine filming, exposure rates may be
higher. Clinicians should realize that the intensity of scatter is higher
during this filming and be especially conscious of radiation protection.

Use of minimum beam-on time reduces patient and personnel exposure. Intermittent fluoroscopy results in less exposure to patient and personnel than constant fluoroscopy because there is less beam-on time. The cumulative timer (5-minute timer) serves to minimize time by making the fluoroscopist aware of the accumulation of beam-on time. The "dead-man" switch minimizes beam-on time by automatically terminating the exposure whenever the fluoroscopist removes his or her foot from the switch.

Milliamperage second, as stated previously, is a measure of the total number of electrons that travel from the cathode to the anode to produce X-rays. Therefore, mAs = mA × seconds.

The kilovoltage level selected determines the energy of the photons. The lower the energy of the photons, the more likely the energy is absorbed by the tissue and never reaches the image receptor. To assure that the photons have enough energy to pass through the tissue and reach the image receptor, a high kilovoltage is recommended. Another factor that affects patient dose is the size of the field being exposed. Primary beam restriction is reduction of the X-ray beam to the area of the patient's body that is of clinical interest, thereby sparing adjacent tissues from unnecessary exposure. Reducing the field also reduces the amount of scattered X-rays produced. For this reason the dysphagia clinician should have an understanding of these factors. Scatter radiation during fluoroscopy is a major source of occupational radiation to personnel. Reduction of personnel exposure can be accomplished by attention to the cardinal principles of time, distance, and shielding. If possible, the clinician should view the procedure on a video screen from remote booth. If not possible, the clinician should wear appropriate lead aprons and try to stand away from the patient during the exposure.

The milliamperage and time multiplied together give the milliamp seconds (mAs), or quantity of exposure. When completing a videofluoroscopy, it is important to keep the total fluoroscopy time to a minimum. Higher kilovoltage will allow the milliamperage to be reduced, with some reduction in patient exposure. However, the kilovoltage should not be so high as to cause a degraded image from the amount of scatter created. Barium studies involving videofluoroscopy of the pharynx and esophagus are usually set between 80 to 95 kVp for sufficient penetration of the tissues without objectionable scatter.

Steps Designed To Ensure Radiation Safety

The federal government has strict guidelines for manufacturers of X-ray producing equipment. The NCRP is composed of experts in the field of radiation who set standards for radiation exposure and radiation-emitting equipment. The NCRP publications are numbered and available through the U.S. Department of Health and Human Services, Public Health Service, Food and Drug Administration, Center for Medical Radiation Development, Rockville, MD 20857. Specific NCRP standards as they relate to fluoroscopic equipment and the personnel who operate them are discussed earlier in this chapter in the discussion of fluoroscopy equipment.

A great deal of variation exists in the regulations imposed by the 50 states. Although each state's regulations must meet the federal standards, the mandates of many states exceed those imposed at the federal level. States require that radiation-emitting equipment be registered with the state and subjected to periodic state inspections. Regulations vary as to whom is allowed to own and operate X-ray equipment. Some states strictly regulate the licensing and testing of those who can operate X-ray equipment, whereas other states have no regulations. The NCRP guidelines indicate that medical fluoroscopy should be performed only by or under the supervision of physicians properly trained in fluoroscopic procedures. Most states that license operators exempt physicians. When considering owning or operating X-ray equipment, it is advisable to check the specific state's regulations.

While conducting a videofluoroscopic swallowing study, it is necessary to provide unique considerations to assure the safety of the patient and the clinician in the radiation-rich environment. The considerations for each are quite different. Following is a discussion of variables that can be controlled and measures that can be taken to ensure safety.

Minimizing Radiation Exposure to the Patient

When considering the radiation dose the patient may receive, there are two considerations. The first is whether the dose associated with the single videofluoroscopic swallowing study a clinician will perform is sufficient to produce any immediate negative effects. The second is whether the single dose is of concern in the broader context of the patient's cumulative radiation dose.

The instrument settings chosen by the fluoroscope operator and the shielding provided to the patient can have a direct impact on the quality of the study achieved and the radiation dose received. Although these are often the responsibility of the fluoroscope operator, clinicians must be aware of their effects.

Fluoroscope Beam Restriction. The area of the patient's body exposed to radiation should never be more than necessary to view the appropriate anatomy. Tightly controlled shutters on the fluoroscopy equipment allow the operator to "cone down," limiting the field to only the necessary structures. In the case of the oropharyngeal swallowing study, in the lateral position the necessary view is from the lips anteriorly to the cervical spine posteriorly, and from the hard palate superiorly to the point just inferior to the upper esophageal sphincter (UES) and the upper trachea. In the anterior–posterior (AP) view, the field should extend from the hard palate to a point inferior to the true vocal cords. The lateral dimension must be wide enough to accommodate the full width of the mandible and the soft tissues of the neck. Enlarging the field of view to include unimportant structures will result in an unnecessary increase in the radiation dose to the patient and an increase in scatter radiation that will fog or gray the image.

Filtration. Filtration is built into the radiologic equipment and reduces the skin dose of radiation to the patient. Standard amounts of filtration are required and will be checked by the physicist or radiation safety officer during required equipment checks.

Protective Equipment Features. Fluoroscopic equipment must have protective lead drapes, a bucky slot cover, and a cumulative timer to alert the fluoroscopist of on-beam time. This timer will alarm after 5 minutes of fluoroscopy time. At this time the operator may cancel the bell but allow the timer to continue timing. At the completion of the study, the clinician will have an accurate measure of total fluoroscopy time.

Shielding of Adjacent Body Areas. The patient's radiosensitive organs should be shielded when possible. In doing studies of the pharynx and esophagus, it is not practical to shield the patient's thyroid or breast. The radiation dose to the eyes, however, can be limited by ensuring that the field of study extends no further in a superior direction than the hard palate. The gonads can be shielded with a lead apron, drape, or with specifically made gonad shield.

Understanding Radiation Output from Fluoroscopy. Fluoroscopy systems typically use very low amperage (1 to 3 mA) compared with conventional X-ray films, which can be several hundred times greater. Although this difference might lead one to expect that fluoroscopy would provide a lower radiation dose, actually the radiation dose received by the patient during fluoroscopy is much higher than that for routine diagnostic films due to the extended period of time the patient is exposed. It is important to note that, when manipulating variables to improve penetration or image quality, an increase in milliamperes, even by 1.0, will significantly increase the radiation dose the patient receives. The dysphagia clinician should also be aware that when he or she asks the fluoroscopist to use the magnification mode in image-intensified fluoroscopy, the radiation dose will at least double.

To put fluoroscopy dose levels into perspective, consider the following. The radiation received by a patient who is exposed to only 1 minute of fluoroscopy at 5,000 mrad/minute would equal the annual dose allowable (50 mGy) for occupational purposes. Only 5 minutes of fluoroscopy would give the patient a significant dose of radiation (25,000 mrad or 250 mGy). In comparison, a typical chest X-ray exposes the patient to 10 to 20 mrad (0.1 or 0.2 mGy) and a computerized tomography (CT) scan might provide 3,000 to 4,000 mrad (or 30 to 40 mGy).

The Food and Drug Administration has established the following thresholds as related to the skin. Erythema is produced after receiving 6 Gy (600 rad) (Burlington, 1994). A threshold of 15 to 20 Gy (2,000 rad) is required to produce moist desquamation, dermal necrosis, and secondary ulceration. Rosenthal et al. (1998) studied 859 catheter ablation cases and found that the mean total fluoroscopy time was 53 minutes. In 22% of their cases, the radiation dose necessary to produce skin damage was exceeded. Total fluoroscopy times are much shorter for the videofluoroscopic swallowing study. Is the amount of radiation that the patient is likely to receive in a 5-minute swallowing study significant in terms of potential skin damage? Although, depending on equipment settings, the radiation dose provided by the direct fluoroscopy beam can be higher, it typically provides between 0.02 to 0.05 Gy/min (2 to 5 rad/minute). If the system produces 5.0 rad/

minute then a 5-minute swallowing study will expose the patient to 25 rad. This is approximately 4% of the dose required to produce erythema and 1.2% of that required to produce necrosis. Consequently, the risk for immediate skin damage in a 5-minute fluoroscopic swallowing study is quite low. Still, there is reason to cautiously limit exposure. Considering that a patient may undergo multiple fluoroscopic swallowing studies as well as barium swallows, chest X-rays, CT scans, and barium enemas, clinicians should also be concerned for the cumulative dose the patient may receive. As a consequence, clinicians should follow the ALARA philosophy in regard to radiation exposure, under which all exposures must be justified and kept "As Low As Reasonably Achievable" (ALARA). This concept applies to workers, patients, and the general public.

Several controls and factors collectively govern the quality of the fluoroscopy image. The first controls that should be adjusted to improve image quality are the monitor's contrast or brightness controls. In completing the examination, the kilovoltage must be set sufficiently high to penetrate the body. Even though a very low setting of 50 to 60 kVp will most often penetrate the pharynx and esophagus, it will do so only at high milliamperage rates. High milliamperage levels increase the dose of radiation that will be encountered by the patient, the fluoroscopist, and the speech–language pathologist. Thus, a higher kilovoltage is desirable to provide adequate penetrating power while reducing the milliamperes necessary to produce it. As stated earlier, 80 to 95 kVp when using barium in the pharynx and esophagus is ideal and will allow a low 1 to 3 mA for most patients. The more the kilovoltage exceeds this range, the more scatter radiation will be produced. Scatter fogs the image, reducing overall contrast, but it is acceptable in this kilovoltage range with average-sized patients. Also, the lower kilovoltage may not fully penetrate the tissue. With very large patients, scatter radiation increases and degrades the quality of the image. Because increasing kilovoltage will further increase scatter, it is not recommended. In this circumstance, the fluoroscopist may need to increase the milliamperes to allow adequate visualization.

Controlling Total Fluoroscopy Time. The total fluoroscopy time required to complete a swallowing study varies depending on the complexity of the study. The study needs to be long enough to allow the critical clinical questions to be answered. One primary way of limiting fluoroscopy time is through thorough preparation for the study; this means knowing the patient, the qustions to be answered by the study, and the protocol sequence that will most efficiently lead to a diagnostic and management conclusion. For example, when direct and significant aspiration of a 5- and 10-cc bolus of an intermediate liquid (60 centipoise) is seen, then it is often unnecessary to evaluate a 15-cc bolus of the same viscosity. Depending on the patient, it may also be unnecessary to evaluate a low-viscosity liquid (1 to 11 centipoise). If the clinician can envision the patient's possible responses and their impact on the study protocol, then the study will proceed more directly toward its conclusion, eliminating unnecessary fluoroscopy exposure for the patient and clinician.

Each fluoroscopy system records the amount of time the system is activated during the study. At the completion of each swallow study, the dysphagia clinician should record total fluoroscopy time as a part of the procedure report. As studies accumulate, these times will offer an excellent data source for process improvement, that is, for reducing the total fluoroscopy time for each study to the minimum that is needed. With these data it will be possible to determine the mean total time for disorder types, specific diagnostic questions, and individual clinicians. When a study varies excessively from the mean, it will be possible to complete a focused review to determine what actions, if any, might have reduced the amount of fluoroscopy time required. This type of introspective approach to process improvement can help to ensure that radiation exposure is kept to an acceptable minimum.

The patient's exposure to radiation also can be reduced when the fluoroscopist uses intermittent fluoroscopy, meaning a light touch on the exposure when it is not necessary to see continuous motion. Light touch, which is accomplished by manually pulsing the fluoroscopy exposure switch, takes advantage of the fluorescence that continues after the radiation has stopped for a short period. The fluoroscopist can touch the exposure switch only after the image begins to fade, rather than constantly holding the switch in the on position. For example, when a patient masticates whole meat, it is not necessary to witness the entire episode to form a judgment regarding mastication ability. Units with pulsed fluoroscopy capability perform this intermittent function at a reduced dose. Herrmann et al. (1996) and Aufrichtig, Xue, Thomas, Gilmore, and Wilson (1994) demonstrated that fluoroscopy that pulsed at a rate of 12 to 15 pulses per second yielded a minimum reduction in radiation dose of approximately 50%. When in the pulse mode, there is some compromise in the quality of motion visualization related to the pulse rate. Not all fluoroscopy systems have pulse capabilities. Another technique employed by Martin and Hunter (1994) demonstrated that the settings selected by the Automatic Exposure Control (AEC) could result in as much as a 20% to 50% reduction in the radiation received by the patient.

Minimizing Occupational Radiation Exposure

The operator of the radiologic equipment should never be exposed directly to the primary radiation beam. The primary beam is the area of exposure coming directly from the X-ray tube before it interacts with a body part. The operator's exposure usually comes from secondary or scattered radiation, which occurs from the interaction of the radiation with the body and scatters radiation exposure in many directions. Scattered radiation is not as penetrating as incident radiation but will cause a graying effect on the image and will provide the operator with additional exposure.

In regard to occupational exposure, three basic factors must be considered: time, distance, and shielding. When the clinician operates with these factors in mind, occupational exposure will be kept to a minimum. The actions taken to reduce occupational exposure will also benefit the patient through reduced radiation exposure.

Fluoroscopy Time. Any procedural steps that will reduce the amount of fluoroscopy time will reduce exposure to the fluoroscopist and dysphagia clinician, in addition to the patient. See the previous discussion of steps that can be taken to reduce total fluoroscopy time.

Distance. The further the fluoroscopist or viewers are from the primary beam, the less exposure they will receive (see Figure 3.5). The relationship of radiation dose to distance is governed by an inverse relationship known as the inverse square law. Speech–language pathologists are familiar with this concept as it relates to the intensity of sound. In the case of radiation, it means radiation intensity varies inversely with the square of the distance from the source. For example, if a clinician who is 24 inches away from a radiation source repositions so that he or she is 48 inches away, then exposure will be reduced by a

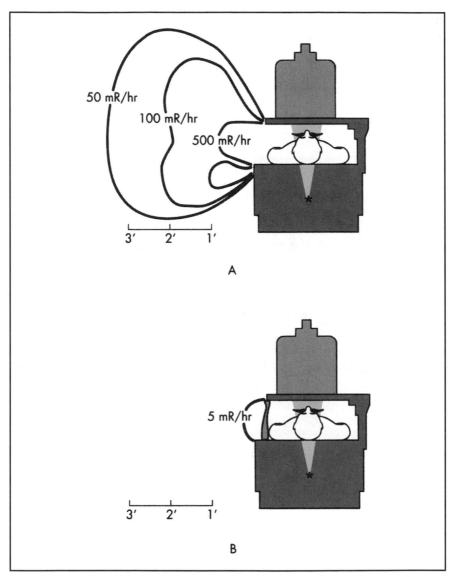

Figure 3.5. A depiction of unshielded radiation exposure. From *Radiologic Science for Technologists* (6th ed., p. 512), by S. C. Bushong, 1997, St. Louis: Mosby. Copyright 1997 by Mosby. Reprinted with permission.

factor of 4. Thus, radiation exposure will be reduced by 75%. In orthopedic procedures that are fluoroscopically guided, the clinician who is within 24 inches of the beam receives significant radiation exposure, whereas one who is 36 inches or greater away receives extremely low amounts (Mehlman & DiPasquale, 1997). The reduction of dose for personnel is best accomplished by maintaining a maximum distance from the patient during exposure.

This relationship between dose and distance is a simple yet very important factor for dysphagia clinicians to remember. It is reflected in the following practice considerations. Having provided a bolus of test material, the clinician should take at least two full steps back from the patient before the fluoroscope is activated and the command to swallow is given. Also, even though the clinician's hand is not in the field of view, he or she should avoid holding a cup of liquid test material while the patient's straw drinking is viewed. Just because the clinician's hand is not visible in the fluoroscopy image does not mean that it is not being irradiated. Holding a cup in this manner places the clinician in close proximity to the beam and in a location where scatter radiation levels are high.

Shielding. The safest place for the fluoroscopist or dysphagia clinician to stand during the videofluoroscopic swallowing study is within the shielded control area where maximum shielding from radiation is provided. Many times it will not be possible for the clinician to perform the study from this remote location. The inability of geriatric or pediatric patients to cooperate, to hold a cup of test material, to swallow on command, or to perform compensations and maneuvers by verbal command most often requires the clinician to be in the fluoroscopy suite near the patient. It is important then, for the fluoroscopist and dysphagia clinician to employ shielding to reduce their occupational exposure. The most commonly used shielding devices are protective aprons, lead gloves, thyroid shields, and lead glasses.

Protective Aprons. Anyone in the fluoroscopy room during the examination, including the fluoroscopist, dysphagia clinician, observers, dietitians, and family members, must wear a lead apron (Figure 3.6). Only the patient is exempt from this requirement. NCRP Report #102 states that protective lead aprons that have at least 0.5-mm lead equivalent shall be worn by each person in the fluoroscopy room. Most aprons protect the wearer from shoulder to shoulder and from clavicles to the

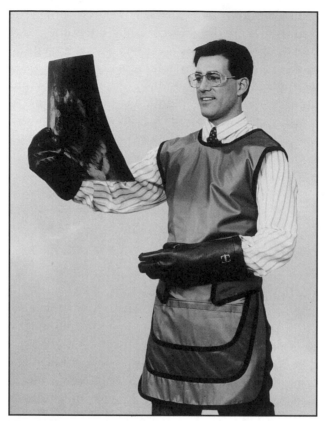

Figure 3.6. Protective barriers: the lead apron and gloves. Photograph courtesy of E-Z-EM, Inc.

knees, but only when the wearer is facing the radiation source. The back of most aprons provides little or no protection. Sometimes the patient, test materials, and video-recording system are arranged in such a way that it is mandatory that the clinician turn his or her back to the radiation source while the beam is on. This provides unprotected exposure of the back and gonads to scatter radiation. To avoid such an arrangement, the clinician and fluoroscopist should step through a mock swallow study, making such positioning errors apparent and allowing them to be corrected in a radiation-free environment.

Thyroid Shields. As stated previously, the thyroid gland is sensitive to radiation. Although no data are available for fluoroscopic swallowing studies, measurements gathered during cardiac catheterization and other fluoroscopic procedures indicate that the radiation dose to the thyroids of clinicians is higher than the dose that is registered by the dosimeter at the level of the shirt collar. Dysphagia clinicians who work in the fluoroscopy suite should wear a thyroid shield when performing procedures. The shields are not uncomfortable to wear, allow free movement, and provide protection where the apron cannot. If a radiation badge is worn attached to the shirt collar and a thyroid shield is worn, then the wearer needs to check to see that the badge is on the outside of the shield. If it is not, the cumulative dose readings will be inaccurate.

Lead Gloves. NCRP Report #102 states that the fluoroscopist's hand shall not be placed in the useful (primary) beam unless the beam is attenuated by the patient *and* a protective (0.25-mm lead equivalent) glove is worn (see Figure 3.6). Although lead gloves are bulky and make holding a Styrofoam cup or operating a catheter-tip syringe a challenging task, they are mandatory if the clinician's hand will enter the field of study. When a bolus is delivered via syringe to a patient who is unable to delay the swallow until commanded, then a lead glove can be used in a different way to provide shielding. If the glove is positioned between the fluoroscopy beam and the clinician's hand, it can serve a shielding function without being worn. For a patient in the supine position, the glove is laid lateral to the patient's neck and extending to the edge of the fluoroscopy table. In this way it is possible for the clinician to position his or her hand and the syringe to avoid the direct radiation coming from the tube located below the table's surface. Although this procedure will likely expose the hands to some scatter radiation, the extremities are relatively more resistant to radiation effects than other parts of the body.

Lead Eyeglasses. Lead crystal glasses (Figure 3.7) offer protection to the eyes, another susceptible organ. Such glasses are expensive and can be purchased as prescription or nonprescription. It is useful to note that even standard eyeglasses afford some protection from X-ray exposure to the eyes.

Radiation Exposure Monitoring

Facilities that operate X-ray and fluoroscopy equipment are required to have a radiation exposure-monitoring program in place. Under this

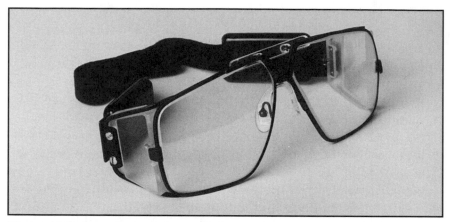

Figure 3.7. Protective lead glasses. Photograph courtesy of E-Z-EM, Inc.

program each worker who is potentially exposed to radiation must wear a personal radiation-monitoring device. Three types that are in general use are the film badge, thermoluminescent dosimeter, and pocket dosimeter.

Film Badge. Shortly after Röntgen's discovery of X-rays, he demonstrated with the aid of his wife's hand, that X-ray could be recorded on photographic film. The film badge in Figure 3.8 is composed of a small piece of radiographic film inside a holder. After an interval, usually a month or a quarter of a year, the film is extracted and processed. The film's image density is measured and can be directly correlated with an amount of radiation exposure received.

Thermoluminescent Dosimeter. Thermoluminescent dosimeters (TLDs) are composed of a crystal of lithium fluoride inside a holder. When the crystal is heated, it emits light which, when measured, corresponds to a given amount of radiation exposure. These are slightly more reliable in measuring radiation dosage than the film badge and are a little more expensive.

Pocket Dosimeter. Pocket dosimeters offer an immediate reading of radiation exposure, but are not routinely used in monitoring programs. They are most useful where a one-time exposure reading would be useful. The dosimeter may be used to document exposure of individu-

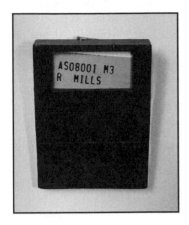

Figure 3.8. A film badge used in radiation monitoring programs.

als not in the formal monitoring program (e.g., students, observers, or family members).

Radiation Monitoring Reports

The institution's radiation safety officer will check the periodic reports of radiation monitoring and post them in a visible location. The clinician should check these reports to be aware of his or her interval and cumulative dosage. A reading of "M" is given when "minimal" or no exposure has been detected on the monitor. Otherwise, exposure for the period on the monitor will be given in milliSievert (mSv) values. As shown in Table 3.2, the maximum occupational exposure is 50 mSv for a year. Most reporting systems provide monthly, quarterly, yearly, and lifetime totals on each report. If the values are high, then the clinician should seek the counsel of the radiation safety officer to determine means by which exposure can be reduced. When changing employment, the cumulative totals of radiation exposure should be transferred to the new employer to maintain accurate lifetime totals. These reports are permanent records and are to be maintained indefinitely.

Important Factors in the Radiation Monitoring Program

For the monitoring program to work effectively, clinicians must follow these rules. Each individual who is regularly exposed to radiation during occupational duties must be included in the radiation monitoring program. Radiation badges, TLDs, and pocket dosimeters must be worn on the collar outside the lead apron and thyroid shield during each and every study that is performed. Monitoring devices must be changed after an assigned period (usually 1 to 3 months) and should not be worn outside of the radiation work environment. Finally, it is the employee's responsibility to review the monitoring reports and understand his or her exposure.

Contrast Agents

X-rays penetrate matter according to the material's density and the penetrating power of the X-ray beam. X-ray films and fluoroscopy exhibit the penetration or lack of penetration by the beam differently. On X-ray film tissue that lacks significant density appears as dark areas on the film. Tissue such as bone that has significant density shows up as light areas on the film. Dark areas are termed *radiolucent* and light areas are *radiopaque*. If a piece of metal such as a necklace or belt buckle were in the radiographic film image, it would appear as white due to the inability of the X-ray to penetrate the material. In viewing the fluoroscopic image, this concept is typically reversed, with radiolucent areas showing up as light and radiopaque areas showing up as dark.

Often body tissues and organs are difficult to visualize because they do not differ from the densities of surrounding tissue or are overshadowed by other, more dense body parts. In these cases a negative or positive contrast agent may be used to render these tissues more visible.

Positive Contrast Agents

Positive contrast agents produce areas that are radiopaque and appear black on the fluoroscopy image. Predominantly, the contrast material used has a barium sulfate ($BaSO_4$) base. Barium is quite suitable as a positive contrast agent because of its high molecular density. Barium is opaque to X-rays and is effectively inert in the body. It is not absorbed or metabolized and is eliminated unchanged by the body. Barium sulfate–based materials are available in liquid, powder, and paste forms. The liquids are commonly mixed with H_2O or other dietary liquids to produce liquid test materials with varied viscosities. Powder $BaSO_4$ is suitable for mixing with foods such as mashed potatoes and applesauce to render them radiopaque. Barium paste is frequently used to coat solids such as Lorna Doone cookies. Some flavored contrast materials are available; they make H_2O more palatable, but result in some unusual flavors when mixed with dietary items.

Barium products are labeled w/w (weight/weight), w/v (weight/volume), or both. The higher the w/w or w/v number, the more dense the mixture and, therefore, the greater the radiodensity. For some fluoroscopy studies, the dysphagia clinician needs to coat the lumen of a structure, such as the esophagus. In this case a contrast material with a high w/v or w/w value is chosen. Its high viscosity will ensure adequate tissue coating. If, on the other hand, the clinician needs to fill a lumen or cavity, then a less viscous material may be selected. A large variety of products is offered, even including barium sulfate tablets used to detect minimal esophageal strictures.

The use of barium-based contrast agents is contraindicated for patients with known or suspected gastrointestinal tract perforations. If swallowing studies are required on these patients, an iodine-based contrast media may be considered. After any study using barium in the gastrointestinal tract, it is important to rehydrate the patient to prevent barium impaction. The patient should be encouraged to increase water intake following completion of the study. The use of cathartics may also be required, especially in patients with a history of constipation.

Iodine is often used as a contrast medium by injecting it into a vein or artery. It is readily absorbed by the body and is excreted through the kidneys. It comes in different concentrations depending on use. The only product available for oral use in swallowing studies is Gastrografin (Squibb). Gastrografin has a viscosity that is very much like H_2O and, therefore, it does not coat the walls of the pharynx or esophagus very well. This material has a distinct and somewhat unpleasant taste that some patients find objectionable. Patients with known allergies, especially to shellfish or other iodine products, may have a severe reaction to any iodine-based product. A careful medical history should be taken from the patient before administering Gastrografin. An emergency cart should be available to cope with possible reactions, even for patients with no known allergies.

Negative Contrast Agents

Air is the only negative contrast agent used today. In the past, substances such as CO_2 were used as well. In the gastrointestinal tract, air may be injected following the administration of thick barium in what is termed a double-contrast study. The barium coats the mucosal surfaces and the air dilates the esophagus for improved visualization.

Summary

The environment encountered by dysphagia clinicians when they perform radiographic swallowing studies is unique to their practices. Within that environment the videofluoroscopic swallowing studies performed can be of immense benefit to the patient; however, through ignorance of the environment, there is potential for damage to both clinician and patient. With the information provided in this chapter and local guidance from the radiologist, radiation safety officer, and radiologic technologist, the clinician can function safely and reap the greatest benefit for the patient.

References

Aufrichtig, R., Xue, P., Thomas, C. W., Gilmore, G. C., & Wilson, D. L. (1994). Perceptual comparison of pulsed and continuous fluoroscopy. *Medical Physics, 21,* 245–256.

Brill, A. B. (1982). *Low level radiation: A fact book.* New York: Society of Nuclear Medicine.

Burlington, B. (1994, September 30). *FDA Public Health Advisory: Avoidance of serious X-ray–induced skin injuries to patients during fluoroscopically-guided procedures.* Rockville, MD: Center for Devices and Radiological Health, Food and Drug Administration.

Bushong, S. C. (1997). *Radiologic science for technologists* (6th ed.). St. Louis: Mosby Year Book.

Doody, M. M., Mandel, J. S., & Boice, J. D. (1995). Employment practices and breast cancer among radiologic technologists. *Journal of Occupational and Environmental Medicine, 37,* 321–327.

Herrmann, K., Helmberger, T., Waggershauser, T., Schatzl, M., All-mendinger, H., & Reiser, M. (1996). Initial experiences with pulsed fluoroscopy on a multifunctional fluoroscopic unit. *Rofo-Fortschr-Geb-Rontgenstr-Neuen-Bildgeb-Verfahr, 165,* 475–479.

Howe, G. R., & McLaughlin, J. (1996). Breast cancer mortality between 1950 and 1987 after exposure to fractionated moderate-dose-rate ionizing radiation in the Canadian fluoroscopy cohort study and a comparison with breast cancer mortality in the atomic bomb survivors study. *Radiation Research, 145,* 694–707.

Johnson, C. J. (1984). Cancer incidence in an area of radioactive fallout downwind from the Nevada test site. *Journal of the American Medical Association, 251,* 230–236.

Land, C. E., McKay, F. W., & Machado, S. G. (1984). Childhood leukemia and fallout from the Nevada tests. *Science, 223,* 139–144.

Martin, C. J., & Hunter, S. (1994). Reduction of patient doses from barium meal and barium enema examinations through changes in equipment factors. *British Journal of Radiology, 67*(804), 1196–1205.

Mehlman, C. T., & DiPasquale, T. G. (1997). Radiation exposure to the orthopedic surgical team during fluoroscopy: How far away is far enough? *Journal of Orthopaedic Trauma, 11*(6), 392–398.

National Council on Radiation Protection, Food and Drug Administration. (1987). *Ionizing radiation exposure of the population of the U.S.* (Report No. 93). Rockville, MD: Author.

National Council on Radiation Protection, Food and Drug Administration. (1989). *Medical X-ray, electron beam and gamma-ray protection for energies up to 50 MeV (equipment design, performance and use)* (Report No. 102). Rockville, MD: Author.

Ron, E., Lubin, J. H., Shore, R. E., Mabuchi, K., Modan, B., Pottern, L. M., Schneider, A. B., Tucker, M. A., & Boice, J. D., Jr. (1995). Thyroid cancer after exposure to external radiation: A pooled analysis of seven studies. *Radiation Research, 141,* 259–277.

Rosenthal, L. S., Mahesh, M., Beck, T. J., Saul, J. P., Miller, J. M., Kay, N., Klein, L. S., Huang, S., Gillette, P., Prystowsky, E., Carlson, M., Berger, R. D., Lawrence, J. H., Yong, P., & Calkins, H. (1998). Predictors of fluoroscopy time and estimated radiation exposure during radio-frequency catheter ablation procedures. *American Journal of Cardiology, 82,* 451–458.

Singer, S. J. (1989). Radiation safety. In K. Kandarpa (Ed.), *Handbook of cardiovascular and interventional radiologic procedures.* Boston: Little, Brown.

Williams, D., Pinchera, A., Karaoglou, A., & Chadwick, K. H. (Eds.). (1993). *Thyroid cancer in children living near Chernobyl: Expert panel report on the consequences of the Chernobyl accident.* Luxembourg: Commission of the European Communities.

Yochum, T. R. (1995). 1895–1995: Diagnostic imaging in its first century. *Journal of Manipulative Physiological Therapeutics, 18,* 618–625.

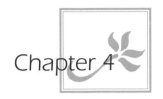

Chapter 4

Increasing the Precision of the Videofluoroscopic Swallowing Examination

Russell H. Mills

Mills discusses ways in which the dysphagia clinician can structure the video-fluoroscopic swallowing study to meet the needs of the patient. He focuses on controlling patient positioning, test material selection, bolus viscosity, and method of test material delivery.

1. *Viscosity-accurate liquid test materials for the VFSS can be prepared by use of the dilution curves that Mills provides. Prepare three samples using a dilution curve for the barium sulfate you use in the VFSS to ensure that you understand how the curves are used.*

2. *Mills states that it is important to test natural methods of test material delivery, such as cup drinking. As it is normally used, cup drinking does not reveal the amount that the patient has swallowed. How can the clinician determine bolus volume from a cup-drinking task?*

3. *Mills does not provide the reader with a complete VFSS protocol. Why did he choose not to do so?*

⁂ ⁂ ⁂

Clinicians have adopted a variety of technologies for use in the evaluation of dysphagia. Each has strengths and weaknesses. The videofluoroscopic swallowing study (VFSS) has several demonstrated strengths. Although the clinical examination does not reliably detect aspiration, the VFSS can do so (Khoo, Buller, & Wong, 1996; Kidd, Lawson, Nesbitt, & MacMahon, 1993). The results of the VFSS have proven valuable in treatment planning (Wright & Jordan, 1997). It has also been demonstrated that, when the VFSS is used, some aspects of outcome are improved (Logemann et al., 1992). Further, use of the technique can reduce the cost of patient care and speed recovery (Logemann, 1997).

While the expansion in the breadth of knowledge across the subspecialty of dysphagia is important, equally significant is the increase in the depth of knowledge regarding the VFSS as the primary instrumental diagnostic technique. Clinicians now have more knowledge with respect to how the VFSS is performed, for whom, with what materials, and with what measurements. It is now clear that a variety of factors must be controlled if meaningful results are to be achieved. If these factors are allowed to vary freely, it is likely that faulty conclusions will be drawn from the study. Having arrived at faulty diagnostic conclusions, clinicians are likely to develop management plans that are flawed. In an era when the focus is on outcome, clinicians must do all possible to ensure that accurate results are obtained from the VFSS so that management goals can be reached.

Clinical experience indicates that VFSS examinations do not always provide the illuminative data required by the clinician. Consider this familiar scenario. A patient is referred from a medical ward. The nursing staff reports that the patient is choking on liquids. A VFSS is completed and the results fail to show evidence of significant aspiration. What interpretations will explain the inconsistency between the complaint and the VFSS results? It is possible that

1. The choking was a result of penetration and not aspiration.

2. The patient's swallowing was temporarily improved at the time of the VFSS due to improved mental status, absence of fatigue, altered medication, or other reason(s).

3. The patient experienced long-term improvement in his or her acute medical condition that is reflected in improved swallowing.

4. The requirements of the VFSS did not represent the patient's real-world swallowing.

Any of these four explanations could apply to a patient who failed to demonstrate functional abnormality when the VFSS was conducted. First, some patients seem to be hypersensitive to material that enters the laryngeal vestibule; the resultant cough may be taken as evidence of aspiration but in reality only represents penetration. Second, other patients may show fluctuations in behavior from day to day and sometimes from hour to hour. Fluctuations may be due to fatigue, medication effects, or other factors. The variability in those factors that led to the consultation request and VFSS evaluation may account for an inconsistency. Third, patients do make gains from acute disease; that is, their medical condition and functional abilities improve. This certainly is true of patients who have experienced acute cerebrovascular accidents. If any of the first three reasons holds true for a patient, then the VFSS results showing no evidence of significant aspiration were correct.

When the fourth possibility is true, then the VFSS has failed to provide the clinician with the needed information. If, by failure in design or execution, the VFSS does not detect a problem that in reality exists, then a false negative error has been made. In this condition, the patient may have been asked to perform swallowing under conditions that are not representative of real-world swallowing for this patient. Warms (1998) pointed out that the VFSS cannot completely simulate the clinical (on the ward) feeding situation. The VFSS is a *simulation* of actual feeding and as such will never be a perfect replication. Still, important variables can be controlled that will increase the precision of VFSS examinations. According to Bisch, Logemann, Rademaker, Kahrilas, and Lazarus (1994), the VFSS should systematically evaluate the effects of variables known to affect the swallow including bolus volume, texture, and method of delivery. A failure to control any of these variables may account for failure to detect an existing dysphagia.

The prominent textbooks, diagnostic manuals, and national workshops in the area of dysphagia diagnostics have attended to image interpretation, compensation testing, testing of maneuvers, and so forth. These books and manuals include those by Groher (1984), Logemann (1986, 1998), Murray (1999), and Perlman & Schulze-Delrieu (1997). Because of their excellent and extensive coverage, this chapter limits its focus to how clinicians can design and conduct a VFSS examination with precision. Performing the precise VFSS examination requires that several variables be recognized and controlled.

Factors To Consider in Patient Selection

Dysphagia clinicians have a variety of diagnostic choices: the clinical examination, VFSS, Fiberoptic Endoscopic Evaluation of Swallowing (FEES), electromyography, manography, scintigraphy, pH monitoring, and others. FEES (Langmore, Schatz, & Olsen, 1988) has been an important addition for the dysphagia clinician (see Chapter 5 of this text). Both VFSS and FEES can provide valuable diagnostic information regarding dysphagia, but each excels in certain respects. When clinicians require information about the oral or esophageal stage, oral or pharyngeal movements need to be visualized and perhaps timed, and VFSS is the best choice. Although these data are important, FEES also has strengths. An important one is that FEES allows the examiner to view the actual anatomic structures rather than a two-dimensional black-and-white representation. In some respects, FEES proves more flexible than stationary fluoroscopy with patients who are difficult to transport or position, although some can be accommodated with specialty seating. Patients located in intensive care units are typically connected to oxygen, humidification, intravenous drips, and so on. Moving patients to the fluoroscopy suite for a study can be very difficult, often with results that are less than satisfactory. Also, it is usually difficult to position a badly contracted patient for a satisfactory VFSS result. In these circumstances the clinician may have the option of providing an examination at the bedside in the form of a FEES or a fluoroscopy examination using a mobile C-arm system.

Purposes of the Videofluoroscopic Swallowing Study

At the outset, the reader might wonder why I include as a topic the *reason* for completing the VFSS. Obviously, clinicians want to visualize the patient's swallowing so that appropriate recommendations can be made. However, I acknowledge three distinct purposes for the VFSS examination. These purposes are fulfilled as the three stages of the VFSS are completed.

Stage I: Demonstrating the Swallowing Problem

If a swallowing abnormality exists, the first purpose of the examination is to demonstrate that disorder. The proper management of dysphagia must proceed from diagnosis to treatment planning that is based on an understanding of the patient's altered physiology (Huckabee & Pelletier, 1999). To accomplish effective treatment planning and management, it is important that the dysphagia be demonstrated. If the dysphagia cannot be demonstrated, then it cannot be understood. If it cannot be understood, then it cannot be properly managed. Attempts to demonstrate the dysphagia cannot be pursued with abandon. Clinicians must at all times be aware of risks that are present and respond with the patient's welfare in mind. While dysphagia clinicians seem quite attuned to the risks associated with significant aspiration, there are also risks associated with failing to detect a problem that indeed exists. Failing to detect a swallowing problem may allow a patient to continue with unsafe swallowing practices.

As it is often performed, the VFSS may betray this first purpose in a subtle manner. Often the VFSS is performed in positions and with bolus volumes and consistencies that are considered ideal, with no appreciation given to the patient's real-world feeding situation. For example, consider an impulsive, long-term care patient who experiences difficulty (perhaps aspiration) while self-delivering solid and liquid bolus volumes of 20 to 30 ml in a semireclined position. Such a patient may do quite well when delivered ⅓-teaspoon bites and sips by the examiner while seated in a 90-degree upright position in the fluoroscopy suite. The result may well be a false negative error, as the patient is returned to the floor with a clean "swallowing bill of health" only to continue to have difficulty. Because ward personnel are told that coughing may not necessarily mean aspiration, the patient's continuing difficulty may no longer be pursued until he develops systemic complications such as malnutrition, dehydration, or pneumonia. For these reasons, when patients who are receiving PO (per oral) feeding are seen for a VFSS, the examination should be completed with a consideration for the real-world feeding status of each patient. For the patient who is NPO (nothing per oral), the study should attempt to demonstrate the swallowing disorder under conditions that will likely exist if the patient is returned to PO status.

Answering the Stage I questions reinforces the critical importance of the information to be gathered in the history taking, interview, and clinical examination, as described by Groher in Chapter 1 and Zenner in Chapter 2. In particular, the meal observation will provide the clinician with the needed information regarding feeding position, self-feeding versus assisted feeding, impulsive tendencies, and so on. With this information the clinician can then design a study that will have the best opportunity of demonstrating the dysphagia under conditions that approximate real-world conditions.

Stage II: Understanding the Cause of the Problem

Stage II of the VFSS is predominantly a cognitive exercise that takes place simultaneously with Stage I test material administration. It is the process by which the clinician moves beyond the recognition of symptoms. Huckabee and Pelletier (1999) recognized the importance of this step, observing that the plan of management must not be based on symptomatology but rather on the underlying physiology. For example, it is not sufficient to base a management plan on the presence of aspiration because aspirations that occur before the swallow, during the swallow, after the swallow, and across differing viscosities and bolus sizes have different causes. The management plan must differentially address those causes. The identification of the physiologic changes that cause the dysphagia will enable the clinician to propose appropriate remedies.

Stage III: Evaluation of Potential Intervention

Once the clinician has observed the swallowing disorder and understands its causes, then he or she can begin with the systematic modification of variables that may improve swallowing performance. By the time this point of the study has been reached, the effects of bolus volume, viscosity, and method of delivery should be known. Stage III testing should then focus on the effects of positional compensations and swallowing maneuvers on the adequacy of the swallow. These have been shown to have a powerful effect in the management of dysphagia (Logemann, 1993).

Patient Safety Issues

As stated previously, examination of a patient's swallowing must be conducted with patient safety in mind. The first obligation of the clinician is to do no harm. How can clinicians demonstrate a swallowing problem in the fluoroscopy suite without placing the patient at undue risk? Precedents can be found in the means by which other disorders are evaluated.

One diagnostic test frequently performed in cases of suspected cardiac difficulty is the treadmill test, in which the patient is connected to cardiac monitors and his or her cardiac system is stressed by having the patient walk and then run on a treadmill as the incline of the treadmill is increased. This test carries risks for some patients. A small percentage of patients experience a cardiac crisis while completing the test. Cardiologists have found that for most patients the benefits of obtaining critical information outweigh the risks. In cardiac treadmill testing the level of risk is held within acceptable limits in two ways. First, the patient is carefully screened prior to the examination. That screening includes a review of the history and a clinical examination. This provides the physician with an improved ability to predict who might not be an appropriate candidate for the test and who, if accepted for the test, might be most likely to encounter difficulty. Second, recognizing that complications can sometimes occur, the examination facility is always equipped with a crash cart and personnel trained to use it.

In the case of the dysphagia evaluation, the same two factors hold. Risks can be reduced through a thorough knowledge of the patient's medical and swallowing history, results of the clinical examination, and the meal observation. For example, patients with a history of repeated aspiration pneumonia, a total lymphocyte count of less than 900, or a history of airway obstruction during eating require the clinician to be especially cautious.

Perhaps the two most important untoward events seen during the VFSS are significant aspiration that requires pulmonary suctioning and airway obstruction. Recognizing that these may occur, albeit infrequently, the dysphagia clinician must ensure that equipment and procedures are in place to handle them. The equipment required to perform pulmonary suctioning should be available. In addition, one of the individuals present during the examination must be privileged to perform the suctioning. Physicians, nurses, and respiratory therapists often have these skills. Although there is currently discussion among dysphagia clinicians regarding whether they should assume this responsibility during the VFSS, a consensus is not yet apparent. Should a dysphagia clinician choose to provide suctioning, then he or she must be privileged to do so. In preparation for the time when airway obstruction occurs in the fluoroscopy suite, those present during the VFSS should be trained in the use of the Heimlich maneuver.

Development of Questions for the Videofluoroscopic Swallowing Study

The quality of information contained in the consult request is highly variable. With the advent of electronic consulting, I have noticed a significant decline in the specificity of the information provided. I have received consults that simply request, "Please evaluate," leaving me to ferret out the nature of the complaint that prompted the request. From the history, interviews, and clinical examination, a clinician must develop the critical questions that will drive the VFSS examination. Table 4.1 provides a list of frequently encountered questions. A review of the questions makes it clear that few can be adequately answered based on the VFSS alone. Information from other sources is often needed to fully address the questions raised. Often the questions asked have to do with the appropriateness of dietary textures, which should be addressed only through the use of dietary food textures. Other questions in the list rely heavily on input from the registered dietitian. Still others tend not to be answerable by use of the VFSS. In preparation for the VFSS the clinician must develop a very specific list of diagnostic questions. These questions will drive the design and conduct of the examination.

Positioning the Patient for the VFSS Examination

The least satisfactory visualization of the swallowing structures is often obtained when the patient is in a supine position for the VFSS. Supine studies allow primarily an anterior–posterior (AP) view of the

Table 4.1
Frequently Encountered Diagnostic Questions

Questions Related to Swallowing Safety

Is the patient safe for per oral (PO) intake?
What diet consistency can this patient safely consume?
What consistency is appropriate to avoid airway obstruction?
Will the use of compensations or maneuvers improve the safety of the swallow?

Questions Concerning Dietary Texture

What dietary texture is most appropriate for the patient's swallowing pattern?
Should the patient's diet consistency be changed?
Should the patient chew adequately for a whole texture diet?

Questions Regarding Thickened Liquids

Will thickened liquids help the patient avoid episodes of aspiration?
Will thickened liquids compound a stasis problem?
What viscosity of thickened liquids is appropriate?
Should the viscosity level of thickened liquids be changed?
Should thickened liquids be discontinued?

Nutritional Status

Is the patient's weight loss due to a swallowing problem?
What can be done to improve this patient's nutritional status?
What diet textures might encourage intake to prevent the patient from losing more weight?
Is the patient's loss of interest in eating due to a swallowing problem?
What can be done for the patient who refuses to consume the diet consistency provided?

Alternate Avenue of Intake

Should tube feeding be instituted?
Should the patient's tube feedings be discontinued?
Should the patient be NPO?
Should this patient have PO intake for pleasure?

Repeat VFSS Examinations

The last VFSS was negative. Why is the patient still coughing or choking?
Was the patient's pneumonia caused by aspiration?
Does the patient's changed condition require a change in his or her dysphagia management
   plan?

swallow, which proves more difficult for the interpretation of common parameters. In addition, although fluoroscopy tables have the ability to be tilted from 0 to 90 degrees with retaining straps to support the patient, even with the supporting straps in place, tilting the patient beyond approximately 25 degrees is difficult. Thus, if the examiner wants an examination that approximates an upright position, it is unlikely that it will come from a study performed in this manner.

The results achieved with the standard supine position can be improved somewhat by positioning the patient for a slightly oblique view of the swallowing mechanism. This is done by use of foam wedges that are placed between the patient's shoulder and back on the left or right. The oblique view shifts the superimposition of the trachea and esophagus, aiding in the identification of aspiration. Still, such a position is less than ideal.

For most fluoroscopy systems, only limited space is available between the upright table and the fluoroscopy camera. Standard wheelchairs are most often too wide for use in this space, and they fail to position the patient high enough for the clinician to view esophageal transit. Standing for the study is not an option for many adults with dysphagia. For such patients specialty seating can offer a real advantage. These devices can improve the quality of the study results while ensuring patient safety.

The VESS Chair

Perhaps the most widely known specialty chair is the VESS Chair (see Figure 4.1). The chair is narrow (15.5 inches wide), allowing it to fit into the limited space between the upright table and the fluoroscopy tower. The chair is manufactured of molded plastic in an ergonomic shape and is radiolucent so that views are unobstructed, including the AP view. The angle of the torso can be changed quickly via a crank mechanism. The VESS chair sits on rotating casters that will allow it to be used as a transport vehicle. In this way a patient can be moved directly from bed into the VESS chair, taken to the radiology department for the VFSS, and returned to the ward without leaving the chair. The patient can be positioned for a lateral view to initiate the study and then easily rotated for an AP view. A variety of attachments, including medical chart holders and oxygen tank holders, are provided. It has proven to be very successful with clinicians.

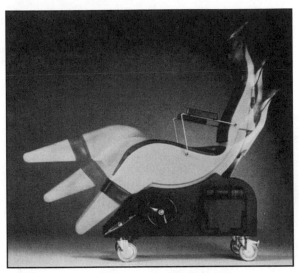

Figure 4.1. The VESS Chair. Photo courtesy of VESS Chairs, Inc.

The Hausted Video-Imaging Chair

The Steris-Hausted company manufactures gurneys, examination tables, and specialty chairs for use in the medical center environment. The Hausted Video-Imaging Chair, shown in Figure 4.2, can assume either a gurney or chair configuration. It allows patient transport personnel to slide the lying patient from the bed to the chair while it is in its gurney configuration and then reconfigure it for a seated study. The chair is equipped with a foot-operated hydraulic system that will raise or lower the unit's overall height to match that of the patient's hospital bed (27 to 34 inches). The chair back is tapered to fit the confined space between the upright table and the fluoroscopy camera. The back angle is fully adjustable, is radiolucent, and has a width of 14 or 16.5 inches. Pivoting from a lateral to an AP view is easily accomplished.

The Ferno Aviation Chair

Those who have traveled on commercial airliners may have seen a narrow chair used to transport nonambulatory passengers to their seats. This chair, commonly called the airline aisle chair, is manufactured by

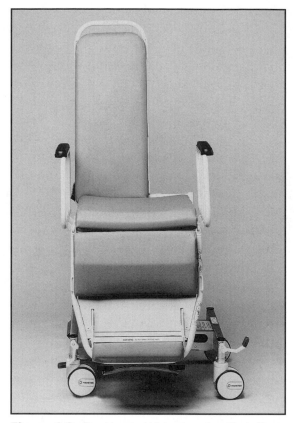

Figure 4.2. The Hausted Video-Imaging Chair. Photo courtesy of Steris-Hausted, Inc.

Ferno Aviation (see Figure 4.3). The restricted width enables this chair to be used in the VFSS because it fits between the table and the tower. Because of the front skid plate and rear wheel arrangement, shifting from lateral to AP views is more difficult than with the two dedicated specialty chairs previously mentioned. Safety straps are provided for the patient's security. There are two primary limitations. First, the chair is not offered with a reclinable back. Consequently, studies can be performed only in a 90-degree upright position. Second, a horizontal bar at the back of the chair is not radiolucent and is visible during AP views. The placement of the bar is high enough that for most patients it crosses the skull well superior to the swallowing mechanism. The

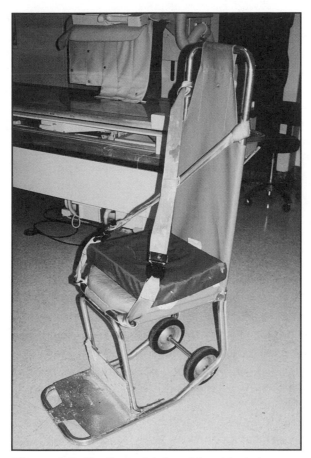

Figure 4.3. The Ferno Aviation airline aisle chair.

primary advantage of this chair is its low cost. Whereas the dedicated chairs can cost up to $6,000, the aisle chair can be acquired for less than $1,000. A hospital maintenance shop may be able to modify the chair to allow adjustment of the back, yielding a very cost-effective seating solution.

Before purchasing a positioning system, the clinician needs to consider exactly how it will be used to support the dysphagia program. The scheduling and flow of VFSS examinations will have an impact on how positioning systems can be used and how many will be required. A pivotal question is whether the patient will be transported to and from the ward in the chair or be positioned in it upon arrival in the radiology department. Videofluoroscopic swallowing studies are often scheduled back to back to maximize use of the equipment and staff. With this type of scheduling, it is necessary for the second patient to arrive as the first patient is completing an examination. If only one chair is acquired, then delays will result while the team waits for the first patient to be returned to the ward and the second patient picked up and brought to the department. If these delays are not acceptable, two chairs may be needed to avoid downtime. Another consideration is storage for the chairs when they are not in use for VFSS examinations.

Selection and Creation of VFSS Test Materials

Characteristics of Barium Sulfate

In Chapter 3, Edwards and Hawkins discuss the nature of contrast agents. The agents used by dysphagia clinicians in the VFSS are negative contrast agents. Although an iodine-based material, Gastrografin (Squibb), is available, the vast majority of VFSS examinations are performed by use of contrast agents that have barium sulfate ($BaSO_4$) as a base. Barium sulfate is mixed with water (H_2O) or other dietary liquids to produce the test material. When viewed under the fluoroscope, these test materials appear darker than the surrounding tissues. The degree of blackness seen on the screen is a direct result of the inability of the radiation beam to pass through the dense contrast material. This is termed *radiodensity* and it is a feature that makes barium an excellent choice. Commercial barium sulfate–based contrast materials are provided in dry powdered and liquid forms. Dry materials are rendered useful by adding a liquid to them, usually water or a thin dietary liquid. Liquid products may be used in their undiluted forms or mixed with water or dietary liquids to reduce their viscosity.

Suspensions Versus Solutions

When mixed, the barium sulfate is held in a suspension; it does not form a true solution. This is an important distinction because suspensions have a tendency toward sedimentation; that is, the barium sulfate particles tend to separate, ending up at the bottom of the container.

How rapidly this occurs depends on a variety of factors, including particle size, particle uniformity, and the suspending agents added by the manufacturer. Pure barium sulfate is a powder and not recommended for use in the VFSS because it has no suspension agents and is prone to rapid sedimentation. Although powdered commercial products have suspending agents, they are not recommended for use in the creation of liquid test materials because the mixing methods used can alter the contrast material that is produced. Rapid mixing can carry the absorbed cushion of air into the suspension, affecting texture and viscosity. Careful and slow mixing is often required to displace the absorbed air that attaches to the surface of barium particles. Therefore, it is recommended that liquid test materials be prepared using a commercial liquid barium sulfate and that its viscosity be adjusted through the addition of water or other thin dietary liquid.

Even when a liquid commercial agent is used, sedimentation remains an important problem. Sedimentation depends, in part, on the amount of barium in the solution created. Low-viscosity test materials (thin liquids) have low proportions of barium sulfate and are most prone to sedimentation. To a lesser degree, sedimentation is also a problem with more viscous preparations (thick liquids). The relevance to the dysphagia clinician is that liquid test materials must be stirred frequently to redistribute the barium particles. If they are not, then sipping from the cup will provide the patient with a thinner test material than is intended. Straw drinking, on the other hand, will deliver material that is appreciably more viscous than intended. In either situation, a diagnostic error is possible. Whether the test material in question is of high or low viscosity, it is important that it be reagitated by spoon stirring immediately before it is given to the patient. Viscosity also is temperature dependent. Decreasing the temperature increases the viscosity, whereas increasing the temperature decreases its viscosity. A change in temperature will have its greatest effects on viscous samples.

Without specific training and guidance, dysphagia clinicians tend to select a contrast material for the VFSS from those that are available in the fluoroscopy suite. A random selection may not provide optimal results because some agents tend to work better for certain purposes. Thin barium (low-viscosity) preparations tend to fill cavities well but coat the mucosa poorly. A very thick liquid (high-viscosity) preparation coats well but may not fill. It is recommended that clinicians use three separate contrast agents to produce their test materials. For the preparation of liquid test materials, they should use a premixed commercial barium sulfate liquid. This material can be combined with water or a thin dietary liquid to produce desired viscosity levels. A method for preparing viscosity-accurate liquids is described in the next section of this chapter. For pureed and minced foods that contain high percentages of liquid, a barium powder such as EZ-HD (EZ-EM) powder should be sprinkled on and mixed into the food. A paste such as Esophatrast (EZ-EM) should be mixed into stiff purees, minced, and ground items, or spread on whole foods such as whole meat, bread, and cookies.

Dietary Items as Test Materials

Some clinicians use a $BaSO_4$ liquid, a thick $BaSO_4$ paste, and a cookie as test materials. However, a review of the list of questions in Table 4.1 reveals that a wider range of test items is often helpful. Questions such as, "Is it appropriate to advance the patient from a pureed to a minced diet?" and "Should the patient receive thickened liquids?" are easier to answer if a wider range of test materials is available to the clinician. Further, because the VFSS purports to evaluate the swallowing of dietary items, then, where possible, dietary items should be used. A listing of the test materials I recommend using is provided in Table 4.2.

For the patient who is NPO, food-based test materials are prepared, primarily from pureed menu items. When a dietary upgrade is being considered, test materials should include food at and above the patient's current dietary level. Consequently, if the patient is receiving a pureed diet, test materials will include pureed, minced, ground, and possibly whole foods. In my clinical practice, a registered dietitian attends each VFSS and is responsible for acquiring the appropriate dietary items from the hospital kitchen and readying them for use in the study.

Bolus Viscosity

The viscosity of test materials used in diagnostic examinations and of foods and liquids consumed by patients with dysphagia is a very important variable. Failure to control viscosity in swallowing examinations may produce diagnostic errors and lead to inappropriate management recommendations.

Table 4.2
Test Materials for Use in the Videofluoroscopic Swallowing Study

Test Material	Viscosity	Components
Thin liquid	10.0 cP[a]	HD-85 and H_2O
Thick liquid	60.0 cP[a]	HD-85 and H_2O
Ultra-thick liquid	240.0 cP[a]	HD-85 and H_2O
Thin puree	As available	Applesauce[b]
Stiff puree	As available	Mashed potatoes[c]
Minced	As available	Vegetables, meat[c]
Ground	As available	Vegetables, meat[c]
Whole	As available	Whole meat[c]
Bread	As available	Bread with crust[c]

Notes. cP = centipoise.
[a]Viscosities at a shear rate of 11s⁻¹. [b]Powdered $BaSO_4$ added. [c]$BaSO_4$ paste added.

Fundamental Viscosity Concepts

Viscosity is a property of all dietary and nondietary liquids and may be defined as the material's resistance to flow (Miller, 1972). Viscosity is roughly equivalent to the liquid's thickness. Water is an example of a thin dietary liquid and has a viscosity of approximately 1.0 centipoise (cP) at room temperature. Buttermilk is an example of a thick dietary liquid and has a viscosity of approximately 52.0 cP at room temperature. Table 4.3 provides viscosities of common dietary liquids.

A review of the clinical literature clearly indicates that bolus viscosity is an important variable in the swallow. Bolus viscosity has been shown to affect the oral (Pouderoux & Kahrilas, 1995), pharyngeal (Bisch et al., 1994; Dantas, Dodds, Massey, & Kern, 1989; Lazarus et al., 1993), and esophageal (Kim et al., 1994) stages of the swallow. Various authors have reported an increased risk for direct aspiration when thin liquids are consumed by dysphagic patients (Curran & Groher, 1990; Groher, 1991; Logemann, 1998; Martin, 1991; Siebens & Linden, 1985; Stanek, Hensley, & Van Riper, 1992). Further, Logemann (1983) reported that patients with reduced pharyngeal peristalsis levels of stasis may increase as more viscous materials are swallowed.

Table 4.3
Viscosities of Common Dietary Liquids[a]

Dietary Liquid	Viscosity
Thin Liquids	
Coffee	1.0
Water	1.0
Tea	1.0
Clear broth	1.0
Clear juice	1.1
Skim milk	1.1
2% milk	1.2
Whole milk	1.2
Thick Liquids	
Nectar	50.6
Buttermilk	52.2
Tomato juice	65.6
Ultra-Thick Liquid	
Cream soup	240

[a]Measured at 25 degrees Centigrade with a shear rate of $11s^{-1}$.

Note. From *Revisiting a Critical Issue: Viscosity Control in Videofluoroscopic Swallowing Examinations,* by R. H. Mills, C. R. Daubert, D. Y. Stewman, and C. Church, 1997, paper presented at the meeting of the American Speech-Language-Hearing Association, San Antonio.

Belief in the importance of viscosity has had a significant effect on management practices. Groher (1984) recommended that clinicians restrict patients' intake of thin liquids as an aspiration precaution. Logemann (1983) recommended that patients alternate liquids and semisolids to aid in pharyngeal clearance. Furthermore, a number of diets have been designed to meet the specific needs of the dysphagic patient, including a reduction in the risk of aspiration (Curran & Groher, 1990; Finestone, Greene-Finestone, Wilson, & Teasell, 1995; O'Gara, 1990). Clinicians' recommendations have led care facilities to order and use commercial food thickeners for a large number of patients.

A review of published studies suggests that some investigators have not exercised precision in the control or reporting of viscosity in their studies. In articles that have used the VFSS, some authors did not report the viscosity values they used (Crary, 1995; DePippo, Holas, & Reding, 1994; Johnson, McKenzie, & Sievers, 1993; Neumann, Bartolome, Buchholtz, & Prosiegel, 1995; Strand, Miller, Yorkston, & Hillel, 1996). Others described their barium as "liquid" (Feinberg, 1993; Shannahan, Logemann, Rademaker, Pauloski, & Kahrilas, 1994), "thin" (Croghan, Burke, Caplan, & Denman, 1994; Logemann et al., 1993), or "high-density" (Rubesin, 1995). Brown, Mills, Daubert, and Casper (1998) demonstrated that there is virtually no agreement in the meaning clinicians attach to such labels. Whether the viscosities go unreported or are reported in subjective terms, the net effect is the same; interpretation of the findings and replication of the studies become difficult, if not impossible.

Certain authors have provided a degree of specificity by stating brand names and weight/volume (w/v) percentages of the materials used. In the w/v measure a specific weight of barium powder (e.g., 40 g) is used and enough water is added to create 100 ml of suspension. In this case the w/v would be given as 40%. Ali et al. (1996) reported using E-Z HD, and Palmer, Rudin, Lara, and Crompton (1992) used an 80% w/v suspension of barium sulfate powder in apple juice. Still, even if a clinician knows that testing was completed with a contrast agent that has a specific w/v, management questions such as the following remain difficult to answer: "Is the patient safe for PO intake of thin dietary liquids?" and "Exactly how much should liquids be thickened to be considered safe?" For the VFSS test materials to be useful in making appropriate diagnostic recommendations, they must be related to the viscosities of the liquids that patients consume.

It cannot be said that all liquids exhibit only one viscosity. A liquid's viscosity may be influenced by a variety of factors, including temperature and a factor called shear rate. A liquid's viscosity may be changed by its rate of flow. When this occurs the liquid is said to be shear thinning. In this case, a liquid's apparent viscosity decreases (becomes thinner) as the speed with which it moves over a surface, between two plates, or through an orifice increases. Such shear thinning liquids are classified as non-Newtonian. Fluids whose viscosities remain constant regardless of their rate of flow are called Newtonian. The vast majority of dietary liquids and the barium sulfate test materials used in the VFSS are non-Newtonian. To varying degrees, they exhibit the shear thinning phenomenon.

A viscometer measures viscosity and the effects of flow rate on viscosity. When measured with a viscometer, the liquid's viscosity can be plotted as rotational speeds of the viscometer are varied. These rates are expressed in reciprocal seconds and are written as xs^{-1}. Thus, a viscosity achieved at a shear rate of 11 reciprocal seconds would be expressed as $11s^{-1}$. Viscometers used in food science applications routinely measure viscosities as the shear rate is varied from $1s^{-1}$ to $100s^{-1}$.

The present understanding of the exact shear rates found in the swallow is limited, with estimated shear rates falling across a wide range of values. It is likely that there is no single shear rate for swallowing. The oral cavity, pharynx, and esophagus most certainly exhibit different shear rates. The effect of the presence of oropharyngeal dysphagia on shear rate is also unclear. Given this limited state of knowledge, it is important that investigators report data in such a way that they can be interpreted at a later time when more precise information is available. Toward this end, data in this chapter are reported, plotted, and discussed at a shear rate of $11s^{-1}$. To aid with future interpretations, the appendixes at the conclusion of this chapter provide tabled data for viscosities of dietary liquids (Appendix 4.A), viscosities of VFSS test materials (Appendix 4.B), and dilution curves for Barium Sulfate contrast agents (Appendix 4.C) at three different shear rates: $11s^{-1}$, $36s^{-1}$, and $58s^{-1}$.

The Viscosities of Test Material Currently Used

The data presented in this section concerning viscosity is a portion of that prepared by Mills, Daubert, Stewman, and Church (1997). In their study they established viscosity target values for thin and thick liquids that are based on the viscosities of common dietary liquids and then determined how well dysphagia management teams (DMTs) approximated those targets as they prepared test materials for use in VFSS examinations. Finally, a method based on the use of dilution curves was created to aid clinicians in preparing viscosity-accurate liquid test materials.

Viscosities of Dietary Liquids. When the viscosities of the dietary liquids in Table 4.3 were measured, Mills et al. (1997) found that they fell into three groups. The viscosity groupings of these liquids are shown in Figure 4.4. The first group of liquids, shown at the left of the figure,

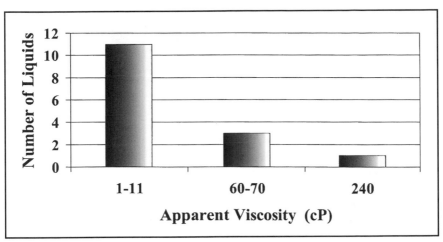

Figure 4.4. Viscosities of common dietary liquids. *Note.* cP = centipoise.

had a mean viscosity value of 1.1 cP and included water, coffee, tea, milk, and clear juice, all commonly recognized as thin. A smaller cluster of liquids (nectar, tomato juice, and buttermilk) had a higher mean viscosity of 56.1 cP. The authors classified these as thick dietary liquids. A cream soup was the most viscous liquid tested (240.0 cP) and was labeled by the authors as an ultra-thick liquid. These data showed that, in this sample, thin dietary liquids were by far the most numerous. Also, few naturally occurring thick or ultra-thick dietary liquids were in this sample.

Viscosities of VFSS Test Materials. A total of 20 DMTs provided Mills et al. (1997) with samples of the thin and thick liquid test materials that they use when conducting a VFSS examination. All samples were agitated and temperature stabilized. The viscosities were then measured with a BohlinVOR rheometer.

    Viscosities of Thin Liquid Test Materials. The data in Figure 4.5 are based on usable thin liquid test materials submitted by 16 DMTs. DMTs have been placed on the *x*-axis and numbered from 1 to 16 according to the increasing viscosity value of the thin liquid sample submitted. The 1.1-cP target for thin liquids is represented by a horizontal line very near the baseline of the graph. The thin liquid test materials used by all of the teams to varying degrees exceeded the target value, with a mean viscosity of 57.2 cP (*SD* = 69.7). The target value was significantly

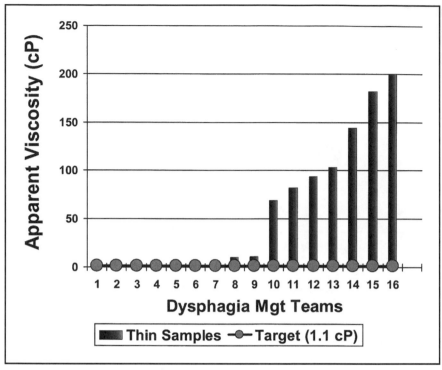

Figure 4.5. Viscosities of thin liquid test materials. *Note.* From *Revisiting a Critical Issue: Viscosity Control in Videofluoroscopic Swallowing Examinations,* by R. H. Mills, C. R. Daubert, D. Y. Stewman, and C. Church, 1997, paper presented at the meeting of the American Speech-Language-Hearing Association.

different from the test samples ($t = 3.681$; $p = .0022$). Although the dietary target for thin liquids approximated the viscosity of H_2O, on average the DMTs submitted samples that were often more viscous than thick dietary liquids (i.e., like nectar or buttermilk). The mean value of the test samples was 52 times greater than that of real thin dietary liquids. The large standard deviation reflects the wide variation in what the DMTs use to measure thin liquid swallowing.

On closer inspection it can be seen that two groups of thin liquid samples appear. DMTs 1 through 9 developed thin liquid test materials that had a mean value of 4.6 cP. These values are so small that they are obscured by the target value line in Figure 4.5. While these preparations are slightly thicker than dietary thin liquids, they behave very much like the thin dietary liquids sampled in this study. Despite the lack of full information regarding the sensitivity of the swallowing mechanism to changes in viscosity, these are considered to be appropriate for thin liquid testing. In contrast, DMTs 10 through 16 used samples that had a mean of 124.8, or 113 times the thin liquid dietary target. These were not considered to be appropriate.

Viscosities of Thick Liquid Test Materials. Figure 4.6 presents the data for thick liquid test materials with dysphagia teams ordered as they were in Figure 4.5. The horizontal line across the graph gives the thick liquid target of 60.0 cP. The mean value of the 17 usable thick liquid samples was 689.7 cP (SD = 330.2 cP). The samples were significantly different from the target (t = 5.368; $p < .0001$). The mean of the thick liquid test samples was fully 11 times greater than the dietary target. Ninety-four

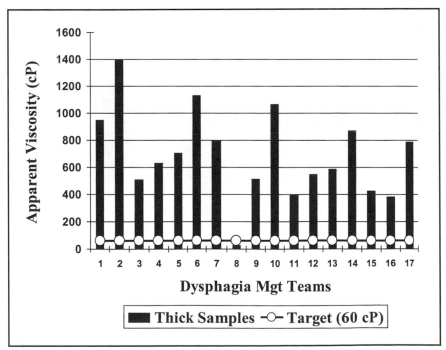

Figure 4.6. Viscosities of thick liquid test materials. *Note.* From *Revisiting a Critical Issue: Viscosity Control in Videofluoroscopic Swallowing Examinations*, by R. H. Mills, C. R. Daubert, D. Y. Stewman, and C. Church, 1997. Paper presented at the meeting of the American Speech-Language-Hearing Association.

percent of the teams used thick liquid test samples that were even more viscous than the study's only ultrathick liquid. None of the thick liquid test materials submitted accurately reflects the viscosities of naturally occurring thick dietary liquids.

Interpretation of Viscosity Results. The DMTs that participated in the Mills et al. (1997) study reported mixing their test materials by visual approximation. That is, they mixed $BaSO_4$ and H_2O until they thought it looked to be the right viscosity. It is clear from the data presented in this study that visual approximation fails to produce viscosity-accurate test samples. Glassburn and Deem (1998) also found this method flawed when nectar- and honey-thickened liquids were prepared by clinicians. In Mills et al.'s study it was shown that the method did not work when preparing VFSS test materials, either. For a large minority of thin liquid samples and nearly all of the thick liquid samples, the participating DMTs used materials that were substantially more viscous than their dietary liquid counterparts.

Probable Diagnostic Error Patterns. Mills et al. (1997) concluded that a test material was inappropriate if its viscosity resembled the viscosity not of the intended class of liquids (thin or thick) but of an adjacent class. For example, when a thin liquid test material had a viscosity of a thick dietary liquid, it was considered inappropriate. Thick liquid test materials were considered inappropriate if they resembled the viscosities of either thin or ultra-thick liquids as identified in this study. Based on the above-stated criterion, 69.6% of the samples submitted by DMTs were inappropriate and may pose risks for false negative errors. Stated another way, the use of test materials that were too viscous may lead to conclusions that a patient can safely drink thin or thick liquids when, in fact, he or she cannot. When patients are cleared for the consumption of liquids that they may not be able to safely swallow, then their welfare and the outcomes of management strategies are in jeopardy.

Overall, DMTs appear to have used far more $BaSO_4$ than is necessary to achieve the needed visual contrast. In so doing most increased the viscosity of their test materials to the point that they are no longer representative of any of the dietary liquids sampled. This is a case where more is definitely not better. A means of producing viscosity-accurate test materials is needed.

A Method for Producing Viscosity-Accurate Test Materials

There are three ways in which accuracy might be achieved in preparing test materials for the VFSS exam. The first requires that each DMT equip itself with a viscometer and the expertise to use it. In this way each team could test both the dietary liquids provided to patients and the test materials produced. The reality is that viscometry can require expensive instrumentation and more expertise to operate than most clinicians are trained to provide. A second method requires the purchase of prepared test materials from a contrast agent manufacturer. These are now becoming available in single-use packaging (e.g., Varibar by E-Z-EM, Inc.), but they are more costly than bulk agents and are useful only if the viscosities selected by the manufacturer can be directly related to the dietary items dysphagic patients actually consume.

Mills et al. (1997) recommend the adoption of the third method, which they call the *dilution curve methodology.* They prepared dilution curves for four commonly used liquid contrast agents: HD-85 (Figure 4.7), Liquid E-Z-Paque (Figure 4.8), Liquid Sol-O-Pake (Figure 4.9), and Liquid Polibar (Figure 4.10). For each product the authors created a graph with the x-axis representing product concentration from 10% to 100%. For example, 80 on the x-axis represents a suspension of 80% product and 20% H_2O. The y-axis represents viscosity as measured in centipoise (cP). The contents of a container of a liquid $BaSO_4$ product was agitated and temperature stabilized at 25 degrees Centigrade. The viscosity of the undiluted product was measured and plotted at the 100% concentration point. Next, a second sample was prepared that was 90% product and 10% H_2O. The viscosity was measured and transferred to the graph at the 90% point on the x-axis. This process continued until all deciles had been measured. The points were then connected to yield the dilution curve.

Testing the Visual Approximation Method. Twenty registered dietitians, speech–language pathologists, and dietary technicians were recruited to determine whether the use of the dilution curve methodology would produce more viscosity-accurate test samples than would visual approximation. Each participant was first asked to prepare a sample

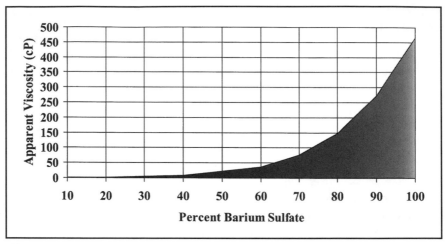

Figure 4.7. Dilution curve for HD-85 contrast material (a product of Lafayette Pharmaceuticals, Inc., Lafayette, IN).

that had the thickness of buttermilk using the visual approximation method. That is, they combined the HD-85 contrast material and H_2O until they believed it looked, stirred, and poured like buttermilk.

For the test of the dilution curve method, each participant was provided with a container of HD-85 and its dilution curve (Figure 4.7), a

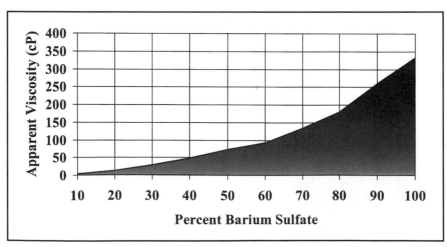

Figure 4.8. Dilution curve for Liquid E-Z-Paque contrast material (a product of E-Z-EM, Inc., Westbury, NY).

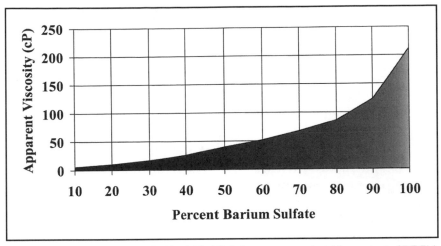

Figure 4.9. Dilution curve for Liquid Sol-O-Pake contrast material (a product of E-Z-EM, Inc., Westbury, NY).

supply of H_2O, a 100-ml graduated cylinder, and a mixing cup. They were also given a description and verbal examples of how to use the curve. The target value for the task was 60 cP, a close approximation of the viscosity of buttermilk, the target in the visual approximation task. Use of a dilution curve is very simple. First, the clinician finds the

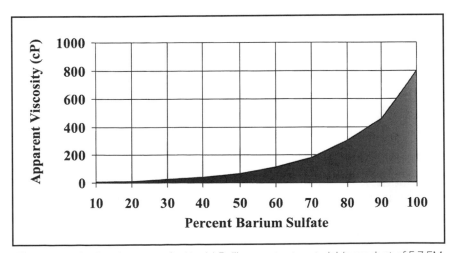

Figure 4.10. Dilution curve for Liquid Polibar contrast material (a product of E-Z-EM, Inc., Westbury, NY).

target (60 cP) on the y-axis and then traces a line horizontally to the right until it intersects the dilution curve. Dropping a vertical line to the x-axis at this point of intersection gives the percentage of $BaSO_4$ product needed. Referring to Figure 4.7, it can be seen that a 60-cP test material will require 55% of HD-85 and 45% of H_2O. Once each subject had created a sample, the samples were individually sealed and returned to the laboratory where viscosity was measured.

The Results of Two Methods of Test Sample Preparation. The test materials produced by visual approximation did not resemble the 60-cP target. The mean viscosity of samples was 182.9 cP ($SD = 111.5$ cP). They were statistically different from the target ($t = -4.928, p < .0001$). The findings indicate that visual approximation–produced test samples were not representative of the dietary thick liquids they were intended to mimic. They were not considered appropriate for use in the VFSS for the testing of thick liquid swallowing.

When the subjects used the dilution curve method, their performance was strikingly different. When attempting to produce a 60-cP sample, the subjects produced a mean value of 61.6 cP ($SD = 6.7$ cP). The samples were not significantly different from the target ($t = -1.035$, $p = .3139$), confirming the fact that the samples produced by the dilution curve method were viscosity-accurate replications and were considered appropriate for use in the VFSS. Although only the preparation of liquids approximating a nectar consistency were tested, there is no reason to suspect that clinicians would perform any differently with less viscous liquids.

When first determining the proper proportions for $BaSO_4$ and H_2O, a 100-ml graduated cylinder can be used for measurement. The required amount of H_2O is measured first and then poured into a styrofoam cup. The level of the H_2O is then marked on the side of the cup. The $BaSO_4$ is then measured and added to the cup. A line is marked on the side of the cup representing the fluid level of the test material in the cup. If the clinician retains this as a master mixing cup, remeasurement will not be required for later studies. It will only be necessary that the two lines be transferred to a new cup and then that the H_2O and $BaSO_4$ be added. If disposable graduated cups are used, line marking is unnecessary.

The dilution curve method does not require special instrumentation or expertise and is easily used in the fluoroscopy suite. A further advantage of the dilution curve method is that the curves are quite forgiving across the 1- to 70-cP viscosity range common to most dietary liquids. Thus, a measurement error of several percent in the $BaSO_4$:H_2O ratio will not produce a major shift in the viscosity of the test material produced. Clinicians should not attempt to apply these dilution curves to other products. The viscosities that result with dilution reflect the particle sizes present, as well as the amount of barium sulfate, liquid medium, suspension agents, and other additives that are included by the manufacturer. A product's unique combination will have a significant effect on viscosities that result with dilution.

Methods of Delivery and Control of Bolus Volume

When performing the VFSS examination, the clinician has several bolus delivery options from which to choose. Most often clinicians use a spoon, syringe, cup, or straw to deliver the test materials. These options vary in terms of their naturalness, efficiency, and precision in measuring bolus volume, and degree of control the clinician maintains over the volume of the bolus delivered. A fundamental premise in this chapter is that the status of variables in the VFSS should, if possible, reflect the patient's feeding environment. This includes method of bolus delivery. The meal observation will tell the clinician what methods of delivery are used. It will also allow the clinician to determine whether the patient or another person is responsible for delivering the foods and liquids at mealtime. If the patient drinks liquids from a cup at mealtime, then, if possible, this mode of delivery should be tested in the VFSS. Once it is known how the patient performs with the current delivery system, then the clinician should treat it as an experimental variable to determine whether another delivery method would yield superior results.

A natural delivery method is one that is commonly used across the population for the ingestion of liquids. A delivery method that is precise allows the clinician to accurately measure the amount consumed. When the clinician has control, then he or she is able to determine the bolus volume delivered. Delivery of liquid via spoon or syringe allows the clinician precise measurement and control of the volume the patient receives. Unfortunately, these methods are not very natural. Few patients, whether dependent or independent for feeding, receive their liquids in this manner. Still, depending on the patient, it may be prudent for the VFSS to first assess liquids delivered by these methods, preferably by spoon delivery. In this way the clinician can exercise absolute control over the volume delivered, being sure that no more material is delivered than is safe. Although a syringe offers this same control of the volume of test material delivered, it should be used with caution. In using a syringe the clinician may inadvertently direct the test material into an open airway. I consider this delivery method to be the last choice. Once the patient demonstrates success with controlled volumes, then the clinician can begin to assess more natural methods, (i.e., cup and straw drinking).

It is clear from the literature that bolus volume produces significant effects on the oral and pharyngeal stages of the swallow. It is important to note that there are large differences between the bolus sizes normally ingested and those that are recommended for testing in some VFSS protocols. Logemann (1986) recommended that testing begin with a ⅓ teaspoon of liquid (about 1.5 ml). The small bolus volume is recommended so that aspiration risk can be controlled and so that the bolus will not obliterate the view of anatomical structures. Palmer, Kuhlemeier, Tippett, and Lynch (1993) provided a protocol for the VFSS in which they begin by testing the swallowing of 5 cc of liquid and then progress to patient-determined cup drinking volumes. Perlman, Lu, and Jones (1997) tested volumes from 3 ml to 20 ml. This trend to assess the swallowing of larger volumes is appropriate in light of the results of Anderhill, Ekberg, and Groher (1989), who evaluated bolus volumes in cup drinking by men and women with dysphagia. They found that, when provided with water, men self-delivered a mean volume of 25 ml, whereas women ingested 20 ml. The authors also found that when volumes were this large they did not obstruct the view of anatomical structures. These data suggest that many patients likely ingest volumes larger than 5 ml. Consequently, it is important to test larger volumes if safety considerations will allow. It is also important to know the volumes the patient uses when self-delivering the test materials.

Although cup and straw drinking do not normally lend themselves to precise measurement of volume, the clinician can approximate bolus size during the VFSS in the following manner. Before the patient drinks from the cup, the clinician marks a level line that represents the top of the fluid on the side of the drinking cup. Once the patient has taken the first bolus, the clinician marks a second level line representing the new fluid level. If additional swallows are taken, a new line is marked for each. At the completion of the study, the clinician can use a 60-ml syringe to add water to the remaining contents of the cup. The clinician records the amount required to return the fluid level to each level line. These amounts represent the volumes for the swallows taken. When successive swallows are tested, as in stress testing, the clinician needs to mark the initial and ending level lines. By reviewing that segment of the videotape, the clinician will know how many swallows the patient took during the stress test. The volume of water required to restore the fluid to the original line is then divided by the number of swallows to yield a mean volume for successive swallows. It is not practical to follow this procedure for every swallow taken by cup and straw. It is usually most meaningful to measure a representative one or two single swallows and then for the successive swallow stress test.

When performing an initial VFSS with a newly referred patient, the clinician should control the bolus volume using a spoon or syringe. If the patient demonstrates an ability to safely handle these, then the clinician should allow the patient to assume control, using a cup or straw, but measure the amount consumed for representative swallows by use of the level-line method. This sequence reflects an awareness of patient safety issues and proceeds, only where possible, to evaluation of the swallowing of bolus volumes that are natural for the patient. This technique offers another advantage. One form of a stress test is to ask the patient to take a slightly larger than normal sip from a cup. Under this condition of an abnormally large volume, the patient may decompensate, perhaps demonstrating aspiration. When decompensation occurs with a larger than normal volume, this method allows the clinician to determine the volume required to produce the breakdown.

It is important to know whether the patient can achieve PO intake of liquids with natural methods because limiting the patient's intake to spooning is problematic. A teaspoon holds 5 ml of liquid. A liter of liquid contains 1,000 ml. Spooning the liquid will require 200 administrations for the patient to ingest 1 liter of liquid. If a caregiver can deliver and the patient can swallow 1 teaspoon each 6 seconds (optimistic for many patients), then it will take 20 minutes to deliver the liquids. Considering that many feeding-dependent patients will be unable to ingest at this rate, that there are also dietary solids to be consumed, and that nursing staffs in many locations experience chronic shortages, achieving the intake of the liquids required to maintain hydration will be difficult.

Use of Protocols in the Videofluoroscopic Swallowing Study

Parameters Governing the Progression of the Study

A VFSS protocol provides the dysphagia clinician with a beginning point and a rationale for progressing through the study of swallowing. It is not a "road map" that will be appropriate for each and every study. In fact, as Perlman et al. (1997) pointed out, it is necessary to tailor the examination to fit each patient and his or her clinical symptoms. Logemann (1986) recognized the need to redesign the protocol "on the fly" and recommended providing at least one or two swallows under her protocol before deciding to deviate. Consequently, I provide starting points and, in Table 4.4, a series of parameters that can be used to direct the progression of the study. As with most published protocols, I begin with lateral and proceed to AP views.

To demonstrate the problem, the study proceeds from current feeding positions to those that may be more ideal. To ensure patient

Table 4.4
Parameters that Guide the Progress of the VFSS

From		To
Lateral view	⟶	Anterior–posterior view
Current positions	⟶	More ideal positions
Clinician-controlled delivery	⟶	Patient-controlled delivery
Small bolus sizes	⟶	Larger bolus sizes
Ultra-thick liquids	⟶	Thick liquid to thin liquid
Liquids	⟶	Pureed, minced, ground, and solid
Current dietary items	⟶	Target dietary items
Uncompensated	⟶	Use of compensations and maneuvers

safety, the study begins with the clinician in control of bolus volumes and then proceeds, as possible, to provide the patient with that control. Bolus volumes progress from small to large and liquid viscosities from ultra-thick to thick and then to thin. Liquids are most often presented before the various textures of foods. When the examination seeks to determine whether a patient can move from a current diet texture to another, then the study proceeds from current items to the potential targets. Finally, the study progresses to determine the effects of compensations and maneuvers on the swallow.

Application of the VFSS Protocol

The VFSS protocol used is individualized according to the diagnostic questions that are asked. The following is a common scenario. It begins with the activation of the video-recording system. The patient is positioned and the image area is adjusted. Then, brief diadochokinetic speech testing to assess lingual, labial, and velar movements takes place. Swallow testing is initiated with parameters set to ensure clinician control and patient safety. The patient is placed as close as possible to the position that is usually assumed for feeding. The fluoroscopic view is lateral. The first bolus viscosity presented is usually an ultra-thick liquid. For many patients this viscosity reduces the risk of direct aspiration compared with less viscous liquids. In addition, for patients who are prone to pharyngeal stasis, this viscosity is often less problematic than foods. The volume of the initial bolus the examiner delivers is 5 ml. If the patient is successful, then a 10-ml bolus of the same liquid is presented. With success, the patient progresses through thick and thin liquids. If the patient is cup or straw drinking liquids in a PO diet, then the clinician tests using cup or straw administration of single swallows as soon as the clinician believes it can be safely done. Level lines are used to estimate bolus size of one or two swallows. The study then progresses through the food items the registered dietitian has prepared. Single rounded teaspoon-sized bites of thin puree (applesauce), thick puree (mashed potatoes), and minced, ground, and whole bites of foods are presented. A bite of a bread slice with crust will be tested last.

If the patient's performance warrants, the clinician will return to the presentation of the least viscous liquid that was safely swallowed for stress testing. As a stress test the patient will be given the cup of that liquid and asked to take three successive swallows. Level lines will be used to determine mean bolus size (total volume/3 = mean bolus volume). Throughout the administration of materials in Stage I, the clinician will be analyzing the accumulating data, seeking to determine the physiology that has resulted in the observed symptoms (Stage II). Because bolus volume, viscosity, and method of delivery will have been tested throughout the study, their effects should be known. The effects of food texture on the swallow will also have been shown. Once the causes are understood, then the clinician moves to Stage III, in which the clinician manipulates variables such as body position, compensations, and maneuvers to improve the swallow. The testing of compensations and maneuvers is generously covered by Logemann (1998).

In the final portion of the VFSS, the patient is turned for the anterior–posterior view and asked to phonate to assess vocal cord adduction. Then the least viscous safe liquid test material at the largest safe volume is presented for swallowing. The clinician looks for asymmetry in the swallowing response and for residue left in the valleculae and pyriform sinuses. Compensations that will show a unilateral deficit or positioning effect are best tested with this view.

Termination of the VFSS Study

The clinician terminates the study under a variety of conditions that are patient specific. It is terminated when the diagnostic questions have been answered. It also may be terminated when significant aspiration is seen. Termination in this case depends on the amount of aspiration and on patient-specific factors. For example, a patient without a history of aspiration pneumonia, who has good laboratory values, including a total lymphocyte count of greater than 1,499 (see Chapter 6) and an intact clearance response, will be treated more liberally than a patient who is compromised. This is one more reason for the dysphagia clinician to know each patient's history and related assessment results prior to initiating the study. Without this information the clinician will be stressed to make an on-line decision without the needed information. Ultimately, the decision to terminate rests with the clinician and must be based on a composite of history, clinical examination, meal observation, and VFSS information.

When presenting dietary foods, the clinician will terminate the sequence based on the patient's current feeding status, mastication, and overall performance with these items. A patient who comes to the study in NPO status will usually have the food portion of the study terminated at the puree or minced level. If the patient is successful with these items, then a puree or minced diet is recommended on a trial basis. It will be followed with a meal observation, clinical examination, and perhaps a repeated VFSS before the diet consistency is upgraded. If the clinician sees that the patient is unable to adequately masticate minced foods, then ground and whole will not be evaluated.

The protocol is routinely modified to fit the patient's needs and to limit radiation exposure to the patient. When a patient fails with a small bolus size within a viscosity category, then usually a larger bolus volume is not administered. If a patient shows significant aspiration on a high-viscosity liquid, then liquids of lesser viscosities are often omitted.

Summary

It is possible to perform the VFSS with little regard to the influence of variables discussed in this chapter. The study can be performed without recognition of the patient's real-world swallowing environment. When the study is performed in such a manner, there is a high likelihood that the results will not reflect the patient's swallowing deficit, abilities, or potential to improve with management. Through this imprecise diagnostic effort, inappropriate management recommendations may be made. When the clinician acknowledges and controls the variables mentioned in this chapter, he or she has a much better probability of arriving at a correct diagnosis and providing management that will result in a positive outcome.

Appendix 4.A

Viscosity Values of Dietary Liquids at Three Shear Rates[a]

Dietary Liquid	Shear Rate		
	$11s^{-1}$	$36s^{-1}$	$58s^{-1}$
Coffee	1	1	1
Water	1	1	1
Tea	1	1	1
Clear broth	1	1	1
Clear juice	1	1	1
Skim milk	1	1	1
2% Milk	1	1	1
Whole milk	1	1	1
Nectar	51	23	12
Buttermilk	52	22	16
Tomato juice	66	28	20
Cream soup	240	96	68

[a]Viscosity values rounded to nearest centipoise.

Appendix 4.B

Viscosity Values of VFSS Test Materials at Three Shear Rates[a]

Dysphagia Management Team	Thin			Thick		
	$11s^{-1}$	$36s^{-1}$	$58s^{-1}$	$11s^{-1}$	$36s^{-1}$	$58s^{-1}$
1	1	1	1	949	394	321
2	1	1	1	1,400	683	523
3	2	1	1	509	286	204
4	2	2	2	630	340	278
5	4	4	4	703	457	389
6	4	2	1	1,130	562	430
7	6	5	5	800	412	313
8	10	8	6	27	23	23
9	11	7	6	515	237	202
10	69	36	28	1,064	522	398
11	82	63	59	397	184	139
12	94	48	38	548	422	384
13	103	78	63	589	310	253
14	144	64	48	868	484	448
15	182	87	66	428	385	312
16	200	92	71	381	168	117
17	—	—	—	787	433	342

Note. Blanks indicate that sample is not suitable for measurement.

[a]Viscosity values rounded to nearest centipoise.

Appendix 4.C

Dilution Curves for Barium Sulfate
Contrast Agents at Three Shear Rates

Shear Rate	Concentration (in percent)									
	10	20	30	40	50	60	70	80	90	100
HD-85 [85% w/v][a]										
$11s^{-1}$	1	2	5	8	23	37	76	147	273	465
$36s^{-1}$	1	1	3	5	10	34	64	121	211	390
$58s^{-1}$	1	1	1	2	8	29	62	114	195	365
Liquid E-Z-Paque [60% w/v][b]										
$11s^{-1}$	5	13	29	49	74	94	135	180	261	334
$36s^{-1}$	2	7	13	20	34	47	62	84	108	146
$58s^{-1}$	1	5	9	14	24	32	42	59	79	102
Liquid Polibar [100% w/v][b]										
$11s^{-1}$	7	13	27	40	68	116	182	306	458	803
$36s^{-1}$	3	8	17	28	45	77	118	209	322	511
$58s^{-1}$	1	6	14	24	37	64	98	178	276	420
Liquid Sol-O-Pake [72% w/v][b]										
$11s^{-1}$	6	10	17	26	40	52	68	86	123	212
$36s^{-1}$	1	5	10	18	26	34	42	65	106	174
$58s^{-1}$	1	3	7	16	23	29	36	58	101	160

[a]Manufactured by Lafayette Pharmaceuticals, Inc., Lafayette, LA.
[b]Manufactured by EZ-EM, Inc., Westbury, NY.

Note. From "Rheology Overview: Control of Liquid Viscosities in Dysphagia," by R. H. Mills, 1999, *Supplement to Nutrition in Clinical Practice, 14*(5), pp. 552–556. Copyright 1999 by *American Journal of Parenternal and Enternal Nutrition*. Reprinted with permission.

References

Ali, G. N., Wallace, K. L., Schwartz R., DeCarle, D. J., Zagami, A. S., & Cook I. J. (1996). Mechanisms of oral-pharyngeal dysphagia in patients with Parkinson's disease. *Gastroenterology, 110,* 383–392.

Anderhill, I., Ekberg, O., & Groher, M. (1989). Determining normal bolus size for thin liquids. *Dysphagia, 4*(1), 1–3.

Bisch, E. M., Logemann, J. A., Rademaker, A. W., Kahrilas, P. J., & Lazarus, C. L. (1994). Pharyngeal effects of bolus volume, viscosity, and temperature in patients with dysphagia resulting from neurologic impairment and in normal subjects. *Journal of Speech and Hearing Research, 37,* 1041–1049.

Brown, A., Mills, R. H., Daubert, C. R., & Casper, M. (1998, October). Establishing labels and standards for thickened liquids in the dysphagia diet. *Consultant Dietitian, 23,* 1, 3–5.

Crary, M. A. (1995). A direct intervention program for chronic neurogenic dysphagia secondary to brainstem stroke. *Dysphagia, 10,* 6–18.

Croghan, J. E., Burke, E. M., Caplan, S., & Denman, S. (1994). Pilot study of 12-month outcomes of nursing home patients with aspiration on videofluoroscopy. *Dysphagia, 9,* 141–146.

Curran, J., & Groher, M. (1990). Development and dissemination of an aspiration risk reduction diet. *Dysphagia, 5,* 6–12.

Dantas, R. O., Dodds, W. J., Massey, B. T., & Kern, M. K. (1989). The effect of high- versus low-density barium preparations on the quantitative features of swallowing. *American Journal of Radiology, 153*(6), 1191–1195.

DePippo, K. L., Holas, M. A., & Reding, M. J. (1994). The Burke Dysphagia Screening Test: Validation of its use in patients with stroke. *Archives of Physical Medicine and Rehabilitation, 75,* 1284–1286.

Feinberg, M. J. (1993). Radiographic techniques and interpretation of abnormal swallowing in adult and elderly patients. *Dysphagia, 8,* 356–358.

Finestone, H. M., Greene-Finestone, L. S., Wilson, E. S., & Teasell, R. W. (1995). Malnutrition in stroke patients on the rehabilitation service and at follow-up: Prevalence and predictors. *Archives of Physical Medicine and Rehabilitation, 76,* 310–316.

Glassburn, D. L., & Deem, J. F. (1998). Thickener viscosity in dysphagia management: Variability among speech–language pathologists. *Dysphagia, 13,* 218–222.

Groher, M. E. (1984). *Dysphagia diagnosis and management.* Stoneham, MA: Butterworth.

Groher, M. (1991). Management: General principles and guidelines. *Dysphagia, 6,* 67–70.

Huckabee, M. L., & Pelletier, C. A. (1999). *Management of adult neurogenic dysphagia.* San Diego: Singular.

Johnson, E. R., McKenzie, S. W., & Sievers, A. (1993). Aspiration pneumonia in stroke. *Archives of Physical Medicine and Rehabilitation, 74,* 973–976.

Khoo, J. B., Buller, A. S., & Wong, M. C. (1996). Modified barium swallow examination in dysphagic stroke patients. *Singapore Medical Journal, 37*(4), 407–410.

Kidd, D., Lawson, J., Nesbitt, R., & MacMahon, J. (1993). Aspiration in acute stroke: A clinical study with videofluoroscopy. *Quarterly Journal of Medicine, 86*(12), 825–829.

Kim, C. H., Hsu, J. J., O'Connor, M. K., Weaver, A. L., Brown, M. L., & Zinsmeister, A. R. (1994). Effect of viscosity on oropharyngeal and esophageal emptying in man. *Digestive Diseases and Sciences, 39*(1), 189–192.

Langmore, S. E., Schatz, K., & Olsen, N. (1988). Fiberoptic endoscopic examination of swallowing safety: A new procedure. *Dysphagia, 2,* 216–219.

Lazarus, C. L., Logemann, J. A., Rademaker, A. W., Kahrilas, P. J., Pajak, T., Lazar, R., & Halper, A. (1993). Effects of bolus volume, viscosity and repeated swallows in nonstroke subjects and stroke patients. *Archives of Physical Medicine and Rehabilitation, 74*(10), 1066–1070.

Logemann, J. A. (1983). *Evaluation and treatment of swallowing disorders.* Austin, TX: PRO-ED.

Logemann, J. A. (1986). *Manual for the videofluorographic study of swallowing.* Austin, TX: PRO-ED.

Logemann, J. A. (1993). Noninvasive approaches to deglutitive aspiration. *Dysphagia, 8,* 331–333.

Logemann, J. A. (1997). Role of the modified barium swallow in management of patients with dysphagia. *Otolaryngology—Head and Neck Surgery, 116*(3), 335–338.

Logemann, J. A. (1998). *Evaluation and treatment of swallowing disorders* (2nd ed.). Austin, TX: PRO-ED.

Logemann, J. A., Roa-Pauloski, B., Rademaker, A., Cook, B., Graner, D., Milianti, F., Beery, Q., Stein, D., Bowman, J., & Lazarus, C. (1992). Impact of the diagnostic procedure on outcome measures of swallowing rehabilitation in head and neck cancer patients. *Dysphagia, 7*(4), 179–186.

Logemann, J., Shannahan, T., Rademaker, A. W., Kahrilas, P. J., Lazar, R., & Halper, A. (1993). Oropharyngeal swallowing after stroke in the left basal ganglion/internal capsule. *Dysphagia, 8,* 230–234.

Martin, A. W. (1991). Dietary management of swallowing disorders. *Dysphagia, 6,* 129–134.

Miller, B. F. (1972). *Encyclopedia and dictionary of medicine, nursing and allied health.* Philadelphia: Saunders.

Mills, R. H., Daubert, C. R., Stewman, D. Y., & Church, C. (1997, November). *Revisiting a critical issue: Viscosity control in videofluoroscopic swallowing examinations.* Paper presented at the meeting of the American Speech-Language-Hearing Association, San Antonio.

Murray, J. (1999). *Manual of dysphagia assessment in adults.* San Diego: Singular.

Neumann, S., Bartolome, G., Buchholtz, D., & Prosiegel, M. (1995). Swallowing therapy of neurologic patients: Correlation of outcome with pretreatment variables and therapeutic methods. *Dysphagia, 10,* 1–2.

O'Gara, J. A. (1990). Dietary adjustments and nutritional therapy during treatment for oral-pharyngeal dysphagia. *Dysphagia, 4,* 209–212.

Palmer, J. B., Kuhlemeier, K. V., Tippett, D. C., & Lynch, C. (1993). A protocol for the videofluorographic swallowing study. *Dysphagia, 8,* 209–214.

Palmer, J. B., Rudin, N. J., Lara, G., & Crompton, A. W. (1992). Coordination of mastication and swallowing. *Dysphagia, 7,* 187–200.

Perlman, A. L., Lu, C., & Jones, B. (1997). Radiographic contrast examination of the mouth, pharynx and esophagus. In A. L. Perlman & K. Schulze-Delrieu (Eds.), *Deglutition and its disorders* (pp. 153–199). San Diego: Singular.

Perlman, A. L., & Schulze-Delrieu, K. (1997). *Deglutition and its disorders: Anatomy, physiology, clinical diagnosis, and management.* San Diego: Singular.

Pouderoux, P., & Kahrilas, P. J. (1995). Deglutive tongue force modulation by volition, volume, and viscosity in humans. *Gastroenterology, 108*(5), 1418–1426.

Rubesin, S. E. (1995). Oral and pharyngeal dysphagia. *Gastroenterology Clinics of North America, 24*(2), 331–352.

Shannahan, T. K., Logemann, J. A., Rademaker, A. W., Pauloski, B. R., & Kahrilas, P. J. (1993). Chin-down posture effect on aspiration in dysphagic patients. *Archives of Physical Medicine and Rehabilitation, 74,* 736–739.

Siebens, A. A., & Linden, P. (1985). Dynamic imaging for swallowing reeducation. *Gastrointestinal Radiology, 10,* 251–253.

Stanek, K., Hensley, C., & Van Riper, C. (1992). Factors affecting use of food and commercial agents to thicken liquids for individuals with swallowing disorders. *Journal of the American Dietetic Association, 92,* 488–490.

Strand, E. A., Miller, R. M., Yorkston, K. M., & Hillel, A. D. (1996). Management of oral-pharyngeal dysphagia symptoms in amyotropic lateral sclerosis. *Dysphagia, 11,* 129–139.

Warms, T. L. (1998). False-positive results on videofluoroscopy. *Dysphagia, 13,* 191–192.

Wright, R., & Jordan, C. (1997). Videofluoroscopic evaluation of dysphagia in motor neuron disease with modified barium swallow. *Palliative Medicine, 11*(1), 44–48.

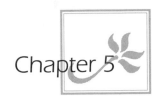

Chapter 5

Fiberoptic Endoscopic Evaluation of Swallowing

Susan E. Langmore

Langmore discusses the use of the fiberoptic endoscopic evaluation of swallowing (FEES). She outlines the equipment required to perform the examination and discusses elements important in patient selection. The diversity of the technique is apparent as she discusses two different protocols, the complete FEES protocol and the Ice Chip protocol.

1. *List the patient characteristics that would make the FEES most appropriate.*

2. *What swallowing characteristics would lend themselves to study by FEES?*

3. *What swallowing characteristics would better be studied by VFSS?*

4. *When would the Ice Chip protocol be more appropriate than the complete FEES protocol?*

❧   ❧   ❧

After the clinical examination of a patient with dysphagia, the speech–language pathologist must decide whether an instrumental examination is indicated. Previous chapters in this text have discussed the clinical and videofluoroscopic examination procedures, including patient selection, the protocol, and decision making. This chapter describes the endoscopic procedure, which is often called the fiberoptic endoscopic evaluation of swallowing (FEES)

(Langmore, Schatz, & Olson, 1988). FEES is an alternative examination that has many of the same purposes and outcomes as the fluoroscopy examination but uses very different technology.

Equipment and Materials

The most basic component of the endoscopic examination is the fiberoptic endoscope. The most suitable type of endoscope is a flexible laryngoscope, such as that used by an otolaryngologist to perform a laryngeal examination. It is also used by speech–language pathologists to examine the velopharyngeal port or the larynx for resonance or voice disorders. The fiber bundle of a laryngoscope is about 3.5 mm in diameter, making it small enough to slide through a nares and to rest in the hypopharynx without disturbing the patient. A flexible pediatric endoscope that is only 2.5 mm in diameter (Pentax Precision Instruments) may be preferable to use with small children.

In addition to the endoscope, a second indispensable element is the light source. One can choose from either a halogen or a xenon light source, but the latter is significantly more expensive. Xenon light sources emit a brighter light, but a halogen light is sufficient for most purposes.

It is possible to perform a FEES exam with only these two pieces of equipment, but just as the fluoroscopy procedure is greatly enhanced by videotaping the study, the FEES procedure is improved when the study is recorded and can be reviewed for detail and archived for later reference. To record the examination, it is necessary to interface a specially designed video chip camera to the endoscope and then connect the camera to a videotape recorder. When the camera is attached to the endoscope, the examiner can no longer look through the eyepiece of the endoscope, but must view the image on a monitor, which needs to be connected to the tape recorder. This has many advantages, as it makes it possible for several people to view the study while it is ongoing, including the patient, the family, and other staff who may be interested in the findings.

Two other useful pieces of equipment are a videocounter/timer and a videoprinter. The counter imprints the date and time (in hundredths of a second) on the tape and is seen on the monitor, and the printer captures any frame in the study and prints a color photograph of the image.

In Table 5.1 the components of a complete FEES system are listed along with commercial sources for this equipment. Other companies sell endoscopes as well, and the reader is encouraged to compare the equipment before purchase. Although it may seem expensive, the total cost is a small fraction of the cost of fluoroscopy equipment. Supplies and materials needed for a FEES exam are also listed in Table 5.1. A topical anesthetic such as lidocaine gel and cotton-tipped applicators are used to anesthetize the nostril that will be entered by the endoscope, if the patient requests anesthetization. Gauze pads and alcohol prep pads are useful for cleaning the tip of the scope if it becomes "gunked" and needs to be removed for cleaning. Gloves are necessary to prevent spread of bacteria to and from the examiner and patient. Food and liquids to be given to the patient must be gathered, along with a bottle of green or blue food dye to color all boli given to the patient, and cups, spoons, straws, plates, and the other items listed in Table 5.1.

All of the equipment and materials are assembled on a cart so that the FEES system can be portable. Shelves, a drawer, and large wheels make the cart easy to move while containing all the small items that are used during the examination.

Training and Competencies

Most new procedures developed require the speech–language pathologist to undergo a period of training before performing them independently. The code of ethics of the American Speech-Language-Hearing Association (ASHA) mandates that speech–language pathologists not practice any procedure that they are not trained and competent to perform and interpret. This precaution was reiterated in ASHA's (1992) policy statement that described FEES and other diagnostic procedures for swallowing as falling within the scope of practice for speech–language pathologists. Unfortunately, some procedures are easier to implement than others and ASHA's mandate to establish competency is sometimes ignored. When it comes to the performance of endoscopy procedures, however, most speech–language pathologists have recognized the need for specialized training. Although inserting an endoscope may seem invasive to the speech–language pathologist who is not used to doing hands-on procedures, it appears much less threatening to the clinician who has already learned to do such things as insert

· **Table 5.1**
Equipment and Materials Needed for a FEES Examination

Equipment[a]

Flexible fiberoptic laryngoscope
Halogen light source
Chip camera
Videotape recorder
Monitor
Microphone to pick up audio signal
Time and date generator (optional)
Video printer (optional)

Supplies

Videotape for recording
Lidocaine 2% viscous gel (optional)
Cotton-tipped applicators (optional)
2 × 2 guaze pads for cleaning endoscope
Alcohol prep pads for cleaning endoscope
Gloves
Lubricating gel for outside of endoscope if not using lidocaine
Medicine cups for holding small amount of lidocaine
Larger cups for holding liquids
Spoons
Plates
Straws
Food and liquids to give to patient
Green (or blue) food color with dropper
Disinfectant for endoscope (as recommended by Infection Control)
Container for disinfectant

---

[a]Sources for equipment: Kay Elemetrics, 1 Bridgewater Lane, Lincoln Park, NJ 07035-1488, phone: 201/628-6200; Olympus America, Medical Instrument Division, 4 Nevada Drive, Lake Success, NY 11042, phone: 800/645-8160; Pentax Precision Instrument Corporation, 30 Ramland Road, Orangeburg, NY 10962-2699, phone: 800/431-5880.

prostheses into a tracheoesophageal stent or perform tracheal suctioning. As clinicians become cross-trained and learn to perform more procedures that deal directly with the patient's medical condition, endoscopy will not appear so unusual.

Clinical privileging is a process that physicians have used for years in every medical institution in the country. Holding clinical privileges means that the professional is competent and able to perform a certain procedure independently in that institution. Until recently, speech–language pathologists did not need clinical privileges because they did not perform any procedure that carried a risk to the patient. As dysphagia management has emerged as a subspecialty of care, that situation has changed. In my view, all diagnostic and treatment procedures associated with dysphagia should be done only after clinical privileges or some equivalent means of approval have been granted.

Clinical privileges are granted by an institution to individual practitioners, based on evidence that the applicant is competent in performing and interpreting the procedure. The evidence is usually submitted in written form and lists the didactic experience the applicant has gained in that procedure (e.g., attending workshops) and some hands-on experience, often under the supervision of a mentor. Clinical privileges do not carry over to another institution, but need to be applied for separately in every institution where the person practices.

In the case of FEES, as with many other procedures, training and competence can be attained in several ways. Frequently, speech–language pathologists learn the technical skill of handling an endoscope from an individual who is already skilled and privileged to perform endoscopy, whether this be for swallowing, voice, or medical purposes. This mentor may be an otolaryngologist, another speech pathologist, or any other professional who performs endoscopy. The knowledge-based skills required to proceed in an examination, identify abnormal findings, and interpret these findings can be attained by attending workshops, reading articles, and working with someone who has experience in dysphagia and knows how to apply endoscopy to this disorder.

ASHA's Special Interest Division—Swallowing and Swallowing Disorders (Dysphagia) has drafted a document outlining the training and competencies needed by any speech–language pathologist who wants to perform a FEES procedure. The reader is referred to this document for further information (ASHA, 1997).

Risks Associated with Endoscopy

With the emphasis placed in this chapter on attaining adequate training and proving competency in endoscopy, one might conclude that the procedure is very risky. In fact, when done properly, nasendoscopy is an extremely low-risk procedure. From the thousands of examinations done over the past 10 years by hundreds of speech pathologists, there is not one reported case where a major complication occurred from the procedure (Langmore, in press; Langmore, Pelletier, & Nelson, 1995).

Five possible complications might occur from a FEES procedure: allergic reaction to the anesthesia, nosebleed, vasovagal response, laryngospasm, and aspiration. In each of these cases, a major complication is preventable. The first possible problem is an allergic reaction to the anesthesia. Certain precautions taken by FEES users significantly lessen the chance of any major allergic reaction. First, lidocaine 2% concentration in gel or liquid form is the anesthesia of choice because it has an extremely low rate of allergic reaction (*Physicians' Desk Reference*, 1995, p. 581). Second, only a small amount is used (approximately 1 ml) and only in one nostril. It is important that a spray not be delivered to the patient so that the pharynx will not be desensitized when assessing swallowing and so that the anesthesia does not travel to the lungs where it could be absorbed into the bloodstream and cause a more systemic reaction.

A nosebleed (epistaxis) is the most predictable complication, and anyone who performs nasendoscopy frequently is bound to encounter this event sometime. The severity of the nosebleed should be minor, however, simply because the examiner always has a view of the path being taken by the endoscope, unlike the nurse or physician who is passing a feeding tube blindly. In the survey taken by Langmore et al. (1995), none of the reported nosebleeds was significant enough to terminate the examination.

A vasovagal response is an episode of fainting in which the autonomic branches of the vagus nerve are overstimulated. Typically, the precipitating stimulus is psychological, meaning that the victim is fearful or anxious and this stimulates an internal reaction that has a predictable course and outcome (Van Lieshout, Wieling, Karemaker, & Eckberg, 1991). In the early stages of a vasovagal response, the person feels hot and sweaty, the heart rate and breathing rate increase, and blood pressure rises. The rise in blood pressure forces more blood flow to the extremities, away from the head, and this in turn causes the person to faint from decreased availability of oxygen to the brain. The act of fainting usually causes the person to fall supine and this restores the needed level; therefore, a vasovagal response is usually self-limiting.

The only danger in fainting is when it occurs in a person with a severe underlying cardiac condition characterized by bradycardia. Because the blood pressure drops and heart rate decreases during the second stage of a vasovagal response when the person actually faints, a person with a very low heart rate could suffer further cardiac damage if he or she faints. The likelihood of a patient fainting during a FEES exam is extremely low and should be prevented by a calm and reassuring examiner and careful monitoring of the patient's status.

An additional complication that could feasibly occur from nasendoscopy is a laryngospasm (Ikari & Sasaki, 1980), an extreme exaggeration of the normal laryngeal adductory response to a stimulus delivered to the larynx or hypopharynx. In a laryngospasm, the stimulus is prolonged and perceived as aversive and unexpected, causing the vocal folds to adduct more tightly for a prolonged period of time, as in a state of spasm. The response is usually self-limiting and there are some indications that the response will never be serious (i.e., no complications) in an awake individual (Ikari & Sasaki, 1980). Laryngospasm is most commonly reported in patients who are recovering from general anesthesia and it has also been reported in sleeping individuals to an event of gastroesophageal reflux that reaches the hypopharynx (Bortolotti, 1989). In the FEES survey reported by Langmore et al. (1995), the only cases of laryngospasm were reported by an otolaryngologist who intentionally touched the true vocal folds to test sensitivity. The unintentional contacts of the scope to the surfaces within the hypopharynx and larynx that always occur during a FEES examination have not been known to trigger laryngospasm. In a FEES procedure, no structures are ever touched deliberately before informing the patient that this will occur.

The final possible complication of a FEES procedure is faced by every clinician who works with patients who have dysphagia: An event of aspiration could cause immediate strangulation, or more commonly, an aspiration pneumonia. The advantage of an instrumental examination is that the amount aspirated can be minimized because the examiner has information that is unavailable to the examiner performing a noninstrumental examination or to a nurse or therapist who is feeding the patient. In this respect, the FEES procedure offers a level of safety unavailable during the clinical examination and can provide information that will hopefully prevent these aspiration-related complications.

Patient Selection for FEES

A major point in decision making is determining whether the patient needs an instrumental examination and, if so, whether a fluoroscopy or endoscopy procedure would be more beneficial. Sometimes, the type of instrumental procedure available to the speech–language pathologist will be the determining factor in his or her decision to continue the assessment beyond the clinical examination. If doing an instrumental examination would require transporting a patient from a nursing home via ambulance to a hospital where fluoroscopy is done, or would require transporting an intensive care unit patient to a radiology suite, this factor may discourage the speech pathologist from making that recommendation. If a FEES system (or mobile fluoroscopy system) is available, the speech pathologist and physician are able to decide whether to proceed with an instrumental procedure based more on clinical needs than logistic factors. An examination that can be taken to the patient at bedside holds some clear advantages over an examination that is done away from the patient's environment and support staff. Sometimes, transportation is not the issue as much as is positioning. For example, some patients with contractures or decubitus ulcers become uncomfortable or experience pain when they are repositioned. Some patients are too obese to fit between the fluoroscopy unit and the table. Patients who are fed in bed should have their swallowing tested in that same environment and in the position in which they will be fed.

If a clinician has access to both fluoroscopy and FEES and there are no overriding practical reasons for choosing one examination over the other, clinical indications should guide the determination of which procedure will be the most beneficial. My experience indicates that the great majority of patients can be tested with either procedure because either will enable the examiner to identify a dysphagia, to understand the nature of the problem, and to make appropriate recommendations. There are many minor reasons for choosing fluoroscopy or FEES and a few compelling clinical conditions that really point to the need for one examination or the other. In Table 5.2, the minor and major indicators for each procedure are listed. The major ones need some discussion here.

A fluoroscopy procedure provides the more comprehensive view of the swallowing mechanism, including the oral, pharyngeal, and esophageal structures. For that reason, whenever a patient presents with vague complaints that might implicate any or all of these regions, a

Table 5.2
Indications for an Endoscopy (FEES)
Versus a Fluoroscopy Examination

Indications for Fluoroscopy

- Oral stage problem needs to be imaged for analysis
- Coordination of oral and pharyngeal movements needs to be imaged
- Need to analyze forces that move the bolus (e.g., tongue posterior thrust vs. laryngeal elevation; cricopharyngeal dysfunction) to assist with differential diagnosis
- Esophageal stage problem or gastroesophageal reflux (GER) is suspected; need to screen esophageal motility and GER (Complete exam of esophageal motility and GER is barium swallow or upper gastrointestinal (GI) study)
- Globus complaints; possible cricopharyngeal dysfunction; possible cervical oesteophytes
- Vague symptomatology from patient; need comprehensive view of all structures

Indications for a FEES Exam[a]

- Fluoroscopy unavailable when the examination is needed
- Transportation to the fluoroscopy suite would put the patient at risk or submit patient to undue stress (the medically fragile/unstable patient); multiple monitors or ventilator in place; additional staff needed to travel with patient
- Transportation to another hospital is problematic (cost of transportation, personnel to accompany patient, strain on patient, patient fearful of leaving familiar surroundings)
- Positioning for fluroscopy study is problematic (e.g., patient has severe contractures, is quadriplegic, wears neck halo, is obese, is on ventilator)
- Concern about excess radiation exposure from fluoroscopy
- Patient has severe dysphagia (i.e., very weak, infrequent, or possibly absent swallow reflex) and/or very limited ability to tolerate aspiration (e.g., brainstem stroke, tube fed for prolonged period, very poor pulmonary or immunologic status), causing concern about aspiration of barium, food, or liquid
- Question of management of secretions
- Postintubation or postsurgery to look for altered anatomy or vagus nerve damage (larynx visualized for signs of trauma or neurologic damage)
- Therapeutic exam when extra time is needed to try out different maneuvers and/or a wide range of food consistencies and a variety of real foods
- Use of endoscopy for biofeedback
- When these clinical symptoms are present: hypernasal voice, velopharyngeal insufficiency; hoarse, breathy, wet voice; rapid respiratory rate, effortful breathing

Note: For many patients who do not fit the listed criteria, either examination will be satisfactory.

[a]The first three indications in this table might not apply if a mobile fluoroscopy unit is available in the facility.

fluoroscopy study is preferred. Similarly, if the patient's complaints point to the oral cavity, the cervical esophagus, or the cricopharyngeal region, fluoroscopy is the procedure of choice. Endoscopy cannot view these regions or capture the temporal relation between oral movements and pharyngeal movements. In my opinion, viewing these structures is most often necessary when the underlying medical diagnosis is uncertain or the nature of the problem is unclear. The typical patient needing a fluoroscopy study is the outpatient who complains of food sticking at the level of the suprasternal notch and who has no known medical diagnosis that could cause pharyngeal dysphagia.

Endoscopy provides a superior view of the hypopharynx and larynx and is the preferred procedure when it is prudent to view this region directly. Patients who have been intubated or who have recently undergone thoracic surgery or neurosurgery that might have damaged the vagus nerve should have a FEES examination to rule out anatomic or neurologic damage to the larynx or surrounding pharynx.

Another type of patient that is better suited to a FEES examination is the one who is tube fed and has not recently eaten by mouth, especially if that patient is suspected of having a severe dysphagia. The endoscopic examination with this patient begins with an assessment of how the patient is handling secretions, which is important because aspiration of contaminated saliva is a major risk factor for pneumonia (Finegold, 1991). Before a decision is made to introduce food during the examination, FEES allows the use of a more conservative test substance such as ice chips to be delivered. The clinician can use this bolus material to evaluate the patient's ability to swallow a relatively benign bolus before barium or more solid food is given that may lead to aspiration.

Although these specific clinical conditions point to the need for fluoroscopy or endoscopy, most of the patients encountered in a hospital, rehabilitation setting, or nursing home can be assessed with either procedure. The poststroke patient who appears to aspirate thin liquids is a good example. In either case, the dysphagia will be identified, the nature of the problem will be understood, and appropriate therapeutic interventions (e.g., increased sensory stimulation, chin-tuck, or thickened liquids) can be attempted and assessed. In the evaluation of the effects of thickened liquids on the swallow, however, FEES will allow delivery of actual liquids that the patient will be drinking, whereas a fluoroscopy procedure is limited to liquids impregnated with barium.

Barium-based test materials may not represent the viscosity, texture, or taste of the actual liquids that will be given to the patient in daily life.

The FEES Protocols

An endoscopic procedure can be completed in a variety of settings and for a variety of clinical reasons. Depending on the particular situation, the protocol will vary. Langmore and McCulloch (1997) provide a detailed description of a comprehensive protocol, and the reader is referred to this source for more information. In this chapter I summarize two different protocols that have proven clinically useful: the full FEES Procedure and the Ice Chip protocol.

Patient and Materials Preparation

Regardless of the protocol to be followed, preparations for the procedure are similar. Outpatients and rehabilitation patients are generally tested while sitting in an exam chair. Inpatients may be tested while sitting in bed if that is how they will be fed. The equipment and supplies needed for the procedure are all contained on a portable cart that can be wheeled to bedside. The first step in patient preparation is to position the patient as desired for the examination and then to anesthetize one of the nares if the patient so wishes. While the anesthesia is taking effect (about 5 minutes), the examiner sets up the equipment (connects the endoscope to the camera, readies the videotape recording systems, etc.). The monitor can be positioned so that the patient can view the ongoing exam, if that is desired.

If the examination is being done with a patient who is currently tube fed (nothing per oral, or NPO), ice chips are prepared by adding blue or green food color to them. If the patient is currently receiving per oral (PO) feeding or if the clinician anticipates that food and liquid will be given, these items are prepared by adding food color to them. The reason for adding food color is simply to make the material uniquely visible and distinct from surrounding mucosal surfaces. Food consistencies typical of the patient's diet are assembled; actual foods from a lunch tray are ideal for the examination of this sort.

The Complete FEES Protocol

The FEES protocol is shown in Table 5.3. There are two major parts to a complete FEES examination. Part I consists of sensorimotor examination of pharyngeal and laryngeal function to assess such parameters as strength, range, symmetry, and briskness of movement. Anatomy is also viewed for its effect on swallowing function. Part II of the exam involves delivery of food and liquid to directly assess swallowing of these materials. Throughout the examination, the endoscopist needs to continually manipulate the endoscope so that the patient is comfortable and the desired view is obtained. Figure 5.1 depicts the placement of the endoscope during a FEES procedure. Figure A.1 shows the view of the hypopharynx when the endoscope is positioned above the epiglottis and Figure A.2 shows the view when the endoscope is lowered to a point within the laryngeal vestibule. Figures A.1–A.5 are located in the Appendix at the end of this book.

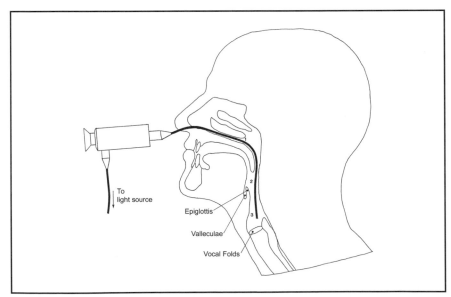

Figure 5.1. Placement of the endoscope during a FEES examination. From "Fiberoptic Endoscopic Examination of Swallowing Safety: A New Procedure," by S. E. Langmore, K. Schatz, and N. Olsen, 1988, *Dysphagia, 2,* p. 217. Copyright 1988 by Springer-Verlag New York, Inc. Reprinted with permission.

Table 5.3
FEES Examination Protocol

I. Anatomic–Physiologic Assessment

A. Velopharyngeal closure

Task: Have patient say 'ee', 'ss', and other oral sounds; alternate oral and nasal sounds (e.g., "duh-nuh").

Task: Have patient dry swallow.

Optional Task: While patient swallows liquids, look for nasal leakage.

B. Appearance of Hypopharynx and Larynx at Rest

Scan around entire hypopharynx to note appearance, symmetry, and abnormalities that impact swallowing and might require referral to another specialty.

Optional Task: Have patient hold breath and blow out cheeks forcefully.

C. Handling of Secretions and Swallow Frequency

Observe amount and location of secretions and frequency of dry swallows over a period of at least 2 minutes.

1 = normal amount

2 = standing secretions in valleculae, lateral channels, pyriforms

3 = standing secretions in laryngeal vestibule transiently over the rating period

4 = standing secretions in laryngeal vestibule throughout the rating period or aspirated without being expelled spontaneously

Task: If no spontaneous swallowing is noted, cue the patient to swallow.

Go to Ice Chip Protocol if rating is 3 or 4, and dry swallows do not clear secretions.

D. Base of Tongue, Pharyngeal Muscles

Task: Have patient say "earl, oil" or other postvocalic "l" words.

Task: Have patient retract tongue while you lightly resist by holding it.

Tasks: Have patient say strained loud, high 'ee'; grunt; cough.

E. Laryngeal Function

1. Respiration

Observe laryngeal structures for rest breathing.

Tasks: Have patient sniff, pant, or alternate 'ee' with light inhalation.

2. Phonation

Task: Have patient say 'ee'.

Task: Have patient repeat "hee-hee-hee" 5 to 7 times.

Task: Have patient glide upward in pitch.

(continues)

Table 5.3 *Continued.*

---

3. Airway Protection

Task: Have patient hold breath lightly.

Task: Have patient hold breath very tightly.

Task: Have patient hold breath to the count of 7.

Optional: Have patient cough, clear throat.

F. Sensory Testing

Note patient's response to presence of scope.

Optional Task: Lightly touch tongue, pharyngeal walls, epiglottis.

Optional Task: Perform formal sensory testing with air pulse.

Note: Additional information about sensation will be obtained in Part II; formal testing can be deferred until the end of the examination if desired.

II. Swallowing Food and Liquid

Dye all foods and liquids green or blue with food coloring.

Consistencies

Try various consistencies, depending on patient needs and problems observed. Suggested consistencies to try:

1. Ice chips—usually ⅓ to ½ teaspoon; dyed green
2. Thin liquids—milk, juice, formula (Milk or other light-colored thin liquid is recommended for visibility)
3. Thick liquids—nectar or honey consistency; milkshakes
4. Puree—applesauce consistency; pudding consistency
5. Semisolid food—mashed potato, banana, pasta
6. Soft solid food (requires some chewing)—bread & cheese, soft cookie, casserole, meat loaf, cooked vegetables
7. Hard, chewy, crunchy food—meat, raw fruit, green salad
8. Mixed consistencies—soup with food bits, cereal with milk

Amounts/Bolus Sizes

If measured bolus sizes are given, a rule of thumb that applies to many patients is to increase the bolus size with each presentation until penetration or aspiration is seen. When that occurs, repeat the same bolus size to determine whether this pattern is consistent. If penetration or aspiration occurs again, do not continue with that bolus amount. The following progression of bolus volumes is suggested:

1. < 5 cc—only if patient is at high risk for aspirating and pulmonary clearance is poor
2. 5 cc (1 teaspoon)
3. 10 cc
4. 15 cc (1 tablespoon)

(continues)

Table 5.3 *Continued.*

---

5. 20 cc (heaping tablespoon, delivered)

6. Single swallow from cup or straw, monitored

7. Single swallow from cup or straw, self-presented

8. Free consecutive swallows, self-presented

9. Feed self food at own rate

General Guidelines

The usual progression for a patient who is currently eating per oral (PO) is to begin the assessment by letting the patient self-feed and observe the patient's ability to swallow a variety of bolus sizes and consistencies as he or she would do naturally. (In other words, do not deliver measured bolus volumes.) Do not intervene until a problem is noted; at that time, choose the intervention(s) that are appropriate and will answer the clinical questions. Sometimes, intervention will prevent the clinical questions (e.g., Would the patient eventually sense the residue and clear it before it is aspirated?) from being answered so it is important to intervene expeditiously. Use the strategy appropriate for the observed problem, including limiting bolus volumes, delivery of food or liquid instead of letting patient self-feed, other change in bolus delivery, postural changes, use of swallow maneuver, or other swallow or feeding strategy.

Patients who are currently (NPO) or who are medically unstable generally need a more structured examination, with more intervention from the examiner. Use your clinical judgment!

Patients who are tracheotomized, who are dependent for feeding, who need to be repositioned to eat, or who need dentures to eat may need an examination that determines swallowing function in its current state *and* under optimal conditions. Again, the clinical questions will guide the protocol.

Note. From *Endoscopic Evaluation and Treatment of Swallowing Disorders,* by S. E. Langmore, 2000, New York: Thieme Medical. Copyright 2000 by Thieme Medical. Reprinted with permission.

Part I: Anatomic–Physiologic Assessment. The sensorimotor examination is conducted in order to understand the underlying anatomic or physiologic cause of the dysphagia. Although endoscopy cannot reveal all underlying causes of a swallowing problem, it is able to reveal some problems much better than fluoroscopy can because of the nature of the tool and the image. The ability to view anatomy directly is one strength of endoscopy. The appearance of all the pharyngeal and laryngeal structures is observed and their effect on swallowing function is determined. Edema is one common finding after intubation that can account for a temporary dysphagia due to reduced sensation and mobility of the affected structures. Suspicious growths or unusual appearance of the mucosal surface alerts the speech pathologist to a possible medical pathology, allowing a referral to otolaryngology. Abnormalities of tissues and structures are often not as easily appreciated via the fluoroscopic view. Using the FEES protocol, the examiner assesses pharyngeal and laryngeal function via a series of tasks, such as having the patient repeat "kuh-kuh-kuh" (for back of tongue movement), dry swallow (velopharyngeal closure), hold the breath (true vocal fold adduction), hold the breath tightly (true and false vocal fold adduction and complete arytenoid medial contact), sustain breath holding for several seconds, and sniff (laryngeal abduction). All of the tasks relating to airway protection are tested in detail because this function is so critical in the prevention of aspiration.

Throughout Part I of the examination, the examiner observes the status of any standing secretions, the ability of the patient to swallow or clear these secretions, and the frequency of spontaneous dry swallows. The presence of excess, standing secretions is an important clue to a dysphagia and has been shown to be an excellent predictor of aspiration of food and liquid (Murray, Langmore, Ginsberg, & Bromberg, 1996).

Next in the protocol, the examiner assesses laryngeal and pharyngeal sensation. An indication of intact sensation may already have been revealed by the patient's response to the presence of the endoscope (verbalizations, increased salivary flow, increased swallowing, etc.), but if this is in question, it can be directly tested by lightly touching the back of tongue, lateral pharyngeal walls, base of tongue, and epiglottis tip. By leaving the laryngeal structure (epiglottis) to the end, and only touching it if the patient is insensate to the touch of other structures, an adverse reaction should be avoided. Recently, a special endoscope has been developed (Pentax Precision Instrument Corporation) to directly test and quantify sensory threshold. This endoscope has a second channel, which can deliver a calibrated pulse of air to the structures of interest. Preliminary research with this instrument suggests that it may have great clinical utility (Aviv, Martin, et al., 1996; Aviv, Sacco, et al., 1997).

Part II: Swallowing Food and Liquid. After the anatomic and physiologic functions of the pharynx and larynx have been evaluated, the FEES exam progresses to the delivery of food and liquid so that a swallowing function can be directly evaluated. A variety of bolus volumes and consistencies are generally given to the patient, and his or her ability to swallow them safely and adequately is noted. Abnormal function is indicated if residue, spillage, laryngeal penetration, or aspiration of material below the true vocal folds is observed. Pharyngeal delay time is also calculated and reduced or delayed epiglottic retroflexion is noted. Special attention is paid to timing of airway closure with bolus flow. As soon as a problem is identified, the examiner intervenes with appropriate therapeutic alterations to observe their effect on swallowing. These alterations might include instructing the patient to assume another posture such as chin-tuck, teaching the patient a swallow maneuver such as the controlled breath-hold prior to swallowing, or adjusting the bolus consistency, size, or method of delivery. The examination ends when the examiner understands the nature of the problem, has determined which bolus amounts and consistencies can be swallowed effectively and safely, and has decided what therapeutic alterations facilitate swallowing.

Whenever possible, the patient, the family, and the nursing staff who feed the patient are involved in the examination and participate in decision making regarding possible treatment for swallowing problems that are observed. In my clinical experience, education of and collaboration with these significant persons are the most effective means of developing realistic and meaningful treatment goals and ensuring compliance with the treatment plan.

The FEES Ice Chip Protocol

Patients who have not eaten PO for several days, weeks, or months sometimes reduce the frequency of spontaneous swallowing. The muscles used in swallowing appear to become "deconditioned" and the swallow, when initially tested, is weak and slow to trigger. Often these same patients are medically fragile and might be unable to clear a large-volume aspiration. For these reasons, I prefer to test their swallow initially with a small, relatively benign bolus that will not harm the lungs if it is aspirated.

Table 5.4 summarizes the FEES Ice Chip protocol. It begins with the same tasks listed in Part I of the comprehensive FEES protocol. Part II begins with the delivery of about ½ teaspoon of ice chips. The patient's response to the ice chips is noted. That is, the examiner notes whether the ice chips stimulated a quicker, stronger swallow. It is

Table 5.4
The FEES Ice Chip Protocol

I. Anatomic–Physiologic Assessment

1. The Ice Chip Protocol is similar to the FEES Protocol, with special attention paid to anatomy, sensation, and airway protection.

2. Rate status of secretions from 1 to 4:

   1 = normal amount

   2 = standing secretions in valleculae, lateral channels, pyriforms

   3 = standing secretions in laryngeal vestibule transiently over the rating period

   4 = standing secretions in laryngeal vestibule throughout the rating period or aspirated without being expelled spontaneously

3. Stimulate dry swallows (verbal request, thermal stimulation, etc.). Is patient successful? What is the effect of the swallow on standing secretions?

   Note: You can stop the exam here, or go on to Part II.

II. Delivery of Ice Chips

1. Give ice chips if the patient is alert. Note the following:

   • Patient's ability to swallow ice chips

   • Effect of swallowing ice chips on stimulating further dry swallows

   • Effect on clearing or thinning of secretions

   • Effect on stimulating a cough if aspirated

2. If patient does not swallow first ice chip well (aspirates it), repeat *at least* once. Usually deliver ice chips five times before stopping.

3. Go on to pureed food, thin liquid (milk), solid food, thick liquid only if the patient is able to swallow ice chips well.

4. Try *appropriate* therapeutic interventions.

Usual Recommendations/Follow-up

1. If ice chips were never even partially swallowed, recommend aggressive management of secretions and oral hygiene.

2. If ice chips were beneficial (stimulated more frequent swallows, cleared or thinned the secretions, etc.), recommend delivery of ice chips in regulated amounts, several times a day.

   Note: Repeat FEES exam (either FEES Examination Protocol or FEES Ice Chip Protocol, depending on patient's performance) before beginning food or liquid PO diet.

Note. From *Endoscopic Evaluation and Treatment of Swallowing Disorders*, by S. E. Langmore, 2000, New York: Thieme Medical. Copyright 2000 by Thieme Medical. Reprinted with permission.

important to observe whether aspiration occurred, whether the patient was sensitive to it, and whether he or she responded with an effective clearing cough. No matter what the response is to the initial delivery of ice chips, a second and usually a third bolus are given to account for the "warm-up" effect that is often witnessed. After three or more trial swallows of ice chips, the examiner decides whether to proceed with test boluses of food or liquid, depending on the success with this initial consistency.

Another type of patient who is given the Ice Chip protocol is the one who presents initially with excess secretions in the hypopharynx or larynx, regardless of whether he or she is eating PO. As Murray et al. (1996) reported, excess secretions, especially those within the laryngeal vestibule, are often indicative of a severe dysphagia and likely aspiration of food or liquid. The examiner can see whether the delivery of ice chips facilitates a swallow and whether that same swallow helps to clear the secretions. If the ice chips help the patient to swallow, they are often recommended as a therapeutic strategy to help stimulate swallowing of saliva over the day.

Repeat Protocols

Repeat evaluations can be completed more frequently with FEES than with fluoroscopy, simply because FEES examinations are logistically easier to perform and there is no concern about excess radiation. These examinations are done to answer specific questions such as "Is the patient now safe with thin liquids?" or "Does the patient still need to turn his head to improve bolus clearance?" Obviously, with these questions in mind, the exam is very short and consists of delivery of only certain consistencies in conjunction with certain maneuvers. I often give a patient multiple FEES examinations, often once weekly, and advance the diet as quickly as possible. Leder, Sasaki, and Burrell (1998) also perform serial FEES exams.

Identifying Abnormal Findings of a FEES Examination

The speech–language pathologist who is new to endoscopy will need specific practice viewing and interpreting FEES videotaped studies before attaining competence in identifying abnormal swallows and understanding the nature of the problem. Prior experience with fluoroscopy is an invaluable aid in attaining competence, but some work is still needed to translate the image from one format to the other.

The most salient findings of either the fluoroscopic or the endoscopic examination relate to the fate of the bolus. Specific questions that can be answered based on the observed swallows include these:

1. Did the bolus spill into the hypopharynx prior to initiating the swallow?

2. Did it penetrate the laryngeal vestibule?

3. Was it aspirated?

4. Was excessive residue left in the hypopharynx after the swallow?

Endoscopy is a superb tool for revealing the location, amount, and path taken by the bolus. Abnormality is defined by the same parameters as for fluoroscopy except for some recalibration of the amount of spillage or residue that should be considered "normal." One of the first differences noticed by new users of endoscopy is that this tool is much more sensitive to every small bit of material in the hypopharynx. What appears to be a significant amount of residue from endoscopy may, in fact, look mild to moderate from the fluoroscopic image. An additional advantage of endoscopy is that the residue is localized much better, so that material that appears to be in the lateral channels on fluoroscopy may be seen to lie within the laryngeal vestibule itself when viewed endoscopically.

Spillage of material into the hypopharynx, shown in Figure A.3 in the Appendix at the end of this book is a vivid event when viewed endoscopically. Both the bolus path and the final resting place of the spilled material are clearly seen. After a swallow, residue is clearly seen, as illustrated in Figure A.4. Because endoscopy can witness events unfolding over several minutes, the examiner can passively observe how the patient reacts to residue immediately after the swallow or over time as the residue moves by gravity or builds up over several new swallows. This is valuable clinical information.

Considering that there is a period of time during the swallow when the view is lost (white-out), many new users of FEES wonder how sensitive endoscopy is to events of aspiration. To date, most who have studied this question have concluded that endoscopy is very sensitive when compared to fluoroscopy (Crary & Baron, 1997; Langmore, Schatz, & Olson, 1991; Leder et al., 1998; Willging, Miller, Hogan, & Rudolph, 1996). One primary reason for this is that many events of aspiration occur before and after the swallow, and endoscopy captures these events directly. The time period immediately surrounding the onset of the swallow is especially common for aspiration, and endoscopy maintains a view up until about 63 milliseconds into the onset of the swallow, if this is defined by the moment when the hyoid begins its final elevation. Thus, aspiration occurring just as the swallow begins can often be witnessed endoscopically. However, some aspiration occurs during the height of the swallow, and these events need to be identified from the view that is presented to the examiner after the swallow. Residue of material lying on the subglottic shelf is a sure sign of aspiration, as seen in Figure A.5, whereas residue on the true vocal folds is a sign of *possible* aspiration. By asking the patient to cough (if he or she has not done so spontaneously), material that might have fallen lower in the trachea or into the lungs can be seen as it is expelled into the larynx.

The one published study that did not find endoscopy to be sensitive to aspiration was from a group of investigators who gave only a small amount of blue-tinged water to the patient to detect aspiration (Wu, Hsiao, Chen, Chang, & Lee, 1997). I highly discourage the delivery of water when the purpose of the examination is to detect aspiration. Water is transparent and nearly impossible to visualize. When it is dyed blue or green, it is somewhat more visible in the pharynx, but it is still very difficult to detect subglottally. I recommend using milk or some other very light-colored liquid for a test material and dyeing all test materials blue or green with food coloring.

Although the path taken by the bolus is the ultimate marker for an "adequate" swallow, observations of anatomy, structural movement, and timing of movements help to explain the cause of the dysphagia. Fluoroscopy earns high marks in this regard, with its ability to image movements of the hyoid, larynx, tongue, epiglottis, cricopharyngeus, and other structures during the swallow. Endoscopy does not have such a comprehensive view and it loses the view entirely for about 66 milliseconds at the height of the swallow (the period of white-out). Nonetheless, a few key movements can be observed and many others can be inferred from the resulting bolus misdirection.

Some movements are actually seen better endoscopically, such as velopharyngeal closure (since the sphincteric nature of the closure can be observed directly and assessed in detail). Also, laryngeal closure achieved by vocal fold adduction and medial contact of the arytenoids can only be assessed directly with endoscopy. However, because it occurs relatively late in the swallow, airway protection or laryngeal competence needs to be assessed separately by having the patient hold his or her breath, cough, phonate, or perform some other task that requires laryngeal closure. One other movement that can be assessed endoscopically is epiglottal retroflexion. Although the entire range of movement cannot be viewed, incomplete epiglottal retroflexion is often identified by its *lack* of movement at the onset of the swallow (prior to white-out) and again when the view returns immediately after the swallow. Because epiglottal retroflexion is largely a function of hyoid movement, one can infer reduced hyoid movement from the poor epiglottal movement.

Many clinicians believe that the single most useful temporal measure of a dysfunctional swallow is a prolonged pharyngeal delay. This measure is defined fluoroscopically with liquid bolus swallows as the duration from (a) the moment that the bolus head passes the posterior faucial arches (in a young person) or the base of tongue–ramus of mandible intersection (in an older person) until (b) the hyoid starts its final elevation (Tracy et al., 1989). The same measure can be taken endoscopically in an older person from (a) the moment the bolus head appears in view along the base of tongue until (b) the moment of white-out, or epiglottal retroflexion. These two measures of pharyngeal delay are nearly equivalent, as shown by simultaneous studies of fluoroscopy and endoscopy. In addition to this important temporal measure, endoscopy is an excellent tool to view exactly where the bolus head travels during the pharyngeal delay.

When dysphagia is due to a structural abnormality in the pharynx or larynx, endoscopy is the superior tool to reveal the problem. Some common findings are edema, malformed structures, altered structures secondary to surgery, or mucosal changes. The adverse effect of a large-bore feeding tube on movement of the arytenoids and epiglottis can be seen as well as the effects of a tracheotomy tube on reduced laryngeal movement.

Interpreting the Findings: The Underlying Anatomic–Physiologic Basis for the Dysphagia

To understand the nature of a patient's dysphagia, the examiner must move from individual findings related to swallowing events to an interpretative level. One useful classification paradigm might be to characterize dysphagia as caused by (a) inadequate bolus propulsion, (b) inadequate airway closure, (c) mistiming of bolus propulsion and airway protection, (d) inadequate sensation, and (e) abnormal anatomy. Although fluoroscopy and endoscopy excel in revealing different patterns, the vast majority of pharyngeal dysphagias can be correctly identified and understood by either instrument. Following is a brief discussion of the performance of fluoroscopy and FEES as they address each of these five elements.

Inadequate Bolus Propulsion

Failure to propel the bolus sufficiently is usually caused by inadequate amplitude of movement of any or all of the structures that move the bolus from the mouth through the pharynx into the esophagus. Fluoroscopy can directly assess the range of movement of the tongue, hyoid, larynx, pharynx, and cricopharyngeus. Endoscopy can see parts of epiglottal retroflexion and pharyngeal shortening, but otherwise must infer incomplete bolus propulsion from excess residue left behind after the swallow. Depending on where the bolus remains, endoscopy infers which regions within the hypopharynx are more impaired (Dejaeger, Pelemans, Ponette, & Joosten, 1997; Olsson, Castell, Johnston, Ekberg, & Castell, 1997).

Velopharyngeal valving helps to direct the bolus down the pharynx and keep it out of the nose. Endoscopy can assess the competence of this valve directly during a swallow, whereas fluoroscopy infers it from bolus misdirection during the swallow.

Inadequate Airway Protection

Failure to protect the airway is caused by incomplete laryngeal closure during the height of the swallow. Fluoroscopy infers this from bolus aspiration during the swallow. Endoscopy infers this from evidence of aspiration after the swallow and from direct assessment of laryngeal competence in tasks such as breath holding, phonation, and cough.

Mistiming of Bolus Propulsion and Airway Protection

Mistiming errors can occur because of poor oral containment of the bolus or delay in initiating the swallow (pharyngeal delay). Either endoscopy or fluoroscopy can reveal this problem directly by observing the bolus movement in relation to the onset of the swallow. Oral containment versus pharyngeal delay can be sorted out by giving the patient instructions such as "hold it in your mouth and don't swallow it until I tell you" versus "Swallow it now." Bolus spillage is the marker for impairment at this level.

Reduced Sensation

A reduction in sensation can be inferred with both endoscopy and fluoroscopy from the lack of patient awareness or response to residue, penetration, or aspiration. Endoscopy is able to assess sensation somewhat better simply because a person with an intact nervous system is sensitive to the presence of the endoscope in the pharynx and will react by increasing salivary flow and swallowing spontaneously in reaction to this. A new endoscope has been manufactured (Pentax, Inc.) that will even measure sensory threshold in the pharynx exactly.

Abnormal Anatomy

Both endoscopy and fluoroscopy allow the examiner to assess anatomy. When viewed via endoscopy, the examiner is able to visualize the problem much more clearly if it involves the larynx or pharynx. Other structural problems are also better appreciated endoscopically, such as presence of a feeding tube, edema, or surgically altered structures. Cervical oesteophytes are one anatomical problem that is imaged better fluoroscopically.

Using the Results of the Examination To Manage the Patient

After performing a FEES examination, the examiner reviews the tape carefully to answer the following questions:

1. Was evidence of a dysphagia seen?

2. What was the nature of the problem, or its defining characteristics?

3. Was it consistent with the complaints or the medical diagnosis and history?

4. What was the severity of the dysphagia?

5. What bolus volumes and consistencies were swallowed safely?

6. What diet is recommended, or should the patient be NPO?

7. What behavioral interventions were used, did they ameliorate the problem in question, and are they recommended?

8. Were any problems noted that need further evaluation and by whom?

9. What type and level of behavioral intervention will be provided by speech–language pathology?

10. What is the prognosis for recovery or improvement of the dysphagia?

A comprehensive FEES examination will provide the answers to all of these questions in the vast majority of patients. The questions regarding the presence, type, and severity of the dysphagia are answered from scoring the swallows and interpreting the abnormal findings in terms of the five underlying patterns described earlier. If any question remains, or the findings are not consistent with the medical diagnosis or the patient's complaints, a further evaluation should be performed. That may be a fluoroscopy, manometry, or other diagnostic study.

Recommendations for management of the patient follow directly from the FEES exam in conjunction with the clinical examination and knowledge of the patient's medical, social, and psychological status. Dietary recommendations are much easier to make from a FEES examination because real foods and liquids are given during the exam without needing to impregnate them with barium. Barium-based materials often do not match the viscosity, taste, and texture of real dietary items.

Other behavioral interventions such as altering the bolus volume, rate delivered, taste, or food temperature can also be tested much more thoroughly in a FEES procedure because of the more generous time allotted to the exam. Use of postures or maneuvers by the patient can also be evaluated during the FEES exam. Further, the patient can practice the maneuvers or postures while viewing the swallows on a monitor to get real-time feedback on the effect of the behavioral change.

One aspect of the FEES yet to be discussed is the active participation of the patient, family, and other staff in the procedure. The examination is done in the patient's environment, usually in his or her bedroom, and other caregivers who care for the patient are generally nearby. They are encouraged to view the examination on the monitor as it is being performed. It is not unusual for four or five people to be in the patient's room during a FEES procedure, with everyone watching the monitor. If the patient is cognitively alert enough to benefit from being involved in the decision making, the monitor is usually set up so that he or she can also view the examination. This feature of the FEES examination naturally facilitates patient, family, and staff education, as the results of each swallow are discussed as they occur. When therapeutic interventions are tried, everyone tends to get involved, with their own opinions as to what will work, what is realistic, what the patient is willing to do, and so forth. As a result of this total involvement, the recommendations represent a consensus of the significant people who will be needed to carry them out. In my experience, because of this involvement, compliance is significantly better after a FEES procedure than after the fluoroscopy procedure, where test results are transmitted in written form on a medical chart.

Reevaluations and Use of Endoscopy as a Therapy Tool

After the initial evaluation, unless the patient's swallow was normal, there is often a period of follow-up and need for some modifications in feeding and swallowing behavior and some dietary modifications.

When the time comes to consider a change in diet or behavioral modifications, the speech–language pathologist must decide whether instrumentation is needed to verify the effectiveness of the proposed change. If an instrumental evaluation is desired, FEES can be done much more efficiently; there is no need to schedule a time slot in radiology, the examination is less expensive, use of personnel is reduced, and there is no radiation exposure. If and when the time comes to consider yet another change, the speech–language pathologist must again decide whether to use instrumentation, and so the process continues.

Often a repeat examination is performed to determine the need for continuing a modified diet. In this case, the consistency in question is given to the patient, new consistencies are tried, and the examination is over. If the question is whether the patient needs to continue using a posture or whether the patient can learn a new maneuver effectively, endoscopy can be used in a biofeedback mode and the procedure becomes entirely therapeutic. Virtually all postures and maneuvers can be practiced with endoscopy. Use of volitional breath holding before the swallow or the full-fledged super-supraglottic swallow requires endoscopy to determine whether the vocal folds are adducted completely during a breath-hold maneuver (Martin, Logemann, Shaker, & Dodds, 1993).

Because repeat FEES examinations can be done relatively quickly and easily, they are often done more frequently than fluoroscopy exams. It is the opinion of many users of FEES that this ability to use the tool on the day it is indicated and to use it repeatedly enables patients to progress as swiftly as possible in regard to their dysphagia until they are discharged (Leder, 1998). Conversely, if there is a worsening condition, the FEES examination can be done promptly and more conservative measures taken accordingly. Either way, evidence suggests that health complications of dysphagia such as aspiration pneumonia may be reduced when the primary assessment tool is FEES (Spiegel, Selber, & Creed, 1998).

The Clinical Decision-Making Process: A Case Study

Management of patients with dysphagia is difficult at best. The decisions clinicians make lead to significant changes in patients' lives. In this chapter, endoscopy has been described as a tool that can help the speech–language pathologist assess and manage the problem. Every patient does not need a FEES examination; no single instrument serves every patient and sometimes a noninstrumental clinical examination meets the needs of the patient and clinician. The competent speech–language pathologist needs to draw on knowledge of dysphagia and medicine, as well as the personal history of each patient, to help guide the best course for that particular patient.

Some steps in this decision-making process are illustrated in the following example of a patient who was referred to speech pathology for a swallowing evaluation. The patient was in the surgical intensive care unit (ICU) after having undergone a coronary artery bypass graft, which was complicated by failure to wean from the ventilator. After a prolonged intubation of 2 weeks, a tracheotomy tube was placed. Within days, the patient began weaning from the respirator and consideration was given to feeding him by mouth (PO). At the urging of the nursing staff, thoracic surgery requested an evaluation to determine what the patient could safely consume.

The speech–language pathologist visited the patient in the thoracic ICU and began with a clinical examination. She noted that the patient was disoriented and somewhat lethargic, displayed effortful breathing, had a rapid respiratory rate, and had a breathy voice quality, even when the tracheotomy tube was occluded. Articulation was clear but dentate status was compromised by several missing teeth. A review of the medical chart revealed no other relevant medical problems or any neurologic complications such as stroke. Written progress notes by nursing indicated that the patient coughed when given water to drink. As a preliminary step in the evaluation of the patient's voice and swallow function, the speech–language pathologist placed a Passy-Muir one-way valve (Passy & Passy, Inc.) on the tracheotomy tube to redirect exhaled air through the glottis, up the pharynx, and out the nose and mouth. The patient tolerated this well and his voice became slightly louder over a period of a few minutes.

The next decision was whether to proceed with an instrumental examination. The speech–language pathologist did not believe she could make firm dietary recommendations using only a clinical examination. The nurse's observation suggested that thin liquids were not safe, but it was always possible that the patient could handle pureed foods adequately. In a healthier, more active and alert patient, trials of food given at bedside might have been trusted, but because of this patient's extremely fragile medical status, no amount of aspiration could be easily tolerated. Therefore, an instrumental procedure was deemed necessary to determine the safety of different food and liquid consistencies.

There were two primary reasons why a FEES procedure was the instrumental examination of choice to evaluate this patient's swallowing ability. First, the appearance of the larynx was of great interest because of the history of prolonged intubation and the bypass surgery. Laryngeal trauma and recurrent laryngeal nerve damage were both possible causes of the suspected dysphagia and would alter the course of treatment. Second, a FEES was preferred for practical reasons because the patient was in the ICU with several cardiac and respiratory monitors in place, a specially trained nursing staff within reach, and physicians nearby. It would have placed the patient at some risk and put the staff at great inconvenience to transport him out of the ICU to the radiology suite for a fluoroscopy examination at some scheduled time in the next day or two. Instead, the speech pathologist and her student trainee returned with the FEES cart within 10 minutes to perform the exam in the patient's room.

The patient's nurse and other staff members, including the senior resident and a respiratory therapist, were present for the examination. The patient was too tired to fully attend to the picture on the monitor for this initial exam, but he was engaged as much as possible. The small risks associated with the FEES examination were far outweighed by the safety of having full monitoring equipment, full emergency resuscitation equipment, and all the trained personnel at hand should he experience a respiratory or cardiac event. Finally, because of his fragile state and prolonged period without eating, barium was not the preferred bolus to reintroduce him to PO feeding.

A small amount of lidocaine was rubbed in one of the patient's nostrils to make the passage of the endoscope more comfortable. The patient was seated at about 45 degrees for the examination. This initially caused him some subjective stress but he accommodated to the change within a few minutes. In the past week, the patient had been confused and in this altered state, he had pulled out the nasogastric (NG) tube several times. His physician had dealt with this by attaching a bridle to a small-bore nasogastric tube. This catheter was fed in one nostril, looped around the nasal septum posteriorly, and came out the other nostril. Because the NG tube was attached in several places to the bridle, it prevented the patient from pulling on the NG tube. In spite of tubing in each nostril, the endoscope was passed through the nostril easily, alongside the tubing.

Upon passing the endoscope past the nasopharynx and into the hypopharynx, the larynx was viewed and was noted to be edematous, especially in the region of the arytenoids. The effects of the intubation were obviously still in effect. Excess secretions were visible throughout the hypopharynx and in the laryngeal introitus. The patient was not bothered by the presence of the endoscope and did not react by swallowing spontaneously, indicating a depressed sensory state. He was instructed to swallow spontaneously, but he could not achieve this, stating that his mouth was dry. To facilitate swallowing, green-tinged ice chips were given to him on a spoon (half a teaspoon). He was instructed to chew the ice chips, move them about with his tongue, and then to "swallow them all at once." The first bolus was not swallowed in a coordinated fashion, but instead leaked a little at a time over the base of the tongue and down the lateral channels, descending to the pyriform sinuses before the swallow was initiated. A second bolus was given and a similar pattern was noted, with a little of this bolus spilling between the arytenoids into the laryngeal vestibule where it was aspirated during the swallow, as evidenced by coughing and expectoration after the swallow. A small amount of water and secretions remained in the pyriforms after these two swallows. On the third, fourth, and fifth bolus deliveries, swallowing appeared to improve; there was less spillage and no evidence of aspiration. By this time, all of the secretions had been swallowed along with the ice chips, suggesting that bolus clearance was fairly effective. The patient then appeared fatigued and the examination was terminated. His bed was lowered, and the Passy-Muir valve was removed to allow him to rest completely.

The impression from this examination was that a dysphagia was present, and appeared to be moderately severe at this point in his recovery. Laryngeal edema was present from the previous intubation and sensation was reduced. The initiation of the swallow was delayed, as evidenced by the spillage of bolus deep into the pharynx before white-out. The swallow appeared to be slightly weak, but this could not be assessed adequately with ice chips because they do not leave much residue. Epiglottal retroflexion, a sign of hyolaryngeal elevation, was difficult to assess because the endoscope was displaced to one side by the tubing in the nose.

The underlying causes of the dysphagia in this patient were structural (edema, tracheotomy tube), reduced pharyngeal–laryngeal sensation (secondary to edema and diverted airflow through the trachea over the past few weeks), delayed initiation of the swallow, and perhaps inadequate bolus propulsion secondary to general weakness and disuse atrophy. Prognosis was considered to be good to excellent for recovery of swallowing, because all of the underlying causes were viewed as temporary. The patient was not swallowing spontaneously, but ice chips facilitated swallowing. The swallows were effective in moving the secretions into the esophagus and reduced the amount that was aspirated.

Recommendations were made to the nursing staff to give the patient ice chips whenever he was seated at 45 degrees and awake, to stimulate swallowing. A reevaluation would be completed in a few days, depending on his medical condition and apparent readiness to tolerate other liquids and food. No behavioral recommendations were made at this point, since the patient was too ill to try any exercises or maneuvers and none was necessary with ice chips.

When the repeat FEES examination was completed a few days later, no excess secretions were observed upon entry. The amount of edema had subsided considerably and the patient was observed to swallow spontaneously when the endoscope was passed. Ice chips were swallowed safely and so puree food and liquids were given. The swallow initiation was still delayed, causing some risk of aspiration with thin liquids. Puree food left a moderate amount of residue, but the patient sensed the residue and swallowed spontaneously to clear. Obviously, swallowing function was returning to normal. After this examination, the recommendation was made that the patient begin PO intake with puree food as snacks only, including precautions for him to be fed slowly and to deliver small bolus amounts. No thin liquids were allowed at this time, since they were at risk for being aspirated. However, the patient was allowed ice chips when he was not taking anything else by mouth. Medications were still to be given via the NG tube or could be crushed in applesauce, but they were not to be given with water.

A third FEES examination was completed a week later when the patient was noticeably stronger and had been moved out of the ICU to a general surgical ward. This examination revealed a generally stronger swallow and improved function. The patient was advanced from PO snacks to a PO diet of mechanical soft foods and thickened liquids, and the NG tube was removed. Within a few days, thin liquids were allowed, beginning with sips of water between meals and quickly advancing to thin liquids with meals. As the patient requested it, he was advanced to a regular diet and discharged from the speech–language pathologist's care.

Summary

In the institution where I work, FEES is used regularly with intensive care, acute care, rehabilitation, and outpatients. Other clinicians have reported the effective use of FEES with nursing home patients (Spiegel et al., 1998). I find that endoscopy is a superb tool for assessing dysphagia and for guiding treatment and I would feel handicapped and less competent without it. It provides the necessary information to diagnose dysphagia and it guides the course of treatment. In managing patients, FEES helps to achieve meaningful goals of improved eating function, good health, and better quality of life by enabling the evaluation and reevaluation of swallowing function in a safe and familiar environment and in an efficient manner, as soon as clinical indications are present.

References

American Speech-Language-Hearing Association. (1992, March). Instrumental Diagnostic Procedures for Swallowing. *Asha, 34*(Suppl. 7), 25–33.

American Speech-Language-Hearing Association, Special Interest Division—Swallowing and Swallowing Disorders (Dysphagia) (1997, June). *Competency and training guidelines for performing endoscopic swallowing evaluations.* Draft of document.

Aviv, J. E., Martin, J. H., Diamond, B., Sacco, R. L., Keen, M. S., Zagar, D., & Blitzer, A. (1996). Supraglottic and pharyngeal sensory abnormalities in stroke patients with dysphagia. *Annals of Otology, Rhinology and Laryngology, 105*(2), 92–97.

Aviv, J. E., Sacco, R. L., Thomson, J., Tandon, R., Diamond, B., Martin, J. H., & Close, L. (1997). Silent laryngopharyngeal sensory deficits after stroke. *Annals of Otology, Rhinology and Laryngology, 106,* 87–93.

Bortolotti, M. (1989). Laryngospasm and reflex central apnea caused by aspiration of refluxed gastric content in adults. *Gut, 30,* 233–238.

Crary, M. A., & Baron, J. (1997). Endoscopic and fluoroscopic evaluations of swallowing: Comparison of observed and inferred findings. *Dysphagia, 12*(2), 108.

Dejaeger, E., Pelemans, W., Ponette, E., & Joosten, E. (1997). Mechanisms involved in postdeglutition retention in the elderly. *Dysphagia, 12,* 63–67.

Finegold, S. M. (1991). Aspiration pneumonia. *Review of Infectious Diseases, 1*(Suppl. 9), 737–742.

Ikari, T., & Sasaki, C. T. (1980). Glottic closure reflex: Control mechanism. *Annals of Otology, Rhinology, and Laryngology, 89,* 220–224.

Langmore, S. E. (in press). Endoscopic evaluation and treatment of swallowing disorders. New York: Thieme.

Langmore, S. E., & McCulloch, T. M. (1997). Examination of the pharynx and larynx and endoscopic examination of pharyngeal swallowing. In A. Schulze-Delrieu (Eds.), *Deglutition and its disorders* (pp. 201–226). San Diego: Singular Press.

Langmore, S. E., Pelletier, C., & Nelson, R. (1995, October). To FEES or not to FEES? Panel discussion presented at the annual meeting of the Dysphagia Research Society, McClean, VA.

Langmore, S., Schatz, K., & Olson, N. (1988). Fiberoptic endoscopic evaluation of swallowing safety: A new procedure. *Dysphagia, 2,* 216–219.

Langmore, S., Schatz, K., & Olson, N. (1991). Endoscopic and videofluoroscopic evaluations of swallowing and aspiration. *Annals of Otology, Rhinology and Laryngology, 100,* 678–681.

Leder, S. B. (1998). Serial fiberoptic endoscopic swallowing evaluations in the management of patients with dysphagia. *Archives of Physical Medicine and Rehabilitation, 79,* 1264–1269.

Leder, S. B., Sasaki, C. T., & Burrell, M. I. (1998). Fiberoptic endoscopic evaluation of dysphagia to identify silent aspiration. *Dysphagia, 13,* 19–21.

Martin, B. J. W., Logemann, J. A., Shaker, R., & Dodds, W. J. (1993). Normal laryngeal valving patterns during three breath-holding maneuvers: A pilot investigation. *Dysphagia, 8,* 11–20.

Murray, J., Langmore, S., Ginsberg, S., & Bromberg, J. (1996). The significance of excess hypopharyngeal secretions in patients with dysphagia. *Dysphagia, 11,* 99–103.

Olsson, R., Castell, J., Johnston, B., Ekberg, O., & Castell, D. O. (1997). Combined videomanometric identification of abnormalities related to pharyngeal retention. *Academic Radiology, 4,* 349–354.

Physicians' Desk Reference (49th ed.). (1995). Montvale, NJ: Medical Economics Data Production Co.

Spiegel, J. R., Selber, J. C., & Creed, J. (1998). A functional diagnosis of dysphagia using videoendoscopy. *Ear, Nose, and Throat Journal, 77*(8), 628–632.

Tracy, J. F., Logemann, J. A., Kahrilas, P. J., Jacob, P., Kobara, M., & Krugler, C. (1989). Preliminary observations on the effects of age on oropharyngeal deglutition. *Dysphagia, 4,* 90–94.

Van Lieshout, J. J., Wieling, W., Karemaker, J. M., & Eckberg, D. L. (1991). The vasovagal response. *Clinical Science, 81,* 575–586.

Willging, J. P., Miller, C. K., Hogan, M. J., & Rudolph, C. D. (1996). Fiberoptic endoscopic evaluation of swallowing in children: A preliminary report of 100 procedures. *Dysphagia, 11*(2), 162.

Wu, C.-H., Hsiao, T.-Y., Chen, J.-C., Chang, Y.-C., & Lee, S.-Y. (1997). Evaluation of swallowing safety with fiberoptic endoscope: Comparison with videofluoroscopic technique. *Laryngoscope, 107,* 396–401.

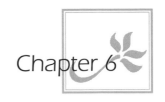

Chapter 6

Nutritional Evaluation and Laboratory Values in Dysphagia Management

Virginia Zachary and Russell H. Mills

Zachary and Mills provide a discussion of how the Laboratory Assessment Battery for Dysphagia (LAB-D) can provide insight into the patient's overall health status and the impact that the dysphagia may have. They discuss tests that reveal protein status, blood sugar, metabolic waste filtering, hydration, immune system status, infectious disease, and more.

1. *The presence of malnutrition is evidenced by tests that measure the status of protein stores. What tests can reveal the presence of malnutrition?*

2. *What test results can provide indications of the presence of dehydration or overhydration?*

3. *How would the presence of overhydration influence the interpretation of an albumin level of 3.8 g/dl?*

4. *The authors' case study highlights two patients whose videofluoroscopic swallowing study results looked very similar, but were very different when the LAB-D values were compared. Review the results in Table 6.3 and 6.4. How would the LAB-D differences between the two patients influence your management decisions?*

⁕　　⁕　　⁕

The importance of adequate nutrition to overall health has been well documented in the literature across various disciplines. Equally well documented is the fact that nutritional needs increase with illness and disease (Mahan & Arlin, 1992; Prescott,

Harley, & Klein, 1990; Zeman, 1991). Although much of the focus in dysphagia management has been on the reduction in the risk for aspiration, the maintenance of adequate nutrition must be recognized as a basic principle in the evaluation and treatment of patients with dysphagia.

This chapter is intended to acquaint the reader with the components of the nutritional evaluation process, and to introduce the elements in laboratory data that relate to nutritional status. It is crucial, however, that individuals not trained as clinical dietitians understand that no single laboratory value is indicative of nutritional status (Skipper, 1989; Weinsier, Heimburger, & Butterworth, 1989). The expertise of the registered dietitian in evaluating various elements of laboratory data in conjunction with physical characteristics and medical conditions exhibited by the patient is paramount in the accurate assessment of nutritional status.

The importance of the role of the registered dietitian as a member of the multidisciplinary team for evaluation of swallowing disorders will become increasingly clear as the complex relationship of laboratory values to disease processes is explained. Failure to involve the dietitian upon receipt of a dysphagia referral and throughout the evaluation and decision-making processes can result in inappropriate or ineffective patient management decisions.

Malnutrition

The primary function of the nutritional assessment is to identify patients who are nutritionally compromised and at risk for malnutrition, which is a strong predictor of patient morbidity and mortality. An estimated 30% to 50% of hospitalized persons are malnourished, either from undernutrition or overnutrition (obesity) (Porth, 1990). In infants and children malnutrition impedes physical growth, prevents proper mental development, and in the severest cases results in premature death. In geriatric populations, composed of those who have complex medical problems, malnutrition is especially lethal, often contributing to an irreversible downward spiral involving major organ system failure, which results in death (Sullivan & Walls, 1994). The three classifications for protein–calorie malnutrition commonly used are marasmus, kwashiorkor, and marasmic kwashiorkor.

Marasmus (or *cachexia*) is the result of a long-term calorie deficit over many months or years. It is characterized by extreme muscle wasting and loss of fat stores, and is easily recognized by the patient's starved appearance. Despite the deficiency in calorie intake and a morbid physical appearance, normal or only slightly reduced serum proteins are revealed in laboratory testing. Cautious nutritional support which avoids overly aggressive feeding can often reverse the marasmic condition (Weinsier et al., 1989).

Kwashiorkor is a consequence of a short-term protein deficit. It can develop within only a few weeks when the patient is severely stressed by illness or physical trauma. With this condition, fat and muscle stores appear normal on physical examination and there may be only a slight decrease in body weight, giving the appearance of adequate nutrition. Physical signs may include skin breakdown and decubitus ulcers, poor wound healing, edema, and easy hair pluckability. In kwashiorkor, laboratory tests indicate depleted protein stores and depressed immune function, and these findings necessitate immediate nutritional intervention to reverse the situation and replace the body protein stores. Kwashiorkor compromises the patient's ability to recover from acute or chronic disease, and delays or prevents healing from surgery or infection (Weinsier et al., 1989).

Marasmic kwashiorkor is a combination of protein and calorie malnutrition that results from a chronically undernourished individual (marasmus) who undergoes a period of acute stress such as surgery, illness, or chronic disease. This superimposes kwashiorkor onto chronic starvation, resulting in severely depleted fat and muscle stores, extremely low serum protein levels, and seriously compromised immune function. With a greater than average risk for infection and poor wound healing, the prognosis is very poor for these patients (Weinsier et al., 1989; Zeman, 1991).

The normal aging process can contribute to malnutrition in older adults, producing changes in taste perception and appetite that may jeopardize nutrient intake. Additionally, complications of illness and disease compound any physical limitations already present, and can result in a severely compromised nutritional status. Reduced calorie and protein intake can compromise body muscle mass, whereas vitamin and mineral deficiencies resulting from inadequate food intake can decrease the effectiveness of medical treatment and delay healing.

Depression often develops in these patients who experience increased physical deterioration, altering their previously independent lifestyle. In the case of any patient, dysphagic or not, it is extremely critical that any degree of malnutrition be addressed, with intervention and compensatory measures designed to provide for correction of nutritional deficiencies (Dwyer, Gallo, & Reichel, 1993; Powers & Folk, 1992; Sullivan & Walls, 1994).

Fluid Status

Water is a vital component of the human body. It maintains body temperature, carries waste products and nutrients in solution, is a major component of the liquid portion of blood, functions as a lubricant, and maintains cell integrity. Sixty percent of the average adult male's body weight is water, compared with 50% in the average adult female (Zeman, 1991). Muscle tissue is 80% water by weight, whereas fat, or adipose tissue, is only 20% water by weight (Skipper, 1989). With increased fat stores and decreased muscle stores, total body water is reduced. Thus, the obese person contains proportionately less water than a person of normal weight. Total body water also decreases with age. The newborn human body is 70% to 75% water, and this percentage decreases throughout life. Even with the maintenance of a consistent adult body weight, the average individual loses about 1 kilogram (kg) of body water per decade of life (Zeman, 1991).

Fluid and electrolyte balance is maintained by homeostatic regulation from the interaction of several systems in the body. The brain, the kidneys, the gastrointestinal tract, and the pituitary gland are collectively involved in balancing water intake with water output. Sodium and potassium are the primary electrolytes involved in maintaining fluid balance. Their concentration in various body compartments determines the movement of water between the compartments. An imbalance of either water or electrolytes results in dehydration (inadequate water) or edema (excessive water).

Dehydration is the state of an inadequate fluid level to maintain the body's fluid balance, and can result from either decreased water intake, excessive water loss, or a heavy solute load (increased serum sodium or other electrolyte) (Mahan & Arlin, 1992; Skipper, 1989). In healthy individuals, temporary dehydration that occurs in response to reduced fluid intake is easily corrected with adequate fluid consumption. However, a physical disorder involving one or more of the fluid-regulating systems mentioned previously, or trauma such as burns, surgery, or respiratory distress will greatly increase fluid replacement needs. Conditions such as diarrhea, vomiting, and fever, which produce excessive body water losses, will increase the need for providing adequate fluid to prevent dehydration.

In the patient with dysphagia, dehydration is often a direct consequence of the impaired swallowing mechanism. In an effort to prevent the coughing or choking that can occur with fluid consumption, the patient or the caregiver may inadvertently cause dehydration by avoiding fluids. A decreased thirst sensation in older adults, which is a normal part of the aging process, often prevents an adequate fluid intake and can contribute to dehydration.

The physical examination may reveal evidence of dehydration. Poor skin turgor, an increased pulse rate, abnormal blood pressure, and lethargy may be signs of inadequate fluid. In the absence of kidney disease, decreased urine output usually indicates dehydration. A rapid weight increase (within a few days) is generally a sign of fluid retention, and a sudden drop in body weight reflects a loss of body water through diuresis (excessive urine production and elimination).

In addition to physical signs of dehydration, several laboratory tests are fairly accurate indicators of fluid status. An elevated blood urea nitrogen (BUN), an elevated BUN-to-creatinine ratio, and an increased serum sodium (Na) level (hypernatremia) usually are present in dehydration (Weinsier et al., 1989). These are discussed in greater detail in the laboratory data section later in the chapter. Serum osmolality, a laboratory test that is calculated from serum sodium, blood glucose, and BUN, gives an estimation of hydration status. Serum osmolality is increased in dehydration and decreased in overhydration or volume overload (Fischbach, 1992).

Fluid status is an important component of the nutritional assessment, and becomes even more critical in the evaluation of the patient who, because of impaired swallowing ability, may also be at increased risk for dehydration. Therefore, it is imperative that the management plan for the patient with dysphagia include the provision of adequate fluid intake.

Assessment of Nutritional Status

Nutritional assessment is the evaluation of nutritional status by determining adequacy of nutrient intake. It combines the findings of actual nutrient intake, the elements of physical and mental status, and the controlling environmental factors that determine the type and quality of an individual's diet. The essential components of nutritional evaluation, also known as the ABCDs of nutritional assessment (Dwyer et al.,1993), are as follows:

A—Anthropometric measurements
B —Biochemical data
C—Clinical evaluation
D—Diet history

Anthropometric Measurements

Anthropometric measurements include the patient's height, current weight, and weight history, noting any recent weight changes. They can include triceps skinfold measurement or arm muscle circumference, if available. Height and weight measurements are used to evaluate the appropriateness of current body weight. These measurements are compared to charts (based on life insurance mortality statistics) of "ideal body weight" for adults (Mahan & Arlin, 1992). Infants' and children's height and weight measurements are compared to growth charts which help to determine normal growth patterns (Zeman, 1991). While not infallible, these methods usually reflect a reasonably accurate picture of past nutritional intake.

Biochemical Data

The clinical dietitian employs laboratory findings of many blood components in evaluating nutritional status. Although many laboratory tests can point to a possible nutritional deficit, no single value can be used to determine nutritional status. It must further be emphasized that none of the tests can be used alone to diagnosis any disease or condition. A physician uses laboratory results, findings from the physical examination, information obtained from the patient or family members, and the best clinical judgment to reach a diagnosis. Similarly, the clinical dietitian uses all the components of the nutritional assessment, including the results of laboratory tests, to arrive at a determination of nutritional status. This again attests to the importance of the dietitian as an active member of the dysphagia management team.

The dietitian uses the biochemical indicators of protein status, anemia, and immune function to assist in the determination of nutritional status. When combined with anthropometric measurements, the clinical evaluation, and the diet history, these are generally the most useful values for assigning a nutritional classification. Indicators of protein status most commonly used are tests for albumin, transferrin, and prealbumin. Although the great limiting factor of these values is that all can be influenced by hydration status, dietitians commonly use them in nutritional assessment because they provide valuable insights into the level of protein stores in the body.

Anemia usually indicates compromised nutritional status since it is always a secondary consequence of another abnormal condition or disease. Anemia is often manifested in individuals with chronic diseases such as cancer or renal or liver abnormalities. The blood tests most commonly used to detect the presence of anemia are hemoglobin, hematocrit, and red blood cell count. Additional laboratory studies are required to differentiate between types of anemia. Excessive blood loss, diseases that cause erythrocyte abnormalities, or nutritional deficiency combined with disease can result in anemia. The term *nutritional anemia* is often used to describe deficiencies of iron, vitamin B12, and folic acid. This is because the nutrients found to be deficient can correct the anemia when given in adequate amounts. The proportion of erythrocytes (red blood cells) and leukocytes (white blood cells) usually remains constant at a ratio of 500 to 1. In anemia, the erythrocytes are decreased either in size or number.

The immune system is usually an efficient mechanism to protect the human body from invasion by foreign organisms. However, malnourished individuals become susceptible to infection due to an impaired immune response. Total lymphocyte count is often used as an indicator of immune system function. This measurement is calculated from the leukocyte concentration and the lymphocytes present in the blood. The white blood count in thousands multiplied by the lymph percentage gives the total lymphocyte count (TLC). A TLC of greater than 1,500 indicates adequate immune function, whereas values of less than 1,500 indicate compromised immune defenses.

Clinical Evaluation

A clinical evaluation performed by a physician or other health care provider incorporates the patient's age, medical history including a complete medication profile, and physical examination. Functional status indicators such as ability to chew and self-feed are important to the nutritional evaluation process. For this component, the thoroughness of the physician's examination is extremely critical. Any missing piece of relevant information could compromise treatment planning for the patient's care.

Diet History

The diet history is obtained by the dietitian from an interview with the patient or a caregiver, or from documented records of health care providers, and includes current and past food intake patterns. The completeness of this component is also very crucial in the determination of nutritional status. Information on socioeconomic factors, such as living arrangements, transportation, and financial resources available to obtain or prepare meals, should also be determined. A case manager or social worker may need to be consulted if resources are insufficient to provide adequate nutrition.

Any circumstance that increases nutrient requirements or impairs the ability to receive, absorb, or retain nourishment will compromise nutritional status. Acute and chronic disease, physical limitations, mental alterations, and socioeconomic conditions may all impact the level of nutritional intake. Nutrient requirements are increased with fever, infection, and surgery, and with chronic diseases such as Parkinson's and pulmonary disease. Conditions that reduce intake may include mental impairment, physical limitations, and lack of financial resources to obtain food. Inadequate absorption can result from food–drug interactions or disorders that limit nutrient uptake in the intestinal tract. Diarrhea, vomiting, or metabolic disorders such as liver or kidney disease can cause increased nutrient losses. Table 6.1 lists these and many other conditions that increase nutritional risk.

Table 6.1
Factors Affecting Nutritional Status

Inadequate Intake	Increased Losses
Alcoholism	Alcoholism
Dementia	Blood loss
Drug addiction	Diarrhea
Anorexia	Recurrent vomiting
Poor dentition/edentulous/ill-fitting dentures	Metabolism disorders: hepatic, renal, endocrine
Socioeconomic factors: poverty, isolation	**Increased Requirements**
Loss of taste or smell	Fever
Limited food choices	Infection
Psychiatric diagnoses	Surgery
Depression	Trauma
Stroke with hemiparesis	Pulmonary disease
Inadequate Absorption	Pressure ulcers
Drugs such as antacids, laxatives, anticonvulsants	Parkinson's disease
Gastrointestinal disorders or surgery	Involuntary muscle movement such as tardive dyskinesia
Pancreatic disease	
Pernicious anemia	

Blood Chemistry Tests

Blood is the carrier of all nutrients, oxygen, hormones, electrolytes, and cellular waste products. It is a dynamic reservoir on which every system of the body is dependent for life. In the average individual, 13% of the body's weight is blood volume. Of the approximately 5 liters of blood in the average adult, approximately 3 liters (55%) are plasma and 2 liters (45%) are the solid cellular portion (Hole, 1989; Zeman, 1991). Plasma is the liquid portion of blood and is a complex mixture of approximately 92% water, amino acids, proteins, carbohydrates, lipids, vitamins, hormones, electrolytes, and cellular wastes from various organs and the intestines. Blood cells are solids derived from bone marrow and are suspended in the clear, straw-colored plasma (Hole, 1989).

Blood serves the body by completing numerous vital functions. It transports oxygen to the tissues and removes carbon dioxide. Blood absorbs nutrients from the gastrointestinal tract and transports waste products to the kidneys and liver. It distributes phagocytes and antibodies necessary to fight infections. To stop bleeding, it transports clotting agents. The blood delivers hormones, vital for a variety of functions. Finally, circulating blood provides cooling for the body core.

Blood cells are classified as red cells, white cells, and platelets. Red blood cells, or erythrocytes, are produced in the bone marrow and their primary function is to transport oxygen. Red blood cell disorders are classified as anemias (decreased numbers of circulating red cells) and polycythemias (increased numbers of circulating red cells). White blood cells, or leukocytes, are further subdivided into granulocytes, lymphocytes, and monocytes. Abnormalities involving leukocytes are either leukocytosis (increased number of cells) or leukopenia (decreased number of cells). An increased number of platelets is termed thrombocytosis, and a decreased platelet count is termed thrombocytopenia.

Blood chemistry tests are accepted methods of evaluating blood abnormalities. A blood sample can be compared with established reference levels to evaluate markers of body metabolism; storage levels of vitamins, minerals, and protein; and the function of various organs and systems. Chemistry tests are available to measure blood sugar, lipids, protein, hormones, enzymes, electrolytes, vitamins and minerals, and drug levels.

Understanding Laboratory Data

In preparation for a discussion of individual laboratory tests, two points must be made. First, normal reference ranges given for each laboratory test may vary slightly from laboratory to laboratory. For absolute comparisons, the values to be compared must come from the same laboratory. Although comparisons across laboratories are possible, the reader should be aware that slight differences may exist. Second, the laboratory tests contained in this chapter are not intended to be a comprehensive listing of those available. The tests included here are only those most readily available and useful to the dietitian for consideration in nutritional assessment.

Complete Blood Count

The basic screening test for blood components, the complete blood count (CBC), gives important information regarding a patient's health and nutritional status. The CBC contains many values, not all of which are relevant to the analyses conducted by the clinical dietitian. Therefore, not all are discussed in this chapter. The following are the pertinent tests included in the CBC.

White Blood Cell Count (WBC). The WBC (reference range = 4.8–10.8 K/cmm) is the total count of leukocytes in a volume of blood. Generally an elevated white blood count indicates the presence of infection. Decreased levels (leukopenia) are associated with bone marrow disorders secondary to drug therapy, cancers, and congenital abnormalities.

White Cell Differential (Diff). In understanding the Diff test, it is important to note that all leukocytes are not the same. As an analogy, it is useful to think of the WBC as the number of marbles in a bag. Although it may be useful to know the number of marbles, it is quite another thing to look into the bag to find that the marbles are of several different colors. So it is with leukocytes. There are several different types and the function of each is different. In conditions of health, each can be predicted to constitute a fixed percentage of the total leukocytes. When they vary from their expected percentages, it tells the clinician something about the cause of the leukocytosis or leukopenia. Leukocyte types and expected percentages are listed here.

   Lymphocytes. Lymphocytes (reference range = 20.5%–51.1% of WBC) are responsible for antibody protection, immunologic memory, and cell-mediated immunity. Two types are T-lymphocytes, which are responsible for cell-mediated immunity, and B-lymphocytes, which provide antibody protection.

   Monocytes. Monocytes (reference range = 1.7%–9.3% of the WBC) phagocytize bacteria, viruses, antibody–antigen complexes, inorganic substances, and erythrocytes. Monocytosis is seen in chronic inflammatory disorders.

Granulocytes. Granulocytes (reference range = 42.2%–75.2% of the WBC) are also termed neutrophils by some laboratories. In their immature form they are called band cells. These cells function to phagocytize invading bacteria. When an infection is detected, the bone marrow is stimulated to produce granulocytes which are then transported via the blood to fight the infection.

Eosinophils. Eosinophils (reference range = 0.5%–4.0% of the WBC) phagocytize antigen–antibody complexes and foreign particles. Elevated levels are often found in patients with allergic diseases.

Basophils. (reference range = 0.0%–1.5% of the WBC) These cells respond to hypersensitivity reactions such as anaphylaxis and bronchial asthma.

Red Blood Cell Count (RBC). The RBC (reference range = 4.7–6.1 M/cmm) indicates the number of erythrocytes in blood. Decreased RBC values can indicate anemia, Hodgkin's disease, leukemia, multiple myeloma, or Addison's disease. Increased values are associated with conditions such as dehydration, severe diarrhea, and pulmonary fibroses.

Mean Corpuscular Volume (MCV). The MCV (reference range = 80–94 cu microns) is the calculated ratio of the volume of packed red blood cells to the total number of red blood cells. It is used in the differential classification of anemias.

Mean Corpuscular Hemoglobin (MCH). The MCH (reference range = 26–31 picograms) is the ratio of the hemoglobin level to the number of erythrocytes in a blood sample. It can also be used to differentiate between various types of anemia.

Mean Corpuscular Hemoglobin Concentration (MCHC). The MCHC (reference range = 33–37g g/dl RBC) measures the average concentration of hemoglobin in grams per 100 ml of packed red blood cells and is a reliable indicator of anemia. It is the ratio of the amount of hemoglobin to hematocrit.

Hematocrit (HCT). Also called packed cell volume (PCV), hematocrit (reference range = 42%–52%) is the measure of the volume of cells found in 100 ml of blood centrifuged and separated from plasma. It is expressed as a percentage of the total blood volume. Decreased values indicate anemia. Increased values are seen in severe dehydration and shock.

Hemoglobin (Hgb). Hemoglobin (reference range = 14–18 g/dl) is the measure of the total number of red blood cells (erythrocytes) found in a cubic millimeter of blood. Hemoglobin's main function is oxygen transport. Decreased levels are found in anemia, liver cirrhosis, severe hemorrhage, Hodgkin's disease, and leukemia. Increased levels are found in chronic obstructive pulmonary disease and congestive heart failure.

Platelet Count. The platelet count (reference range = 130–400 K/cmm) is most useful in evaluating abnormal bleeding in liver disease and with anticoagulant therapy. The platelet count is also used to monitor disease processes involving bone marrow, as in leukemia. Increased levels occur in cancer, heart disease, cirrhosis, chronic pancreatitis, and rheumatoid arthritis. Decreased levels are seen with pneumonia and other acute infections, cancer chemotherapy, and HIV infection.

Sequential Machine Analysis

The Sequential Multiple Analyzer (SMA) by Technicon is one of the auto analyzers used in laboratories to perform a wide variety of tests on a single blood sample. This system allows the medical professional to quickly screen patients for several different blood components. Although numerous tests are available, the dysphagia management team of the Alvin C. York Veterans Affairs Medical Center in Murfreesboro, Tennessee, where we work, uses a combination of tests it has labeled the Laboratory Assessment Battery for Dysphagia or the LAB-D. The LAB-D combines those values from the complete blood count (CBC) and the SMA that are most needed by the clinical dietitian to make analyses and dietary recommendations. The SMA test form that is used reports the values of 12 laboratory tests; therefore, the test is called SMA–12. Additional tests are requested for selected patients depending upon information that is gleaned from the medical history, patient interview, dysphagia history, and meal observation. When the LAB-D information is combined with the results from the clinical dysphagia examination and the videofluoroscopic swallowing study (VFSS), the patient benefits from recommendations that are based not only on swallowing behavior but also on indicators of his or her nutritional status. The blood chemistry tests provided by the SMA–12 can be grouped into tests for blood sugar level, metabolic waste filtering, protein stores, electrolytes, lipoprotein status, and enzyme tests. Additional tests that have been found to be useful as supplements to the SMA-12 must be ordered separately; they are denoted by "S" following their names in the descriptions below.

Glucose (Fasting Blood Sugar). The glucose test (reference range = 75–110 mg/dl) measures blood sugar level and is commonly used to screen for and diagnose diabetes, characterized by a fasting glucose level of > 110 mg/dl, a condition called *hyperglycemia*. It is also used as a monitor in diabetes management. Other possible causes of hyperglycemia include Cushing's disease, acute stress (e.g., myocardial infarction or severe infections), pancreatitis, chronic liver disease, chronic malnutrition, or prolonged physical inactivity. Decreased blood sugar levels (*hypoglycemia*) occur most often from an overdose of insulin or inadequate energy (food) intake. When hypoglycemia occurs in Addison's disease, it is accompanied by elevated potassium, decreased sodium, and elevated blood urea nitrogen.

Tests for Metabolic Waste Filtering. The tests in this section are used to evaluate the body's ability to filter waste from the system. They are measures of kidney and liver function.

Blood Urea Nitrogen (BUN). The BUN test (reference range = 9–21 mg/dl) is used as an indicator of urea production in the liver and its excretion by the kidneys. Impaired kidney function prevents adequate clearance of the waste products of protein metabolism, and BUN rises in direct proportion to decreased glomerular function. Increased levels are also associated with shock, dehydration, gastrointestinal hemorrhage, infection, chronic gout, and diabetes. Decreased levels are associated with liver failure, impaired absorption as in celiac disease, and overhydration (excessive intravenous fluids).

Creatinine. A by-product of muscle breakdown, creatinine (reference range = 0.8–1.5 mg/dl) is normally produced at a constant rate. Impaired kidney function will reduce excretion of creatinine, resulting in increased blood levels. Increased levels will also be seen with chronic nephritis, urinary tract obstruction, muscle disease, diabetic acidosis, and starvation. Decreased levels are rare.

Total Bilirubin. Bilirubin (reference range = 0.2–1.3 mg/dl in adults; 1.5 to 12.0 mg/dl in newborns) is a by-product of the hemolysis, or breakdown, of red blood cells and the release of hemoglobin, which is excreted into the bile by the liver. Excessive breakdown of red blood cells or an inability of the liver to excrete usual amounts causes a rise in serum levels. Measurement of bilirubin is important in evaluating liver function, hemolytic anemias, and hyperbilirubinemia in newborns.

Uric acid. One of the end-products of protein metabolism, uric acid (reference range: 3.5–8.5 mg/dl for men; 2.6–6.0 mg/dl for women) is excreted through the kidneys as urine and in the feces. High levels are common in gout and in kidney failure. Increased levels are also seen in leukemia, metastatic cancer, and starvation. Decreased levels are uncommon but are associated with Wilson's disease and neoplastic disease.

Tests for the Status of Protein Stores. Tests that measure the level of protein stores in the body give critical information regarding the patient's long-term intake of essential nutrients. A chronically inadequate consumption of calories and protein forces the body to obtain components for tissue maintenance and repair from its own muscle protein. This depletes the body's muscle mass and places further stress on the compromised nutritional status. Continued depletion results in the types of malnutrition mentioned at the beginning of the chapter. Thus, it is imperative that protein stores be assessed as part of the nutritional evaluation to determine the degree of depletion present, if any.

Albumin. Albumin (reference range = 3.9–5.0 g/dl) is a plasma protein that is normally maintained at constant levels in the blood. Approximately 60% of total protein is albumin, and the rest is globulin. With a half-life of 18 to 21 days, this value is most useful in evaluating long-term nutritional status. It is an indicator of visceral protein stores (the protein stored in the internal organs). With continued inadequate intake of calories and protein, albumin levels decrease, indicating compromised nutrition status due to the deficiency of stored protein. Albumin is also helpful in maintaining normal distribution of water, and so can be directly affected by any condition resulting in dehydration, such as vomiting or diarrhea, resulting in falsely elevated levels. Overhydration such as with excessive administration of intravenous fluids will result in decreased levels. In either case actual nutritional status can also be decreased with severe liver diseases, diarrhea, malabsorption, and third-degree burns.

Globulins. Globulin (reference range = 2.5–3.5 g/dl) is a key building block of antibodies, and so plays an important role in immune function. It also functions in the maintenance of osmotic pressure of the blood. The globulin level is significant in its ratio with albumin as an indicator of total protein stores. The proportion of albumin to globulin is normally in a ratio value greater than 1. As mentioned previously, prealbumin and transferrin are two additional tests for assessing blood protein levels. Because of their shorter half-lives, these are more sensitive indicators of short-term protein deficits.

Prealbumin (S). Prealbumin (reference range = 19–43 mg/dl) is a short-turnover protein synthesized in the liver. A half-life of 1 to 2 days makes prealbumin more useful than albumin in measuring recent changes in protein stores. Like albumin, prealbumin is sensitive to fluid changes, but can be used to monitor the progress of nutritional intervention or to detect early protein deficiency.

Transferrin (S). Transferrin (reference range = 240–480 mg/dl) is a protein with a half-life of 8 to 10 days. It binds to iron and regulates its transport and absorption in the body. This characteristic, known as total iron-binding capacity, can be used to determine the status of iron stores and assist in detecting the presence of anemias. Transferrin will be increased in patients having inadequate dietary iron intake, iron-deficiency anemia due to blood loss, and acute hepatitis, and in women taking oral contraceptives. Decreased levels are seen in malnutrition, hepatic disease, cancer, chronic infection, pernicious anemia, and sickle cell anemia.

Tests for Electrolyte Levels. Electrolytes are elements or compounds that dissociate into ions and are able to conduct electricity when dissolved in water or melted. The human body requires consistent levels of the principal electrolytes, and balance among them must be maintained for normal metabolism and proper function of all body systems. Tests that measure electrolyte levels are critical indicators of acid–base balance. Abnormal levels demand swift and appropriate intervention to prevent serious damage to the body.

Sodium. The most abundant cation, sodium (reference range = 135–145 mmol/L), makes up 90% of the electrolyte fluid. The kidneys and the central nervous system control sodium concentration. The primary functions are to maintain osmotic pressure, acid–base balance, and nerve transmission. The sodium value can be useful in identifying recent water and sodium balance changes. Decreased levels (hyponatremia) usually indicate an excess of body fluid rather than low total body sodium. Reduced levels are also associated with severe burns, severe diarrhea, vomiting, severe nephritis, diabetic acidosis, and edema. Increased levels (hypernatremia) are uncommon, but are associated with dehydration and insufficient water intake, coma, and Cushing's disease.

Potassium. Most potassium (reference range = 3.6–5.0 mmol/L) is concentrated within cells, and the body normally maintains a constant level by excreting excesses in urine, sweat, and stool. Both potassium and sodium ions are important in renal regulation of acid–base balance, but potassium is of primary importance because it is the main intracellular inorganic buffer. Either low levels (hypokalemia) or high levels (hyperkalemia) of potassium may be potentially lethal. Hypokalemia is most frequently caused by gastrointestinal loss, but can also occur with malabsorption, starvation, or liver disease with ascites. Any excessive loss of body water, such as severe vomiting, diarrhea, or diuretic administration will cause a decreased potassium level. Increased levels (hyperkalemia) are most frequently seen in renal failure, acidosis, and Addison's disease.

Chloride. An anion found primarily in combination as sodium chloride or hydrochloric acid, chloride (reference range = 101–111 mmol/L) is helpful in diagnosing disorders of acid–base and water balance. Decreased chloride levels occur in fever, severe vomiting or diarrhea, acute infections such as pneumonia, and diabetic acidosis. Increased levels are seen in dehydration, Cushing's syndrome, and some kidney disorders.

Calcium. Stored mostly in skeletal bones and in teeth, calcium (reference range = 8.4–10.2 mg/dl) is released into the blood by the action of parathyroid hormone on bone in order to maintain stable blood levels. Half of blood calcium is ionized, the rest is protein bound. Only the ionized calcium is used in muscular contraction, cardiac functions, nerve transmission, and blood clotting. Increased levels of total calcium (hypercalcemia) are associated with many disorders, but its greatest clinical importance is as an indicator in cancer, metastatic disease involving bone, Hodgkin's disease, and leukemia. Decreased levels are most commonly caused by hyperproteinemia, indicating reduced albumin. Excessive intravenous fluid administration decreases albumin levels, and will decrease calcium accordingly.

Tests for Lipoprotein Levels. Lipids are fatty substances that exist as cholesterol, triglycerides, fatty acids, and phospholipids in the body. Lipoproteins are large molecular complexes of lipid and protein that transport lipids that would otherwise be insoluble. The measurement of lipoprotein blood components provides important information in the detection of lipid metabolism disorders. These values are also used to evaluate the degree of risk for coronary artery disease.

Cholesterol. Cholesterol (reference range = 140–200 mg/dl) is used as a component in the production of hormones and bile acids, and as a structural component in most cell membrane. It is well established by the medical community that elevated levels of cholesterol are associated with a higher risk for atherosclerosis and coronary heart disease. The primary purpose of the test is to identify those at risk. A very low cholesterol level is associated with long-term inadequate calorie and protein intake.

Triglycerides. The triglyceride level (reference range = 40–199 mg/dl) is a measure of the body's efficiency in metabolizing fat. When elevated levels are seen along with elevated levels of cholesterol, the individual is at greater risk for atherosclerotic disease. An increase is also associated with heavier than normal eating immediately prior to the test, alcohol ingestion, or a high intake of concentrated sweets.

Tests for Enzyme Levels. Enzymes are proteins produced by living cells and act as catalysts for chemical reactions in organic matter. Enzymes that aid in the digestive process are produced in large quantities, whereas enzymes that act within the cell are produced in very small quantities. In many disease processes, certain enzyme levels can help to identify the source and severity of the abnormality.

Inorganic Phosphorus/Phosphate (S). Of the body's total phosphorus (reference range = 2.7–4.5 mg/dl in adults; 4.5–5.5 mg/dl in children), approximately 85% is found in the bone combined with calcium, and the remaining phosphorus is found in the cells. In blood, phosphorus is in the form of phosphate, and is always evaluated in relation to calcium. With an inverse relationship between phosphate and calcium, abnormally high levels of one causes the kidneys to excrete the other. Phosphate is needed for glucose and lipid metabolism, bone production, energy transfer, and acid–base balance. Because phosphate levels are regulated by the kidneys, any renal abnormality will cause elevated phosphate levels. Decreased levels are seen with hyperparathyroidism, rickets (in children) or osteomalacia (in adults), diabetic coma, or intravenous glucose administration in a nondiabetic patient.

Alkaline Phosphatase (S). Alkaline phosphatase (reference range = 20–70 U/L in adults; 20–150 U/L in children) is found mainly in bone and the liver, and is used in correlation with other findings as an indicator of liver and bone disease. Blood levels rise when excretion is obstructed in liver disease and when osteoblastic activity results in increased cell production in bone disease. Increased levels are seen with liver conditions such as obstructive jaundice, cancer, cirrhosis, liver metastasis, and hepatitis, and in bone diseases such as Paget's disease, osteomalacia, rickets, infectious mononucleosis, and leukemia. Decreased levels are seen in malnutrition, hypophosphatasia, hypothyroidism, and pernicious anemia.

Tests for Infectious Disease. Cultures, smears, and stains are among several laboratory tests that are used in the diagnosis of infectious diseases. A culture is a test that uses a culture medium (agar plates or broth) to grow microorganisms obtained from an infected host, which is then compared to a biological "fingerprint" of the suspected pathogen. The biochemical characteristics of a given pathogen conform to a predictable profile, including microscopic appearance, shape, size, texture, and color, when subjected to various stains. A smear is a specimen prepared on a glass slide for microscopic examination. Material to be studied is fixed to the slide either by heat from the flame of a Bunsen burner, or a fixative such as methanol. Stains are useful in differentiating characteristics of various organisms. The staining agents are salts, which contain a positive and a negative ion, with one being the coloring agent. Basic dyes have a positively charged group, and acid dyes possess a negatively charged group. The specimen picks up the colorant and becomes visible under the light microscope. The positive stain colors the specimen, and the negative stain colors the background and leaves the specimen uncolored. There are two primary types of bacterial stains: simple and differential. The simple stain uses only one of the dyes, such as methylene blue, gentian violet, carbol-fuchsin, or safranine. The culture or smear is stained, and the results are compared with the profile for the pathogen.

Differential staining employs the use of two different types of stain applied to the same smear. Developed by the Danish physician Christian Gram, the Gram stain is the most well-known differential staining method, and divides bacteria into gram-positive and gram-negative groups. The first step in preparing a differential stain is to apply the primary staining agent to the smear. This is followed by treatment with an iodine solution that enhances the dye colorant. The smear is then decolorized with an alcohol solution and counterstained with a basic dye in a contrasting color. Based on the analysis of the organism's color and shape, it can be determined whether the organism is a gram-positive rod, a gram-negative rod, a gram-positive cocci, or a gram-negative cocci.

Another important differential staining procedure is called acid-fast staining. It identifies organisms of the *Mycobacterium* genus, which require a harsher treatment method involving heating to colorize the cells. This method is used to identify the pathogens responsible for tuberculosis and leprosy.

Once the determination is made based on the Gram stain, the patient may be started on an antibiotic that is sensitive to organisms in that particular quadrant. The information derived from the Gram stain will not tell the physician which antibiotic is most effective or most cost effective in managing the infection. For this determination culture and sensitivity testing will be performed in the laboratory. When these results arrive, the physician may modify his or her selection of antibiotic for optimal results.

Clinical Case Studies

The following case studies illustrate the usefulness of including laboratory data in the dysphagia evaluation. The profiles presented are similar to many referred to the dysphagia management team of the Alvin C. York Veterans Affairs Medical Center in Murfreesboro, Tennessee. According to established protocol, evaluations performed by this team include the LAB-D and the VFSS examination. Table 6.2 presents the VFSS findings for the two cases, Mr. Carter and Mr. Bills. Although the two have different etiologies and are 12 years apart in age,

Table 6.2
Modified Barium Swallow Results for Two Patients

Patient Name:	Mr. W. Carter	Mr. H. Bills
Age:	84 years	72 years
Primary diagnosis:	Alzheimer's Disease	Multiple CVA
Anterior spillage	Thin Liquid	None
Posterior spillage	None	None
Mastication	Fair	Fair
Oral transit	Delayed	Delayed
Oral stasis	Mild	WNL
Pharyngeal delay	Moderate	Mild
Thin liquid aspiration	Moderate	Moderate
Pen–Asp Score (thin)	7	7
Thick liquid aspiration	Trace	None
Pen–Asp Score (thick)	6	2
Vallecular stasis	Mild	Moderate
Pyriform sinus stasis	Mild	Moderate
Postural compensation	Inconsistent	Inconsistent
Thickened liquids	Inconsistent	Inconsistent
Feeding status	Dependent	Dependent

Note. CVA = cerebrovascular accident; WNL = within normal limits;
Pen–Asp = Penetration–Aspiration Score.

the patients showed significant similarities in their VFSS results. Both patients showed oral stage deficits, evidenced by impaired mastication of solids and delayed oral transit. In addition, Mr. Carter showed some anterior spillage with thin liquids and mild stasis. Both patients exhibited some degree of delay in the trigger of the pharyngeal swallow, Mr. Carter's being consistently greater than Mr. Bills's. Both experienced their greatest difficulty in safely swallowing thin liquids, demonstrating aspiration to a moderate degree on both 5- and 10-ml boli. Both were given a score of 7 on the Penetration–Aspiration (Pen–Asp) Scale (Rosenbek, Robbins, Roeckeer, Coyle, & Wood, 1996), based on the presence of aspiration and a failure to completely clear it from the larynx or airway, although they tried to do so. Perhaps related to his greater delay, Mr. Carter also showed trace aspiration of thick liquid (Pen–Asp Score = 6). Mr. Bills showed no aspiration of thick liquids, but mild penetration (Pen–Asp Score = 2). Following swallows Mr. Carter showed little pharyngeal stasis, whereas it was consistently present to a moderate degree for Mr. Bills. Neither the use of thickened liquids nor postural compensations were consistently effective for either patient. Significant also, as a risk for the development of aspiration pneumonia, is the fact that both were feeding dependent (Langmore et al., 1998). Thus, on the face of it, the VFSS data would suggest a good deal of similarity between these two patients. The challenging issue is how to effectively manage the aspiration risk posed by these two gentlemen. It is difficult to determine, based on the VFSS data, whether one might be at greater risk than the other for the development of complications associated with the dysphagia.

Table 6.3 provides SMA–12 values for these patients and Table 6.4 gives the results of CBC testing for each. With the evaluation of these data, the two patients begin to look very dissimilar. It was known from the medical history that Mr. Carter was diabetic and was under diet control to maintain his blood sugar level. Because his glucose level was above the reference range, he may not have been in good control at the time his blood was drawn. While Mr. Carter showed few other out of range values, he did show a slightly depressed albumin level of 3.5 g/dl. Although this is below the lower reference value of 3.9 g/dl, it is not an uncommon finding in the geriatric population. In fact, a review of sequential referrals to the dysphagia management team at our medical center indicates that a large minority of patients show an albumin level of 3.5 g/dl or lower. Mr. Carter shows elevated cholesterol and triglyceride values, neither of which should be of particular concern in the evaluation of his swallowing disorder. On the CBC (Table 6.4) there is an elevation of his eosinophil level, perhaps associated with an allergic response, not likely a nutritional concern. This patient's white blood count and differential failed to show values suggestive of infection. Applying the formula for TLC, a value of 1,747 was revealed, suggestive of good immune system function.

Mr. Bills's LAB-D data suggest a very different picture. His SMA–12 results show high BUN and uric acid values that suggest the presence of a waste-filtering problem. In addition, his albumin level of 2.4 g/dl is below the lower border of the reference range. In the interpretation of these data, it is important to note that electrolyte levels are

Table 6.3
Laboratory Assessment Battery for Dysphagia Data:
Selected SMA–12 Values

Laboratory Value	Mr. Carter	Mr. Bills	Reference Range
Glucose	168.0 mg/dl (H)	99 mg/dl	75–110
BUN	12 mg/dl	28 mg/dl (H)	9–21
Creatinine	1.2 mg/dl	1.5 mg/dl	0.8–1.5
Uric acid	5.0 mg/dl	8.8 mg/dl (H)	3.5–8.5
Sodium	139 mmol/L	168 mmol/L (H)	135–145
Potassium	4.4 mmol/L	4.9 mmol/L	3.6–5.0
Chloride	98 mmol/L	121 mmol/L(H)	101–111
Calcium	8.4 mg/dl (L)	11.5 mg/dl(H)	8.4–10.2
Albumin	3.5 g/dl (L)	2.4 g/dl (L)	3.9–5.0
Total bilirubin	0.9 mg/dl	1.1 mg/dl	0.2–1.3
Cholesterol	240 mg/dl (H)	141 mg/dl	< 200
Triglyceride	212 mg/dl (H)	110 mg/dl	40–199

Note. SMA = Sequential Multiple Analyzer; BUN = blood urea nitrogen; (H) = High; (L) = Low.

elevated, suggestive of the presence of dehydration. BUN, uric acid, and albumin are all sensitive to the body's hydration status. Normal levels can be expected to rise in conditions of dehydration and fall to below reference range values with overhydration. The elevation in Mr. Bills's electrolytes points to dehydration. Thus, if he is rehydrated it is likely that BUN, uric acid, and albumin values will fall. This could allow BUN and uric acid to return to within the reference range, altering suspicions about the presence of a waste-filtering problem. With rehydration the true albumin level may be revealed as lower than originally thought. Thus, Mr. Bills's protein stores may indeed be very seriously depleted. On the CBC test Mr. Bills shows a clear elevation in his white blood count and granulocyte counts. This combination is often indicative of the presence of infection. When planning treatment it is important to know how well equipped a patient's system is to combat infection. The

Table 6.4
Laboratory Assessment Battery for Dysphagia Data:
Selected Complete Blood Count (CBC) Values

Laboratory Value	Mr. Carter	Mr. Bills	Reference Range
White blood count	8.2 K/cmm	14.2 K/cmm (H)	4.8–10.8
Red blood count	5.42 M/cmm	4.9 M/cmm	4.7–6.1
Hemoglobin	15.2 g/dl	8.1 g/dl (L)	14–18
Hematocrit	43.4%	28.1% (L)	42%–52%
Mean corpuscular volume	88.0 cu microns	96.4 cu microns	80–94
Mean corpuscular hemoglobin	29.1 pg	27.8 pg	26–31
Mean corpuscular hemoglobin concentration	32.5 g/dl	28.9 g/dl	33–37
Platelets	184 K/cmm	247 K/cmm	130–400
Lymphocytes	21.3%	7.0% (L)	20.5%–51.1%
Monocytes	5.6%	7.2%	1.7%–9.3%
Granulocytes	49.1%	82.6%	42.2%–75.2%
Eosinophils	5.1% (H)	0.5%	0.5%–4.0%
Basophils	0.5%	1.0%	0.0%–1.5%

Note. H = high; L = low.

TLC calculation is one way of estimating the immune system status. In this patient's case, the TLC value was 994, well below the 1,500 level, which we use as a benchmark for good immune system status.

The VFSS results provided in these case studies suggest a good deal of similarity in the swallowing behavior of these two patients. Both patients showed a clear tendency toward aspiration of thin liquids. Neither responded consistently to postural changes or viscosity changes that are often employed to reduce the risk of aspiration. What, then, might be the best course of action in managing their disorders? When the laboratory values were added to the VFSS data, the clinician develops a wider understanding of the dysphagia and its potential for systemic effects. When the evaluation data are considered en toto, the results suggest that Mr. Carter's overall status is quite good. One might project that should he experience a decrease in protein intake, or should his system be confronted with an infective process, perhaps a pulmonary infection, then his system is better equipped than Mr. Bills's to handle it.

The overall pattern seen in Mr. Bills's case is not so encouraging. On gross examination of the LAB-D values, it is clear that his protein stores were depleted. In fact, when it is recognized that he may have been experiencing dehydration, then it is very likely that his nutritional status was severely compromised. Mr. Bills's depressed TLC is very significant when coupled with his moderate thin liquid aspiration. The question is, Should he develop a lung infection, will his own defenses be able to fight it off? While the laboratory assessment cannot allow a clinician to answer with a definitive yes or no, it is valuable information that can influence treatment planning. Although data are currently lacking to allow the clinician to determine definitively the degree of peril Mr. Bills faces, the data suggest that a degree of caution is in order as management decisions are made. Mr. Carter may well offer the clinician a margin for error that Mr. Bills may not. The LAB-D data can be a valuable supplement to the data the clinician collects from other diagnostic measures and sources. Its use can provide the clinician with one more tool to aid in making effective management decisions.

Summary

To formulate appropriate recommendations for treating the patient with dysphagia, the clinician must consider results of both the dysphagia evaluation and the nutritional assessment. An important component in the process is the utilization of LAB-D data, which will allow the clinician to begin to view the dysphagia in terms of its possible systemic effects. Patients exhibiting significant aspiration may require an alternate avenue of intake. Patients who can safely continue eating but who are severely compromised nutritionally may require supplemental nighttime tube feeding in addition to routine daytime meals. When PO intake appears safe for a patient, mild to moderate compromise in nutritional status can be managed by increasing the available calorie intake at or between meals using commercial supplements, snacks, or extra portions. Determination of food preferences will be vital with these patients to ensure adequate intake. Patients with nutritional status within normal limits despite oral or pharyngeal dysphagia will require careful monitoring to ensure nutritional stability.

Just as the assignment of compensatory techniques or diet modification is individualized based on the patient's dysphagia characteristics, multiple factors within the nutritional assessment, as well as the results of the dysphagia evaluation, must be considered in making decisions regarding nutritional management. Such decisions require input from all members of the dysphagia management team. However, because of the strong relationship between nutrition and swallowing, appropriate decisions cannot be made without involvement of a dietitian throughout the evaluation process.

References

Dwyer, J. T., Gallo, J. J., & Reichel, W. (1993). Assessing nutritional status in elderly patients. *American Family Physician, 47,* 613–620.

Fischbach, F. (1992). *A manual of laboratory and diagnostic tests* (4th ed.). Philadelphia: Lippincott.

Hole, J. W. (1989). *Essentials of human anatomy and physiology* (3rd ed.). Dubuque, IA: Wm. C. Brown.

Langmore, S. E., Terpenning, A., Schork, Y., Chen, T., Murray, J. T., Lopatin, D., & Loesche, W. J. (1998). Predictors of aspiration pneumonia: How important is dysphagia? *Dysphagia, 13,* 69–81.

Mahan, L. K., & Arlin, M. (1992). *Krause's food, nutrition and diet therapy* (8th ed.). Philadelphia: Saunders.

Porth, C. M. (1990). *Pathophysiology: Concepts of altered health states.* Philadelphia: Lippincott.

Powers, J. S., & Folk, M. C. (1992). Nutritional concerns in the elderly. *Southern Medical Journal, 85,* 1107–1112.

Prescott, L. M., Harley, J. P., & Klein, D. A. (1990). *Microbiology.* Dubuque, IA: Wm. C. Brown.

Rosenbek, J. C., Robbins, J. A., Roeckeer, E. B., Coyle, J. L., & Wood, J. L. (1996). A penetration–aspiration scale. *Dysphagia, 11,* 93–98.

Skipper, A. (1989). *Dietitian's handbook of enteral and parenteral nutrition.* Rockville, MD: Aspen.

Sullivan, D. H., & Walls, R. C. (1994). Impact of nutritional status on morbidity in a population of geriatric rehabilitation patients. *Journal of the American Geriatric Society, 42,* 471–477.

Weinsier, R. L., Heimburger, D. C., & Butterworth, C. E. (1989). *Handbook of clinical nutrition* (2nd ed.). St. Louis: Mosby.

Zeman, F. (1991). *Clinical nutrition and dietetics.* New York: Macmillan.

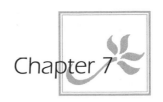

Chapter 7

Dental Aspects of Swallowing

John C. Hudson and Russell H. Mills

Hudson and Mills discuss normal dental anatomy and dental problems that are common in the geriatric population. Because edentulism is so common in the elderly, the authors provide practical information regarding the fitting and use of dentures.

1. *What are the six types of dental problems commonly found in elderly individuals?*

2. *Why is it not possible to predict the degree of mastication impairment by counting the number of teeth missing from the mouth?*

3. *What negative effects do improperly fitting dentures have on mastication?*

4. *How does xerostomia affect the ability to wear dentures?*

꙼ꙛ ꙼ꙛ ꙼ꙛ

Dysphagia, or difficulty in swallowing, is a demoralizing demise for the patient and creates difficulties for their families and health care providers. It presents with a variety of symptoms with varying degrees of severity and may involve multiple distinct anatomic sites. No single treatment modality is considered effective in the management of all of the symptoms of dysphagia. Cooperation among health care disciplines usually offers the best opportunity to share knowledge and arrive at the most effective treatment plan and care. A review of the dysphagia literature reveals that dental issues and dentistry are given only cursory attention, if they are acknowledged at all. As this chapter will establish, dental issues are critical to dysphagia. Dental management will not be appropriate or necessary in every case of dysphagia. However, when appropriate, the evaluation and management of dental maladies will often contribute to a positive outcome for dysphagia and an improvement in the patient's quality of life.

Health care institutions are often organized such that clinical services are functionally isolated from each other. Ross and Beall (1984) observed that the evidence suggests that health care professionals have access to information in their own disciplines, but they know little about other areas. Although literature exists highlighting an interdisciplinary approach to the treatment of dysphagia (Emick-Herring & Wood, 1990; Hutchins & Giancarlo, 1991; Mirro & Patey, 1991; Perlman et al., 1991), the inclusion of dentistry has generally been overlooked. This is reflected in the research undertaken and the clinician education provided. Although investigators and educators have given some attention to certain aspects of the oral and oral preparatory stages of swallowing, a paucity of information remains.

It would seem reasonable that clinicians would understand that the structures and functions of the oral cavity are important to the swallow. After all, under normal circumstances all liquids and foodstuffs enter the body through this orifice. The mechanical and chemical processes that represent the initial stages of digestion actually begin in the mouth. The Department of Veterans Affairs (1998) has recognized that the oral health status of the patient is critical to overall health and quality of life. They state that treatment of health conditions that are prevalent in their patient population without appropriate dental involvement can compromise outcomes. The oral cavity is anatomically and physiologically a part of the complete human body and its malfunction and diseased state will disturb and affect other parts of the systemic system. Patients with dysphagia, as well as those health professionals involved in the management of dysphagia, must realize that dental conditions can have pervasive effects that influence the nutritional, emotional, psychological, and general well-being of the individual.

A large segment of the population with dysphagia is composed of elderly individuals (Shaw, 1981). The literature is replete with epidemiologic studies revealing that the oral and dental health of this population is characteristically poor. Dental health in the elderly is frequently and severely neglected, and this neglect is reflected in a variety of ways that are sufficient to negatively influence per oral (PO) intake and swallowing. Common problems include poor oral hygiene, tooth loss, tooth decay, and periodontal disease. In addition, edentulousness is very common. When dentures are worn, they are frequently defective and are not maintained in a hygienic manner.

A variety of factors function to curtail the dental care that elderly individuals receive. Thines, Karuza, and Miller (1987) suggested that health care practitioners and policy planners share the misconception that dental care is a luxury and that there is little need for it among the elderly population because so many are edentulous. For this reason many dental disorders are not adequately covered by primary medical insurance. Because older Americans most frequently live within fixed incomes, their dental problems often go untreated. Kiwayk (1981) and others have shown that a serious gap exists between the perceptions of dentists and older patients in regard to dental care requirements. Many older individuals believe that "dentistry is just for kids" and that the loss of teeth is inevitable, just a part of normal aging. The elderly dental patients may contribute to the problem by being all too ready to allow a dentist to pull a tooth, not realizing the consequences this action will have on the remaining dentition and their systemic health in the years to come. Undoubtedly, their attitudes influence the care they seek and receive. Evidence has also been noted that negative attitudes by dental providers can influence the extent of dental care that older adults receive (Kiwayk, 1981). For the reasons stated, dental services received by elderly patients have been exceedingly limited. When the patient is not only elderly but also medically compromised, as in the case of many patients with dysphagia , then it is likely that care is even more limited.

The purpose of this chapter is to provide dysphagia clinicians with information on the subject of dentistry and the interrelation between dentistry, the oral cavity, and dysphagia. The chapter provides a discussion of normal dental anatomy and physiology, including saliva production. Common geriatric oral and dental disorders that may have an impact on swallowing are delineated. Mastication and nutritional concerns resulting from mastication impairment are addressed. Significant attention is given to the use of dentures as a management strategy. Finally, the clinician is provided with guidelines to be used when considering a dental referral. The intent is to inform dysphagia clinicians and other interested personnel of some situations in which dentistry may be of assistance when dealing with the elderly patient with dysphagia.

Dental Anatomy and Physiology

The oral cavity and dentition are two of the most forgiving and significant parts of the human body. While most people wish to look nice and want perfectly aligned and brilliantly white teeth, many consistently abuse their dentition. People challenge their tooth structures with extremes of temperature gradients (e.g., ice cream followed by hot coffee), acidic foods, and even highly acidic gastric reflux at times. Many individuals lack acceptable oral hygiene and do not make time for routine dental checkups. Some blame the dentist when a filling is lost, not recognizing that decay and breakdown of the tooth structure as a result of poor dental hygiene may cause it. Humans have been known to use their teeth in attack, for defense, to express emotion, in speech, and in mastication.

Although some of the initial reasons for having teeth no longer exist, man's teeth still serve important functions. Langer (1976) stated that "Man is the only creature that can survive and prosper without his teeth" (p. 64). Still, functional capacity of the oral cavity most often decreases greatly with the loss of any of its component parts. The loss of teeth or of other aspects of oral function often produce negative affects on eating, swallowing, nutrition, communication, and self-esteem. We begin with a discussion of normal dental and oral anatomy and physiology so that the reader can develop a better understanding of the relationship between dental health and swallowing.

The oral system is composed of both rigid and flexible tissues. Rigid elements include the teeth, mandible and maxilla, temporomandibular joint (TMJ), and hard palate. Flexible elements include the muscles of mastication, the tongue, and the soft palate. In addition, the oral system contains multiple major and minor glands, other soft tissues including mucosa, and an elaborate array of vascular and nervous tissue. These components function to serve both nutritive and nonnutritive oral functions. All of these component parts must operate in harmony for function to be optimal.

Anatomy and Physiology of the Mandible, Maxilla, and TMJ

Along with the soft tissues, man is born with a cartilaginous framework on which bone is laid down to form the maxilla and mandible. This beginning bone is termed *basalar bone* and usually remains with the individual until death. As the human undergoes maturation, tooth buds develop within the arches and then erupt as deciduous teeth. Along with the formation of the deciduous teeth, and then the permanent teeth years later, another type of bone referred to as *alveolar bone* is laid down. There are conditions of dental pathology in which the alveolar bone may be lost. Alveolar bone and collectively all the hard and soft tissues that offer support for the teeth are known as the periodontium.

Whereas the maxilla is the stable member of the jaws, the mandible is the moveable part. The maxilla is fused to the skull at fusion lines, and to move the maxilla one must move the entire head. On the other hand, the mandible is one bone, fused in the midline at the mandibular symphysis. It attaches to the skull via the temporomandibular articulation and a sling of muscles. TMJ articulation is via a complicated ginglymoarthrodial joint, with hinge and glide articulation, and with an articular disc or meniscus interposed between the condyle of the mandible and the glenoid fossa of the temporal bone (Ramfjord & Ash, 1971). Mandibular movements involve the entire mandible, and the points of movement are the TMJs. As one side of the mandible moves, the opposite side must move accordingly. Mandibular movements, dictated and limited by the TMJs, the muscular sling, and the occlusion of the teeth, may be classified as masticatory and nonmasticatory. The masticatory movements obviously are the ones necessary for the manipulation and chewing of foods, whereas the nonmasticatory movements entail all other normal and abnormal movements used in speech and oral–facial habits.

Normal Anatomy and Physiology of the Teeth

Most higher mammals, including man, are provided with two sets of dentition. An initial set, the deciduous, primary, or milk teeth, are unerupted yet well developed at birth. The second set of teeth, the secondary or permanent teeth, are developing within the dental arch at the time of birth and, as can be seen in Figure 7.1, continue to develop after the deciduous teeth have emerged. Clinical eruption of the primary teeth begins before the age of 12 months and continues until approximately 24 months. When all have erupted, the full complement of primary teeth includes 4 molars, 4 cuspids, 4 canines, and 8 incisors, for a total of 20 teeth. The primary arch is retained until the age of 6 to 7 years, when shedding begins. When it is time to replace the primary teeth, cells called osteoclasts begin their work. These cells are able to cause the resorption of bone. The osteoclasts reabsorb the roots of the primary teeth, allowing the secondary teeth to erupt through. Loss of the deciduous teeth continues until the age of 11 or 12 years, when the full complement of permanent teeth has erupted. Some individuals retain baby teeth well into their adult years. Third molars may be acquired later, between the ages of 17 and 25 years. Once a tooth erupts into the oral cavity, its working life begins. That is, the tooth is exposed on an hourly and daily basis to the stresses and strains associated with being a tooth. This attrition phase of the tooth's existence lasts throughout life. During this period of time, there is a slow but continual wearing of the teeth at the occlusal orbiting surfaces. As the teeth begin to wear, minute amounts of eruption will help to keep the occlusal surfaces in contact.

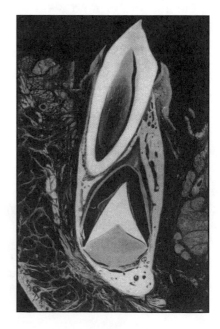

Figure 7.1. A deciduous tooth and a permanent tooth bud within the alveolar arch. From *Speech and Hearing Science: Anatomy and Physiology* (4th ed.), by W. R. Zemlin, 1998, Needham Heights, MA: Allyn & Bacon. Copyright 1998 by Allyn & Bacon. Reprinted with permission.

The human tooth, as shown in Figure 7.2, can be divided into three general sections. In the healthy tooth the crown is the portion that is visible above the gum line. The root is the portion of the tooth that is firmly attached within the alveolar ridge. The neck is the portion of the tooth that connects the crown and root. The largest part of the tooth is composed of dentin, a hard material that is composed of inorganic and animal salts. The exposed surface of the tooth is covered by enamel. It is the hardest material in the human body and is composed of organic salts. The root portion of the tooth is covered by cementum that, in combination with the periodontium, serves to hold the tooth in its socket. The innermost aspect of the tooth contains the soft pulp. The neural and vascular supply is within the pulp cavity, entering through the apical foramen in the root of the tooth.

The hardness of structures in the body can be easily remembered with the first five letters of the alphabet. After eliminating the 'A', their descending order (E, D, C, B) represents tissues ranked in decreasing

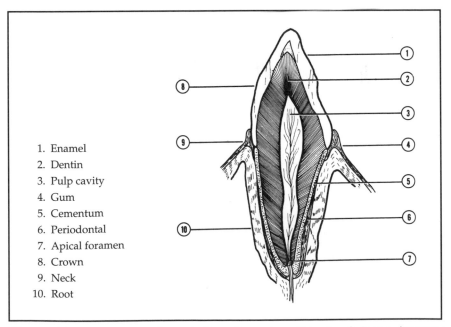

1. Enamel
2. Dentin
3. Pulp cavity
4. Gum
5. Cementum
6. Periodontal
7. Apical foramen
8. Crown
9. Neck
10. Root

Figure 7.2. The anatomy of a tooth. From *Speech and Hearing Science: Anatomy and Physiology* (4th ed.), by W. R. Zemlin, 1998, Needham Heights, MA: Allyn & Bacon. Copyright 1998 by Allyn & Bacon. Reprinted with permission.

hardness. According to this scheme, *enamel* is the hardest human tissue, followed by *dentin, cementum,* and finally *bone.* Thus, the three hardest materials in the human body are located in the oral cavity.

Figure 7.3 shows the adult dental arches with its four types of teeth: incisors, canines, bicuspids, and molars. Each type differs in appearance, the differences reflecting the divergent functions. Together the two adult dental arches contain four central and four lateral chisel-shaped incisors. The flat-blade shape of these teeth reflect their use in cutting. The mouth contains four pointed canine (cuspid) teeth, whose function is best served when tearing foods. There are a total of eight bicuspids. These teeth are capable of grinding foodstuffs, but do not have the large flat occlusal area of the molars. The largest human teeth are the 12 molars. These teeth have a crown that is somewhat rectangular in shape and is ideally suited for grinding solid particles of food before swallowing. The presence of third molars follows no specific rule. Individuals can have no third molars or up to a full complement of four.

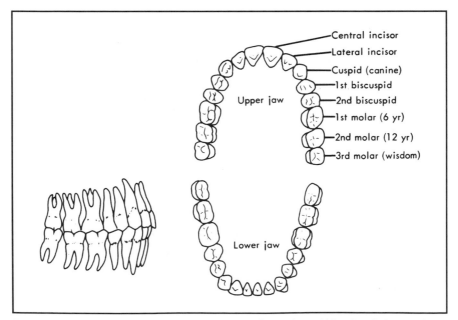

Figure 7.3. The permanent dental arch. From *Speech and Hearing Science: Anatomy and Physiology* (4th ed.), by W. R. Zemlin, 1998, Needham Heights, MA: Allyn & Bacon. Copyright 1998 by Allyn & Bacon. Reprinted with permission.

The diet of primitive man was significantly different from that of modern man. There was a greater reliance on incisors and canines as they were critical for cutting and tearing foodstuffs prior to ingestion. In the modern diet of highly processed foods, man is rarely called upon to tear meat from the leg of a recently killed hyena. Still, the incisors and canines retain their utility for turkey legs, carrot sticks, lengths of thread, cookies, tortilla chips, and so forth. The human diet does continue to require significant amounts of grinding. The bicuspids and first molars perform the main portion of heavy grinding. The loss of these teeth severely impairs chewing ability. Therefore, the premolars and molars remain as significantly important to the consumption of a modern diet.

Oral Mucosa

Lining the inside of the mouth, and continuous with the lining of the pharyngeal spaces, is the oral mucosa. This mucosa is similar in function to the skin that covers the outer body in that it is the first line of defense against infections of the mouth. The oral mucosa is made of three distinctly different types of cells, giving specific function to different areas within the mouth. Generally, the more keratinized tissues with heavy underlying connective tissue firmly attached to the bone provide protection to some areas of the gingiva and mucosa of the hard palate. Mucosa that is less keratinized and lacks the underlying thick connective tissue covers the other areas of the gingiva of the gums, cheeks, and floor of the mouth. Very specialized mucosa covers the dorsum of the tongue. Here taste receptors are abundant and are composed of many different specialized cell types. They are also located throughout other soft tissues of the mouth.

Normal Anatomy and Physiology of the Salivary Glands

The human possesses three major salivary glands and a large number of minor salivary glands. The saliva glands produce saliva, which is important in that it is essential for the maintenance and protection of the oral mucosa, teeth, and epithelium of the intestinal tract. Saliva protects the hard and soft tissues through antibacterial, antifungal, antiviral, hydration, buffering, and remineralization processes. It has lubricating functions that facilitate speech, eating, and swallowing. Saliva also greatly assists taste perception by its cleansing action of taste buds. It has been a common assumption that diminished saliva production is an expected result of the normal aging process; however, several studies suggest that there is no reduction in the volume of saliva production in the normal, healthy elderly adult. Baum (1986) noted that previous suggestions of diminished salivary gland performance correlated with age were primarily reflective of disease and therapy-induced alterations.

Normal Anatomy and Physiology of the Tongue

The tongue is an extremely complex structure composed of intrinsic and extrinsic musculature. It is connected to the hyoid bone, soft palate, pharynx, and epiglottis, but its anterior, lateral, and superior borders are not connected. These muscles are, with one exception, paired. The extensive vascular and neural supply to the tongue allows it to perform very precise movement patterns. Such patterns are necessary for the production of intelligible speech and for bolus preparation and transport. It is covered on its dorsum with a variety of papillae that add texture, increase the surface area, and assist with taste perception and the preparing of foods for digestion. The anchoring of the tongue also plays a supportive role in that it provides anchoring during hyoid elevation and upper esophageal sphincter opening.

Normal Mastication

Davis (1989) provided an excellent overview of the oral preparation stage. After food that requires mastication has been placed into the patient's mouth, the teeth come together and the lips close to form the containment boundaries. The posterior orifice is closed by a downward compression of the soft palate against the back of the tongue. In this way the food is confined to a closed area while preparation of the bolus is completed. The tongue then manipulates the food against the hard palate and the teeth to identify the texture and to place it on the chewing surfaces of the teeth. The tongue, along with the cheek muscles, propel the bolus toward the back of the mouth so the food will be placed on other teeth. The cheeks compress against the mandible and maxilla to prevent food from slipping into the lateral sulcus. The compression of the lips performs the same function for the anterior sulcus.

Most chewing, or grinding, is done by the bicuspids and first molars (Winkler, 1979). The chewing cycle has been identified as occurring in cycles or repeated motions. The food is chewed for several strokes, and then the tongue, cheeks, teeth, and palate all act together to prepare the crushed food, mixed with saliva, into a bolus, of the desirable size to be passed to the posterior of the mouth to be swallowed. As the swallow is initiated, the teeth come together to act as a "stop" for mandibular closing and positioning, and the tongue and hard and soft palates propel the bolus to the point at which autonomic innervation begins the peristaltic action known as swallowing.

Martone (1962) stated that in chewing the tongue serves as a greeter, a moistener, a shock absorber, a bracer, a guide, a taster, a crusher, a sorter, a mixer, and a disposer. Due to the tongue's extensive voluntary innervation, very complex tasks can be performed with very little difficulty. Some tongue functions are fairly obvious, such as its wide range of motions used in speaking and its part in wetting the lips, feeling the front surfaces of the teeth, and licking actions. Other important functions usually go unnoticed but serve immensely important functions that may be involved with dysphagic symptoms. Receiving and distributing food particles for processing, the tongue is responsible for continuously placing chewed foods onto what is called the "occlusal table," the chewing surfaces of the teeth. During mastication food also is pressed against the palate by the tongue to help assist its breakdown. When particles are lost into the sulci, the tongue is used to retrieve them. The tongue also works in conjunction with the teeth and the hard and soft palates to propel the bolus toward the pharyngeal area in preparation for the pharyngeal stage of the swallow. The tongue performs a cleansing action on the teeth and other oral structures, and offers "countering" forces to the lingual surfaces of the teeth opposing the forces created by the facial musculature.

Although the number of teeth that are retained is important in mastication, it is not the most critical factor. The most important element is the number of teeth whose occlusal surfaces meet with an opposing tooth during mastication (Figure 7.4). For example, loss of molars is a common phenomenon in the aging human. If an upper left molar is lost, then the functional effect is the same as if both upper and lower

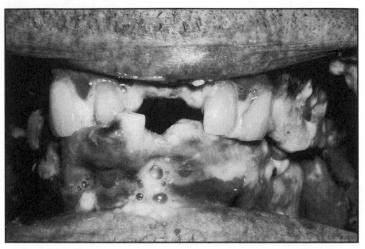

Figure 7.4. A patient with poor dentition and lacking occlusal surfaces.

opposing molars are lost on the same side. Whether one or both are missing, the meeting of occlusal surfaces is lost and mastication will to some degree be compromised. During the oromotor examination the dysphagia clinician should look for loss of matching occlusal surfaces, which can indicate that mastication compromise may exist.

Common Problems of the Oral Cavity

Saliva Problems

One has only to recall the symptoms of his or her own dry mouth in the early morning hours to sympathize with the patient who suffers from xerostomia, or dry mouth. Inadequate amounts or quality of saliva causes the tongue to literally stick to the palate, making talking difficult and greatly affecting the swallowing process. It is uncomfortable for the healthy individual and becomes devastating for the patient with dysphagia. Xerostomia is commonly associated with irradiation of the oral cavity and with certain medications (see Table 1.2 in Chapter 1 of this text). Prolonged xerostomia can lead to the sensation of a burning mouth and tongue, as well as increased oral infections and tooth decay. Xerostomia also creates an extremely harsh environment for denture wearers. Dentures require a coating of saliva on the mucosa to develop the adhesive qualities that secure the dentures to the gums. Not only do dentures not adhere without saliva, but also natural lubrication is lost, leading to sore gums, pressure sores, and actual lacerations of the mucosa. Lubricating agents are available but cannot provide all the functions of normal saliva.

Abnormalities of the Tongue

Tongue abnormalities can cause many severe difficulties. Paralysis of the tongue muscles can have far-reaching effects on mastication and swallowing. A loss of unilateral function often results in a loss of the tongue's ability to seal against the teeth on the affected side. As a consequence, liquids will escape beneath the tongue and into the sulci during processing. Food particles will be lost as they are inexpertly moved to and from the occlusal surfaces on the paralyzed side. Paralysis can affect the posterior seal with the soft palate and result in premature spillage into the pharynx, a potential for aspiration before the swallow. Such impairment can also interfere with the oral stage of the swallow and impair bolus transport to the pharynx. With poor oral hygiene, the tongue will harbor a multitude of harmful agents, ranging from decaying foods and medicines to bacterial and viral components, which affect taste and appetite, and contribute to halitosis. Vitamin deficiencies have been blamed for a burning sensation localized to the tongue. When oral cancer occurs, common locations for the cancerous lesion are at the posterior sides of the tongue and the floor of the mouth. Finally, the size of the tongue relative to the volume of the oral cavity can increase substantially with the loss of the teeth, creating significant problems for the denture wearer.

Common Dental Problems in the Elderly

In addition to the tissue changes associated with aging, elderly individuals can experience six major types of dental problems (Storer, 1985):

1. Elderly patients experience problems associated with normal wear or attrition and abrasion of the teeth.

2. As recounted earlier, tooth loss is common in the elderly population, due either to the presence of decay (caries) or

periodontal disease (disease of the supporting tissues of the teeth). When there is loss of teeth, the patient will likely experience migration of remaining teeth.

3. Migration affects the alignment of occlusal surfaces and may impair the efficiency of mastication. As teeth are lost the remaining teeth tend to drift out of their proper places, causing legions of problems. Food traps develop that lead to poor oral hygiene and eventually pyorrhea, gum disease, or periodontal disease. Carious lesions (breakdowns of the tooth enamel) also occur, which lead to the inability to perform adequate oral hygiene, thus beginning a cycle of tooth decay, pain, abscesses, and the loss of more teeth.

4. Due to a combination of tooth loss and migration, the elderly patient may experience a decrease in the efficiency of mastication.

5. A deterioration in oral hygiene, as shown in Figure 7.5, is common in this age group. Members of the geriatric population frequently are unaware of their dental needs. The lack of hygiene can preclude a complete examination of oral tissues because they can obscure important features. Due to altered pain responses, chronic caries and tooth abscesses are quite common.

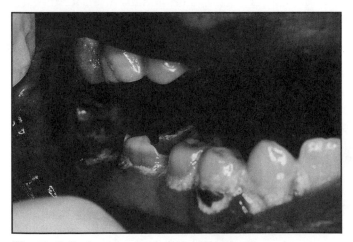

Figure 7.5. An example of poor oral hygiene.

6. For elderly individuals who have been fitted with dentures, problems related to the effect of dentures on the oral tissues are seen.

Tooth Loss and Edentulism

Tooth loss is a significant problem in modern society. Surveys completed in 1957–1958 indicated that 22 million people in the United States, or approximately 13% of the nation's population, had lost all their permanent teeth. In 1960–1962 conservative estimates indicated 20.1 million noninstitutionalized men and women had lost all 32 of their permanent teeth. Nearly 10 million more adults had lost all 16 teeth in either the upper or the lower jaw. This means that at least one in four adults had no natural teeth in either one or both jaws, and one in every two had lost all of his or her teeth (Cheraskin, 1976). Data from Great Britain (Hobdell, Sheihan, & Cowell, 1970), South Australia (Roder, 1975), and Canada (Martinello & Leake, 1971) indicated that the majority of people over age 50 had at least one edentulous jaw, and that more than 50% to 75% of those over 60 were completely toothless. Even though fluoridated water and other extensive preventative measures are much more common in the United States today, still 10% of adults under age 75 and 44% of adults 75 years of age and older are missing all of their teeth ("A Look at Dental Diseases and Treatments," 1997). These statistics are truly alarming because, barring accidents and intentional extractions, tooth loss is completely preventable. Years of poor oral hygiene, gross dental neglect, caries, and periodontal infections produce significant agony. Beyond this, many of the soon-to-be-edentulous will discover that they are entering into serious problems as denture wearers that will last them the rest of their lives.

Dentures

Of all the challenges in the profession of dentistry, treatment for the edentulous or partially edentulous patient overwhelmingly presents the most difficulties for the patient and the dentist. This is especially true for patients who are edentulous. The treatment provided for many of the patients is the preparation of a complete set of pros-thetic teeth, or dentures. Various authors (Bergman & Carlsson, 1972; Ettinger, 1973; and Sheppard, Schwartz, & Sheppard, 1971) have pro-vided evidence that denture failures occur much too frequently and reported that dissatisfaction with dentures ranged from 15% to 45% in the samples studied. They reported that a satisfactory mechanical fit and good occlusion are not the only factors associated with denture success. It appears paradoxical that a good many patients with mechanically stable and satisfactory complete dentures are displeased and unable to function adequately, whereas other denture wearers amaze the practitioner by functioning very well with poor dentures. Basically, dentists strive to obtain the best fit of the denture to the gums and provide a good cosmetic result. Although these objectives are accomplished by emphasizing the design of the denture in accordance with the patient's oral anatomy, many other aspects are obviously involved with patient acceptance and satisfaction. What follows is a discussion of basic denture concepts so that the dysphagia clinician will be able to understand what they are and what problems are com-monly associated with their use.

Design and Construction of a Denture

A denture is a prosthetic device that has several forms. The most com-mon is the complete denture designed for the edentulous patient (e.g., Figure 7.6). For each patient a unique denture is fashioned from acrylic material. Care is taken to produce a prosthesis that will meet the patient's needs and not be traumatic to the oral tissues. It is not an easy task.

The construction of a denture is a highly detailed process. It usually takes several steps to complete, and patient involvement and assis-tance are absolutely imperative. The oral soft tissues (mucosa) should be in good health before the impressions are taken because the denture will incorporate any defect present at the time of construction. It is important to realize that the denture the patient will wear is a rigid appliance that is made to fit the gums of the person at the exact time the master impression is obtained. It is not designed to expand or shrink in the future to allow for changes in the patient's oral tissues. Therefore, if the tissues have been neglected and are thin, or raw and sore, then the

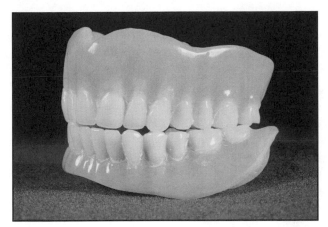

Figure 7.6. A set of complete acrylic dentures. Photo by Robert M. Brown.

new denture will be built to fit the tissues in that state. If the tissues change later (e.g., swelling is reduced), then wearing the denture will likely produce additional trauma to the tissue and will eventually cause much more destruction to the gums and bone. The tissues should be conditioned back to a state of health prior to the fitting of the denture. This can be done by relieving the present denture and adding a soft tissue conditioner for a period of time to allow the tissues to again receive an adequate blood supply and to revitalize themselves.

The purpose of a denture is to restore the lost components of the oral cavity and return the patient to a functional state. These lost components obviously include the teeth, but lost bone and gum tissue must also be replaced. To begin the process, an impression is obtained of the patient's gums and bone structure. A stone cast is then poured to duplicate the oral anatomy. In the dental laboratory the gums are then replicated in wax. The patient then returns for the next step. At this point the patient must be able to open and close the jaw, and complete several jaw movements that allow the doctor to establish the correct position of the teeth, to check for proper tongue, cheek, and jaw movements for speech and mastication.

Family members and many health care providers do not realize the critical part the patient plays in the construction of a denture. Without the patient's cooperation, the whole process becomes a guessing game; in this case, the line of occlusion of the teeth and the physiological rest position of the jaws will most likely not approximate the patient's natural dentition. With errors made in these design elements due to a patient's inability to cooperate, the denture is rendered useless. It can even cause further deterioration of the oral tissues and TMJs, resulting in significant physical and psychological problems.

When the correct parameters have been obtained in the wax occlusal model, the teeth are added and the patient is called for a "try-in" to make sure the teeth are set properly and the lips and tongue can perform their functions. At this point in the process, the wax-up of the gums and teeth are invested in a stonelike mixture. The wax is melted away at very high temperatures and the acrylic poured into the mold space evacuated by the wax. This investment is then cured for several hours in a controlled temperature bath until it is properly hardened. The fully cured denture is then removed from the investment and processed to create a smooth and attractive product that is kind to the oral tissues and functional for the patient. All new dentures should be adjusted two to three times over the first several days or weeks to ensure proper fit and function. This will increase the chance for patient acceptance and will go a long way toward comfort and prevention of pathology.

The Advanced Prosthesis

Despite all the knowledge available today, tooth loss remains common. Carlsson (1984) wrote that conventional denture treatment can offer little to improve the severely reduced masticatory function in edentulous persons. He further stated that the maintenance of a reasonable number of healthy and natural teeth is the best guarantee for good masticatory efficiency with increasing age.

Advancing dental science now provides improved methods to deal with the problems of edentulism. An *overdenture* uses a structure beneath the denture that works in conjunction with alveolar bone to stabilize the denture. It can be fit on the maxillary arch, the mandibular arch, or both. One form of the overdenture makes use of tooth roots to provide that stability. At the time extraction normally would take place, the tooth is ground down so that the roots remain in the bone. Attachments are then affixed to the roots and to the tissue side of the denture. The two are connected and the overdenture becomes more stable because it is connected to the roots embedded in alveolar bone.

Other options include the use of metal dental implants, either positioned on top of the bone but beneath the gums, or placed directly into the bone itself. Both leave appendages extending up through the gum tissues to serve as anchors for prosthetic devices that are placed on them. Although some medical conditions preclude the use of implants, this is the most desirable treatment available. Dental implants and overdentures are very expensive at the present time, but extremely satisfactory results have been obtained. The cost is high for these devices because of the extensive work required to prepare the roots as anchors. Implants may prove to be a viable option with some patients with dysphagia. Carlsson and Lindquist (1994) completed a 10-year study of 28 patients who received complete dentures on osseointegrated implants (CDOI). The results were striking. They found that when the mandibular arch was provided with a CDOI, there was a rapid and dramatic improvement in masticatory function. With traditional complete dentures these subjects produced a mean pressure of 80 Newtons when biting. At all sample points following placement of the CDOI, the subjects had improved bite strength. At the conclusion of the study, the subjects bit with an average force of 250 Newtons, a threefold increase. If such a prosthesis is provided, then good oral hygiene is mandatory. Periodontal disease will affect the implant–bone junction as it would with the root–bone interface.

The Ideal Oral Anatomy for Denture Wearing

Few patients present with ideal physical characteristics to be denture wearers. The primary requirement for a stable fit is adequate amounts of alveolar bone that are correctly contoured on the maxilla and mandible. Resorbed bone makes achieving denture stability much more difficult. It is also important that the muscle attachments on the mandible are properly located. If they are attached too near the apex of the alveolar ridge, then contraction will dislodge the prosthesis. In addition, the patient's tongue, TMJs, and oral mucosa need to be healthy, and the saliva should be of good quality and quantity. Some nonphysical factors need to be considered as well. The patient's recognition of the mental and psychological aspects of wearing a denture prosthesis is important to the quality of the final outcome.

Problems with Dentures

As has been pointed out, most people with dentures are not satisfied and many are unable to tolerate either or both the upper and the lower prostheses. Problems with dentures involve psychological, emotional, and physical factors that have a multitude of origins. These are usually compounded when the patient is dysphagic.

A common complaint is associated with the deterioration of the supporting structures. The mandible is a horseshoe-shaped bone and only a few areas of it can offer support for a denture. The amount of stability provided by the mandible depends on the length of the denture's flange that can be fit. Unfortunately, muscles attach on the facial and lingual sides of the mandible, thus limiting the length of the denture flanges that overlap the alveolar ridges. When the flange is too long and overlaps these muscles, their contractions serve to dislodge the lower denture during mandibular movement. In contrast, the entire width of the roof of the mouth is available to support the upper denture. The muscles that attach to the maxilla do not move the maxilla and thus present much less interference with the denture flanges and usually do not hinder the functioning of the upper denture. Thus, the most frequent problems with denture retention involve the lower appliance.

Bone Resorption. The foremost problem denture wearers experience is bone resorption. The roots of the teeth are the stimulus needed to maintain the alveolar bone, and a progressive loss of alveolar bone is seen after the loss of teeth. Three years after extraction, 50% of alveolar ridge bone is lost and this process continues so that in some individuals absolutely no alveolar bone may be present at all (Heath, 1973). Obviously, the earlier a person looses his or her teeth, the more bone loss can be expected in the future. Thus, in many cases, the decrease in the availability of alveolar bone with which the dentist has to work greatly reduces the probability of achieving denture stability.

Xerostomia. The denture that has been fitted to the edentulous anatomy has no anchor points. It floats, separated from the oral mucosa by a thin layer of saliva. The presence of the saliva is of critical importance in securing the dentures. Without this fluid, dentures are often loose and wobble under the forces exerted by mastication. The poor fit impairs mastication and makes traumatic injury likely. Consequently, fitting the patient who is xerostomic represents a real challenge for the practitioner.

The Effects of Dentures on Nutrition. Several studies have identified a detrimental effect of dentures on nutritional status (Hartsook, 1974; Yurkstas & Emerson, 1964). According to Pilgrim and Kamen (1959), food acceptance results from a complex interaction of biological, environmental, cultural, and behavioral influences. Moreover, these authors found evidence that man usually is not guided by nutritional needs or a reasonable consideration of food availability but by other factors. Especially important are the senses of taste and smell, which promote strong acceptance or rejection responses. Szczesniak and Kleyn (1963) discovered that texture is another important factor influencing food acceptability.

Bates, Elwood, and Foster (1971) found evidence that subjects with neither teeth nor dentures, and those who experience difficulty in using dentures, avoid certain foods. They also found that a substantial proportion of elderly subjects who have dentures do not wear them when eating. Feldman, Kapur, Alman, and Chauncey (1980) established that tooth loss also significantly decreases the swallowing threshold performance and increases the particle size that subjects were willing to swallow. In this study it was evident that older persons required more chewing strokes to prepare foods for swallowing.

Effects of Dentures on Mastication. Although much progress has been made in the construction of dentures since the days of the wood teeth used by George Washington, they still are imperfect mechanical devices that conform to the laws of physics (i.e., the inclined plane and the lever). They are loosely attached, rudimentarily rely on saliva for adhesion and on correct design and shaping to avoid dislodgment by muscle actions, and rest upon a rather thin mucosa covering relatively small amounts of bone for support. For maximum chewing power and desired stability, the forces of mastication should be applied bilaterally and simultaneously upon the long axis of the teeth. Mastication creates multiple forces of various directions that are applied to several different surfaces of the denture teeth and base, and because many of these forces act to dislodge the prosthesis, dentures simply do not stay adequately secured at all times.

Extensive information exists concerning the decreased biting and chewing ability of denture wearers. Studies from Chauncey, Wayler, Kapur, and Loftus (1980), Feldman et al. (1980), and Kapur, Soman, and Yurkstas (1964) confirm that missing teeth, even when replaced by dentures, reduce masticatory ability. Gibbs, Mahan, Mauderli, and Lundeen (1966), in their research into human bite strength, found that the bite force of natural teeth averages 162 pounds, whereas that of the complete denture averages 35 pounds and of the maxillary complete denture–mandibular overdenture is about 51 pounds. Winkler (1979) found that the force necessary to masticate food can vary from 5 to 175 pounds with natural teeth, with the wide range resulting from a person's choice of foods, the condition of the supporting structure of the teeth, and the person's muscular development. The force used in mastication by the denture wearer averaged only 22 to 24 pounds, and the maximum force that could be applied comfortably on a single tooth of a denture was 26 pounds. The bicuspid and first molar area was found to carry the heaviest load and the force exerted in the incisal area only 9 pounds (Winkler, 1979). Thus, it is clear that this decrease in bite force may limit the foods that the denture wearer can consume.

Malpositioning of dentures under these forces creates a "pinching" effect on the gums between the denture and the hard bone beneath. These malpositionings can be acute or chronic in nature and lead to lacerations, bruising, and ulcerations that breech the integrity of the mucosa and create frank portals of entry for infectious agents. The swallowing process also is altered under the anticipated and actually experienced pain of these lesions. Chronic abnormal pressure from dentures causes not only soft tissue damage but also bone resorption. This further compromises bony support for the denture by changing the anatomy for which the original denture was constructed. Therefore, the denture becomes permanently altered in fit, leading to more looseness, mobility, and tissue damage.

Psychosocial Aspects of Denture Wearing. Loose dentures not only cause damage to the delicate oral mucosa, but also can produce extreme mental anguish, disappointment, and depression (Bolender, Swoope, & Smith, 1969; Thines et al., 1987). Many elderly persons, especially those who are medically compromised and institutionalized, have few opportunities for entertainment and pleasurable experiences and therefore place significant emphasis upon eating. In choosing gifts for elderly loved ones, people often select foods thought to be enjoyable. These gifts actually may be problematic for the edentulous group because they may be difficult or impossible to consume.

Denture Maintenance

Two types of denture maintenance activities should be undertaken. The first are those that the patient needs to perform daily. The second are periodic services required of a dental professional.

Denture Wearer Preventative Maintenence Activities. Like natural dentition, dentures require daily attention. It is most important that they be brushed with soap and water and a soft nylon brush. It is necessary to clean obviously dirty areas, as well as any material residing in crevices. Occasionally, the use of any of a variety of over-the-counter cleaning products is recommended. Products that contain alkaline peroxide will produce a bubbling action that will help in removing small particulate matter, but they will not replace the need for daily brushing of the dentures. Deposits that are left on dentures are often plaque (Figure 7.7) and will contain microbial organisms. If not removed, they may produce any of several infections within the oral cavity, often under the dentures.

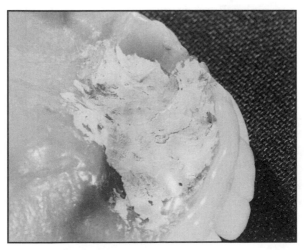

Figure 7.7. Dental plaque coating a denture.

Poor denture and oral hygiene have been associated with oral infections, either independently or in association with denture trauma. A common yeast, *Candida albicans,* is often seen in conjunction with denture stomatitis. In denture stomatitis the mucus along the alveolar ridges or on the roof of the mouth is inflamed and appears edematous and a deep red color. Denture stomatitis is associated with denture trauma due, most often, to poorly fitting dentures. In 90% of patients with this condition, these areas are infected with *C. albicans.* Treatment is threefold. First, if denture trauma is occurring, the denture is adjusted to improve the fit. Second, an antifungal medication may be prescribed. Finally, the patient is provided with education about the importance of proper denture hygiene. One part of that hygiene program may include soaking the dentures overnight in an over-the-counter hypochlorite denture cleaner or 0.1% aqueous chlorhexidine gluconate to kill organisms that may remain after brushing.

Maintenance Provided by the Dental Professional. Many denture wearers assume that having their teeth extracted and being fitted for dentures is a one-time event and does not require checkups by a dental professional. It is not uncommon for a denture wearer to report having worn the same set of dentures for two or more decades. As with any other manmade product, however, dentures do require routine care and periodic maintenance. Most denture wearers probably provide better maintenance for their automobiles than their dentures. Very few individuals still drive the car they drove when they obtained their dentures and most have had their autos maintained or repaired more often than they have returned for routine dental checkups. Dentures have an expected life of only 10 years. Perhaps more important, because dentures place a great deal of stress on the oral mucosa, the denture wearer needs to have routine checkups to assess the adequacy of denture fit. This is necessary because of the normal changes that are associated with aging and especially because of the dynamic changes seen in the alveolar ridges due to bone resorption. Early detection can help to prevent a mobile denture that impairs mastication or causes traumatic injuries. Routine examinations also can detect problems with the prosthetic device. The fractured dentures shown in Figure 7.8 cannot be expected to fit securely and may well cause mucosal trauma.

The dental professional should examine all tissues of the oral cavity and pharyngeal areas, check any denture appliance, and assess the

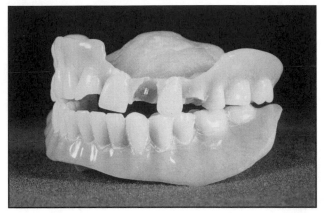

Figure 7.8. A broken and unserviceable denture. Photo by Robert M. Brown.

oral hygiene status. Any prosthesis and remaining teeth should be properly cleaned, and any patient complaint should be addressed and explained in terms the patient and caregiver can understand. Moreover, because informed patients are often the best advocates for their own care, professionals should try to delegate as much responsibility for oral health care to the patient as possible. It is particularly helpful for the patient to notice and report subtle changes in the denture fit that occur over time. Caregivers also should be instructed regarding proper hygiene practice because some elderly patients are unable to practice self-care.

Human tissue constantly undergoes change, but the material of a hard denture is more permanent and basically retains its size and shape. Therefore, as human tissues adapt to their daily environment and demands, the dental prosthetic device must be evaluated for adjustment by trained personnel. Over time, routine oral examinations afford the opportunity for the dentist to provide small, incremental, and systematic adjustments to dental devices. This usually means immediate relief and less acclamation for the patient. When the oral tissues undergo resorption and shrinkage, space is produced between the gums and the tissue side of the denture. This usually can be corrected by relining the undersurface of the denture with a permanent rigid material or with a semiflexible material to help condition the gums back to health. Relining is a procedure in which only a portion of the tissue surface of the denture base is replaced, whereas a rebased denture replaces the entire denture except for the teeth. In the latter case, when the base is completely worn, the teeth typically need replacing or a new denture may be needed. The continuous pressure created by bite forces is transferred through dentures to the underlying hard and soft tissues; therefore, denture wearers should remove the prosthesis for at least 8 of every 24 hours, allowing sufficient rest and recovery for the tissues and opportunity for the tissues to receive needed blood supplies.

Appropriate Referral for Dental Care

The dysphagia clinician needs to refer patients for dental consultation when appropriate. Although most dentists experienced with treating the compromised patient will gladly accept any referral, the results will be better if the clinician can provide the dentist with accurate referral information and expectations for treatment. When the dysphagia clinician can recognize normal oral health, he or she will be better prepared to identify abnormalities. A way for the clinician to learn is to inspect his or her own mouth. When the clinician looks into a patient's mouth, he or she should find the mouth clean, with no debris located on or about the teeth, under the tongue, in the sulci of the maxilla and mandible, or on any dental prosthetic device. If teeth are present, they should be in good repair and their approximation upon occlusion should be noted. Sharp, jagged edges on natural or prosthetic teeth are a source of lacerations to the tongue and lips and should be reported.

As with any tissue of the body, the oral mucosa should not exhibit any of the four cardinal signs of inflammation: redness, swelling, pain, or excessive warmth. The gums are normally pink in color, and their shape should follow the contour of the underlying bone. Dentures should also conform to the general architecture of the alveolar ridges and surrounding musculature and be secure. Severely worn chewing surfaces of the denture teeth, as well as any cracks or fractures of the acrylic, are indications that the denture needs repair. Cracked, red, and sore corners of the mouth indicate overclosure of the jaws and can lead to fungal infections that are difficult to heal.

The amount and condition of saliva should be noted. Although a dry mouth is common upon awaking, persistent xerostomia should be noted and reported. Too little or too much saliva is also an obvious alert. Saliva abnormalities tend to affect the cleansing action of the mouth, resulting in debris left on the teeth, mucosa, and dental devices.

Any swelling warrants a referral to the patient's dentist. Underlying lymph nodes in the oral cavity and neck areas and blocked salivary glands and ducts may swell occasionally, but need attention to rule out more serious conditions. Swelling of the gums may be localized or general and may indicate periodontal disease, leukemia, or other maladies. Any laceration, ulcer, or discoloration may indicate problems with dentures or the beginning of oral cancer. Any jaw shift from midline upon opening and closing of the mouth should be referred for evaluation as it may indicate a TMJ problem. Paralysis of the lips, tongue, or other facial muscles should be referred, because special dental appliances such as obturators or unique denture bases and extensions may be of help.

Observation of the patient during mastication can provide valuable information. This evaluation should take place in the patient's normal environment so that body positioning and other habits may be assessed. Impressions for dental prosthetic devices are obtained with the patient seated in an upright position. The devices tend to malfunction when the person is leaning forward and slumped over or lying down during eating. Head position should also be noted since tipping to one side or the other can have an effect on mastication and swallowing.

Summary

Our intent in this chapter was to inform dysphagia clinicians about the many and varied dental aspects that affect eating and swallowing. The dental professional can offer much to the dysphagia management team and to the dysphagia clinician that will improve patient care. Dysphagia clinicians should seek out dental health providers when oral abnormalities are seen. To enter into this relationship, the clinician needs to be able to recognize normal oral health and refer any oral or dental condition that is of concern. Although nondentists are not expected to identify all oral pathologic conditions, genuine concern and interest should be adequate justification to refer a patient to the dentist. With open communication practitioners will be able to call upon their colleagues to have suspicions identified, confirmed, or ruled out. With this level of interaction, the patient's quality of life will be enhanced for elderly patients with dysphagia.

References

Bates, J. F., Elwood, P. C., & Foster, W. (1971). Studies relating mastication and nutrition in the elderly. *Gerontology Clinics, 13,* 227–232.

Baum, B. J. (1986). Salivary gland function during aging. *Gerodontics, 2,* 61–64.

Bergman, B., & Carlsson, G. E. (1972). Review of 54 complete denture wearers: Patients' opinions 1 year after treatment. *Acta Odontol Scand, 30,* 399–414.

Bolender, C. L., Swoope, C. C., & Smith, D. E. (1969). The Cornell Medical Index as a prognostic aid for complete denture patients. *Journal of Prosthetic Dentistry, 22*(1), 20–29.

Carlsson, G. E. (1984). Masticatory efficiency: The effect of age, the loss of teeth and prosthetic rehabilitation. *International Dental Journal, 34,* 93–97.

Carlsson, G. E., & Lindquist, L. W. (1994). Ten-year longitudinal study of masticatory function in edentulous patients treated with fixed complete dentures on osseointegrated implants. *International Journal of Prosthodontics, 7*(5), 448–453.

Chauncey, H. H., Wayler, A. H., Kapur, K. K., & Loftus, E. R. (1980). Tooth loss and food acceptability: Correlation of subjective and objective masticatory ability [Abstract]. *Journal of Dental Research, 59*(Special Issue A), 373.

Cheraskin, E. (1976). The ecology of the prosthodontic problem. *Journal of the American Dental Association, 92,* 133–139.

Davis, J. W. (1989). Prosthodontic management of swallowing disorders. *Dysphagia, 3,* 199–205.

Department of Veterans Affairs. (1998). *Clinical care guidelines for dental management of the medically compromised patient.* Washington, DC: Veterans Affairs Central Office.

Emick-Herring, B., & Wood, P. (1990). A team approach to neurologically based swallowing disorders. *Rehabilitation Nursing, 15*(3), 132.

Ettinger, R. L. (1973). Diet, nutrition, and masticatory ability in a group of elderly edentulous patients. *Australian Dental Journal, 18*(1), 12–19.

Feldman, R. S., Kapur, K. K., Alman, M. A., & Chauncey, H. H. (1980). Aging and mastication: Changes in performance and in the swallowing threshold with natural dentition. *Journal of the American Geriatrics Society, 28*(3), 97–103.

Gibbs, H. C., Mahan, P. E., Mauderli, A., & Lundeen, H. C. (1966). Limits of human bite strength. *Research and Education, 56*(2), 226–229.

Hartsook, E. I. (1974). Food selection, dietary adequacy and related dental problems of patients with dental prostheses. *Journal of Prosthetic Dentistry, 32*(1), 32–40.

Heath, M. R. (1973). Dental state and bone loss in the elderly. *Proceedings of the Royal Society of Medicine, 66,* 590–594.

Hobdell, M. H., Sheihan, A., & Cowell, C. R. (1970). The prevalence of full and partial dentures in British populations. *British Medical Journal, 128*(9), 437–442.

Hutchins, B. F., & Giancarlo, J. L. (1991). Developing a comprehensive dysphagia program. *Seminars in Speech and Language, 12*(3), 209–215.

Kapur, K. K., Soman, S. D., & Yurkstas, A. A. (1964). Test foods for measuring masticatory performance of denture wearers. *Journal of Prosthetic Dentistry, 14,* 483–491.

Kiwayk, H. A. (1981). Psychosocial factors in dental needs of the elderly. *Special Care in Dentistry, 1,* 22–30.

Langer, A. (1976, December). Oral signs of aging and their clinical significance. *Geriatrics,* pp. 65–69.

A Look at Dental Diseases and Treatments. (1997, February). *Consumers' Research Magazine, 80*(6), 14–20.

Martinello, B. P., & Leake, J. L. (1971). Oral health status in three London, Ontario, homes for the aged. *Journal of the Canadian Dental Association, 37,* 429–432.

Martone, A. L. (1962, March–April). The phenomenon of function in complete denture prosthodontics. *Journal of Prosthetic Dentistry*, 206–219.

Mirro, J. F., & Patey, C. (1991). Developing a dysphagia dietary program. *Seminars in Speech and Language*, 12(3), 218–226.

Perlman, A., Langmore, S., Milianti, F., Miller, R., Mills, R. H., & Zenner, P. (1991). Comprehensive Clinical Examination of Oropharyngeal Swallowing Function: Veterans Administration Procedure. *Seminars in Speech and Language*, 12, 246–253.

Pilgrim, F. J., & Kamen, J. M. (1959). Patterns of food preference through factor analysis. *Journal of Marketing*, 24, 68–72.

Ramfjord, S. P., & Ash, M. M., Jr. (1971). *Occlusion*. Philadelphia: Saunders.

Roder, D. M. (1975). Tooth loss in South Australia. *Community Dentistry and Oral Epidemiology*, 3, 283–287.

Ross, L. N., & Beall, G. T. (1984). *Health promotion and aging: Opportunities for national organizations*. Washington, DC: The National Council on the Aging.

Shaw, J. (1981). Dysphagia in the adult: Its clinical significance, diagnosis, and management: Part III. *British Journal of Clinical Practice*, 35, 73–78.

Sheppard, I. M., Schwartz, L. R., & Sheppard, S. M. (1971). Oral status of edentulous and complete denture-wearing patients. *Journal of the American Dental Association*, 83(3), 614—620.

Storer, R. (1985). The gastrointestinal system—The oral tissues. In J. C. Brockelhurst (Ed.), *Textbook of Geriatric Medicine and Gerontology* (pp. 500–507). London: Churchill Livingstone.

Szczesniak, A. S., & Kleyn, D. H. (1963). Consumer awareness of texture and other food attributes. *Food Technology*, 17, 74–77.

Thines, T., Karuza, J., Jr., & Miller, W. A. (1987). Oral health impact on quality of life: Methodological and conceptual concerns. *Gerodontics*, 3, 100–102.

Winkler, S. (1979). *Essentials of Complete Denture Prosthodontics*. Philadelphia: Saunders.

Yurkstas, A., & Emerson, W. H. (1964). Dietary selection of persons with natural and artificial teeth. *Journal of Prosthetic Dentistry, 14,* 695–709.

Zemlin, W. R. (1998). *Speech and hearing science: Anatomy and physiology* (4th ed.). Needham Heights, MA: Allyn & Bacon.

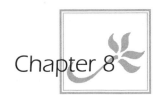

Chapter 8

Evaluation of the Patient with Impaired Pulmonary Function and Dysphagia

Karen J. Dikeman, Marta S. Kazandjian,
and Roperto Chua

Dikeman, Kazanjian, and Chua provide an in-depth discussion of the evaluation of patients with impaired pulmonary function. Central to their discussion is the interrelatedness of pulmonary function and swallowing.

1. *How are obstructive and restrictive pulmonary conditions different from each other?*

2. *What are two noninvasive monitoring tools that dysphagia clinicians can use to evaluate pulmonary function as they manage dysphagia in this population?*

3. *What special considerations should be made for a ventilator-dependent patient who is to undergo a dysphagia evaluation?*

⚹   ⚹   ⚹

Dysphagia researchers and clinicians are discovering that impairments in pulmonary function may have an impact on swallowing even in the absence of obvious neurologic disease. The influence of the respiratory, cardiac, and digestive systems on one another, or *reciprocity,* is related to the shared functions of human anatomical structures. The clearest illustration of this reciprocity between respiration and swallowing is with the evaluation of the patient with pulmonary disease and dysphagia. The clinician needs a thorough understanding of normal pulmonary physiology before he or she can interpret the effects of disease processes and disordered pulmonary function on swallowing. Tracheostomy and ventilatory dependence, a common sequela of pulmonary impairment, further compromises swallowing by changing the dynamics of the upper airway. This creates additional challenges for the dysphagia clinician, the speech–language pathologist, during the evaluation process.

Respiratory Physiology: A Practical Review

The function of the pulmonary system is to deliver oxygen from the atmosphere to the blood and into the cells, and transport carbon dioxide from the cells to the blood and back into the atmosphere. Ventilation is the mechanical movement of air into and out of the lungs in a cyclic fashion. It is accomplished by the action of the respiratory muscles on the thorax. Inhalation is the inward flow of air, whereas exhalation is the outward flow of air from the respiratory tract. *Respiration* is often used synonymously for *ventilation*, but respiration should be used to refer to the exchange of oxygen (O_2) and carbon dioxide (CO_2) in the lungs and at the cellular level. Respiration is the primary function of a lung by which it supplies the body with oxygen and removes the waste product of metabolism, carbon dioxide. To fulfill this function, the lungs must have adequate ventilation. Maintenance of adequate ventilation is controlled partly by chemoreceptors, which are specialized cells (i.e., neural receptors) in the central nervous system that respond to gas levels in the blood, especially CO_2 levels, in order to inform the brain (brainstem) to activate the muscles of inspiration. The peripheral chemoreceptors are located at the bifurcation of the common carotid arteries and in the aortic bodies above and below the aortic arch. There are also neural receptors in the upper airway, lungs, respiratory muscles, and arteries (West, 1990).

Dynamics of Gas Exchange

Gas exchange in the lung is a passive two-way transfer of respiratory gases, O_2 and CO_2, between the alveoli of the lung, blood plasma, and hemoglobin molecules. Gas exchange is mediated by pressure gradients whereby gas molecules move from an area of relatively high partial pressure to an area of low partial pressure. In other words, oxygen diffuses from the alveoli, which have a high partial pressure of O_2 concentration, to the pulmonary capillaries, which have a low partial pressure of O_2 concentration (see Figure 8.1). At this level oxygen combines with hemoglobin in the red blood cells, which is transported to the body tissue capillaries. In these capillaries, O_2 is released from the hemoglobin into the cells. In the cells, O_2 and other nutritive substances are used. This process, known as metabolism, results in the production of energy, water, and CO_2. The CO_2 diffuses from tissue cells into venous blood and is carried in three forms. Some is physically dissolved in plasma (5% to 10%). This is reflected in the usual analysis of blood gases. Another portion of CO_2 is bound to proteins (20% to 30%). The majority of CO_2 is carried as bicarbonate ions after conversion in the red blood cells. Hydrogen ions combine with the bicarbonate ions (HCO_3) in the blood plasma and then divide into water and carbon dioxide. CO_2 diffuses from the plasma into the alveolus and is then eliminated via ventilation.

Homeostasis

The body normally exists in a state of internal equilibrium between multiple body systems known as homeostasis. The dysphagia clinician must understand how a disruption in homeostasis can potentially

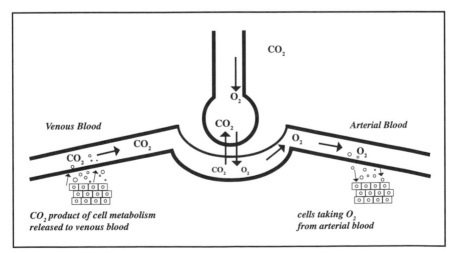

Figure 8.1. Gas exchange (O_2 and CO_2 molecules) over the alveolar capillary membrane. O_2 = oxygen; CO_2 = carbon dioxide.

impact swallowing function. Homeostasis is achieved via an acid–base balance in the blood (West, 1990). The acid–base balance, or pH level, is a measure of alkalinity and acidity. The pH of blood is maintained in a very narrow range (pH = 7.35 to 7.45) by a buffer system provided by the respiratory system (lungs) and the renal system (kidneys). The buffer system returns the pH of the blood to normal when an acid or alkali is added. The respiratory system responds to changes in pH by increasing ventilation (hyperventilation) or decreasing ventilation (hypoventilation), which decreases or increases CO_2 levels, respectively. The renal system, through the function of the kidneys, retains or excretes hydrogen ions and bicarbonate ions in or from the blood to maintain normal acid–base balance. If a patient moves out of the normal pH range, a variety of functions may be disrupted. For example, if a diabetic patient experiences metabolic acidosis (low pH) due to a low bicarbonate level, the respiratory system will compensate by hyperventilation to eliminate CO_2, and return pH levels to a normal range. Thus, a patient's ability to tolerate a dysphagia evaluation, or a meal, can be affected by a disrupted homeostasis that causes this rapid breathing.

The arterial blood gas (ABG) analysis is important in the diagnosis of acid–base balance. The ABG is based on a blood sample analysis, and the blood gas report contains the following information:

pH	7.35 – 7.45	(acidity or alkalinity)
$PaCO_2$	35 – 45 mm Hg	(partial pressure of arterial CO_2)
PaO_2	80 – 100 mm Hg	(partial pressure of arterial O_2)
HCO_3	24 – 26 mEq/L	(plasma bicarbonate)
Sat.%	97% – 98%	(percentage of oxygen saturation)
BE	0 – ± 2 mEq/L	(base excess)

The ABG report provides the medical team with detailed information regarding the patient's metabolic and respiratory condition (homeostasis). Acid–base imbalance is due to either a respiratory or a metabolic disorder or both. Changes in acid–base balance are reflected in the pH of arterial blood. The pH, PaO_2 and $PaCO_2$ values provide information regarding acid–base and respiratory status, whereas plasma bicarbonate (HCO_3) and base excess (BE) provide more information regarding metabolic acid–base status. Although the respiratory care practitioner and physician can use the ABG to identify early cardio-pulmonary disease or to serve as a follow-up for the appropriateness or effectiveness of pulmonary intervention, respiratory status can often be monitored by noninvasive means without resorting to painful arterial punctures.

The ABG and other pulmonary assessment measures are the dysphagia clinician's main source of objective information regarding the possible etiology of a patient's dysphagia. The dysphagic symptoms of patients with metabolic or respiratory disorders may resolve quickly after appropriate pulmonary intervention. The dysphagia clinician will have different expectations for patients in the intensive care unit who are acutely ill but do not have underlying neurologic dysfunction, versus patients who have neurologic impairment as the precipitating factor in their respiratory failure. In the previous example, the diabetic patient with metabolic acidosis experienced respiratory hyperventilation in an effort to normalize the acid–base balance. If this condition progresses without treatment, the patient may experience respiratory failure and require mechanical ventilatory support and nasogastric tube feeding. When the dysphagia clinician is called to the bedside to evaluate the patient's candidacy for resumption of oral feedings, an understanding of the patient's respiratory and medical course will be helpful in guiding the steps of the dysphagia evaluation. There must be communication between the pulmonary physician, respiratory care practitioner, and speech–language pathologist for the interpretation of blood gas results and the subsequent potential impact on the timing of the dysphagia evaluation.

Reciprocity Between Respiration and Swallowing

In addition to understanding normal respiratory physiology, the dysphagia clinician should appreciate the reciprocity between respiration and normal deglutition. The fundamentals of normal function will provide the building blocks for managing pulmonary disease and dysphagia.

The evolution of human anatomy has produced a system in which the structures for speech, swallowing, and respiration are shared. The descent of the larynx in humans places the airway in a direct path with a swallowed bolus. To ensure safety, special airway protective functions were also developed. Even small disruptions in the function or timing of relevant musculature contractions may lead to impairment in swallowing.

The structures and muscles that most significantly participate in both respiration and swallowing include the tongue, epiglottis, pharynx, cartilaginous larynx, and intrinsic and extrinsic laryngeal musculature. The tongue functions in oral preparation, bolus control, and bolus transport, as well as airway maintenance during oral preparation. The tongue and the soft palate function to close the nasal airway, and respiration continues to the point that the bolus is ready to be swallowed. At this point, the tongue assumes its vital role in the generation of positive pressures to drive the bolus through the pharynx. Martin and Robbins (1995), quoting other researchers and exploring the role of the tongue in pharyngeal motility, discussed the importance of this pressure generation as the predominant factor in pharyngeal clearance of a bolus. They concluded that the peristaltic wave created by the pharyngeal constrictors is essentially a secondary clearing mechanism, similar to peristalsis in the esophagus.

Tongue base contraction also contributes to downward epiglottic movement and airway closure. In a classic article, Ardran and Kemp (1967) discussed the protective role of the epiglottis during normal swallowing. The downward excursion of the epiglottis, meeting the arytenoids as the larynx elevates, provides one "level" of airway protection. Laryngeal elevation serves to mechanically move the larynx out of the path of the descending bolus. The aryepiglottic folds, arytenoid cartilages, false vocal folds, and true vocal folds close at other levels to protect the airway. At this point, airflow stops and subglottic airway pressures increase sharply. The rise in airway pressure appears necessary for normal glottic closure and normal "swallowing velocity" as the bolus moves through the pharynx (Eibling & Diez-Gross, 1996). As the larynx closes during the normal swallow, the pharynx shortens via the action of the pharyngeal constrictors, decreasing the distance that the bolus must travel. The cricopharyngeus muscle relaxes, and the upper esophageal sphincter is then pulled open by the combined mechanical traction created by the tongue and larynx, allowing entry of the bolus into the esophagus. At other times, such as during quiet respiration, the cricopharyngeus is in its normal resting posture, tightly closed to resist the entry of inspired air.

The finely timed movements of a normal swallow must occur in a prescribed hierarchy to ensure airway protection. The passageway through which the bolus travels is shared for respiration. Respiration must cease at the moment of the swallow. As the larynx closes, the bolus passes and respiration resumes. Research related to the timing of deglutition and respiration has focused upon both normal individuals and those with pulmonary impairment. In patients with pulmonary disease, disruption of the ability to close the airway at the appropriate time in the swallow can lead to respiratory compromise. Much of the research in the reciprocity of deglutition and breathing has demonstrated a difference in the *timing* of the swallow with respiration for the patient with respiratory disease (Martin, 1994; Nishino, Yonezawa, & Honda, 1995; Shaker et al., 1992; Smith, Wolkove, Colacone, & Kreisman, 1989). Shaker et al. (1992) reported that in most normal subjects, the swallow interrupts expiration; that is, prior to the swallow, the larynx closes and respiration ceases during expiration. The pharyngeal swallow triggers and the bolus moves through the pharynx. When the larynx opens again, expiration continues. The postswallow expiration was theorized to be a pulmonary defense to reduce the risk of aspiration after a swallow. However, in this study, patients with chronic obstructive pulmonary disease (COPD) swallowed more frequently during inspiration than normal age-matched controls. These results would imply that patients with compromised respiratory systems have alterations in the coordination of respiration and swallowing, as compared with age-matched controls. These individuals may also have difficulty in the generation and timing of an effective cough.

The coordination of respiration and swallowing can be influenced by other factors. Bolus size and consistency are two variables that may actually change the pattern of respiration. Martin and Robbins (1995) reported that the apneic interval, the amount of time that the airway is closed during the swallow, increases for large-volume liquid swallows. They stated that "larger volume swallows show longer apneic intervals and a higher incidence of post-swallow *inspiration*" (p. 456). This pattern may pose difficulties for patients with pulmonary dysfunction who are unable to maintain the longer apneic intervals necessary for large-bolus swallows. These patients typically fatigue during a meal and attempt to compensate by reducing bolus size and eating smaller food portions.

Disease Processes

The impact of respiration upon deglutition, and vice versa, mandates that the dysphagia clinician integrate his or her knowledge of the relationship between shared functions and patterns of respiration into the dysphagia assessment. In doing so, the clinician may predict how certain disease processes will affect safe swallowing and therefore guide the evaluation process.

Pulmonary diseases can be divided into two main types, obstructive and restrictive. Conditions such as cystic fibrosis, chronic bronchitis, asthma, bronchiectasis, and emphysema are classified under the term chronic obstructive pulmonary disease (COPD). These are diseases or conditions that cause chronic obstruction to airflow to and from the lungs. Restrictive conditions include neuromuscular diseases and pneumonia. In addition, cardiac impairment, such as congestive heart failure, can also have an impact on pulmonary status. The dysphagia clinician should appreciate the impact of these different diseases and conditions on a patient's overall status and potentially on swallowing function.

Obstructive Conditions

Patients with obstructive lung disease have an increase in resistance to the flow of air through the smaller pulmonary airways. Resistance to flow is greater on expiration than on inspiration. This type of patient needs to take less frequent breaths with longer expirations to more completely empty the lungs. Patients with these conditions are prone to hyperinflation of the lungs with air trapping and subsequent hypoxia and high levels of CO_2.

Patients with obstructive conditions are very sensitive to any increase in the work of breathing. The typical hyperinflation of the lungs causes rapid fatigue and limits the excursion of the diaphragm during respiration. Patients thus commonly report feeling "full" even after consuming only small amounts of food (Dikeman & Kazandjian, 1995; Edgar, 1994). Because CO_2 retention is characteristic for severe or advanced patients, the dysphagia clinician should obtain baseline O_2 and CO_2 levels prior to the swallowing evaluation and monitor these levels for further changes throughout the assessment. Martin, Logemann, Shaker, and Dodds (1994) and Martin (1994) discussed the incidence of dysphagia in patients with a diagnosis of COPD without associated neurologic deficits. The authors identified the discoordination between respiration and swallowing, and the increased work of breathing generated by eating as possible etiologies for the dysphagia.

Restrictive Conditions

The restrictive lung conditions are characterized by reduced expansion of the lungs during inspiration. This leads to a reduction in total lung capacity. In an attempt to meet respiratory demands, patients with this condition have a rapid, shallow respiratory pattern. This pattern is used to maintain adequate ventilation and oxygenation. When the respiratory muscles fatigue and muscle failure occurs, low O_2 saturation and high CO_2 levels signal impending respiratory failure. In most restrictive pulmonary conditions, expiratory muscle weakness is also present. This weakness decreases peak cough flows, reducing the ability to produce a functional cough, which in turn limits the patient's ability to clear secretions from the airway (Bach, 1996b). Bach (1996b) noted that decreased peak cough flow is usually a primary indication of the need for a tracheostomy tube.

Aspiration due to dysphagia can be a precipitating factor in respiratory failure for many patients with weak respiratory muscles (Hoo, Dhanani, & Santiago, 1995). Although it is important for the dysphagia clinician to try to identify aspiration clinically, the patient with weak respiratory musculature should also be monitored for adequate O_2 and CO_2 levels, as well as respiratory rate, throughout the assessment. Increased respiratory rate will indicate that the patient is working hard to maintain O_2 and eliminate CO_2. Energy is being expended to support respiration, and eating poses an additional stress that the patient's respiratory system may not be able to tolerate.

Cardiopulmonary Conditions

The cardiac and respiratory systems are closely linked. The cardiovascular system ensures that blood is adequately circulated to and from the heart through the circulatory system and to body tissues. The respiratory system ensures adequate transfer of O_2 from the lungs to the blood, and removal of CO_2 from the blood via the lungs. In conditions such as congestive heart failure, fluid accumulates in parts of the body. Fluid accumulation in and around the lungs interferes with cardiac and pulmonary function and, if untreated, may result in cardiac–respiratory failure (Eubanks & Bone, 1990). A patient in the early stages of congestive heart failure may experience fatigue and breathlessness during a meal (Frownfelter & Dean, 1996). Dysphagia is also a potential complication of cardiac surgery (e.g., cardiac artery bypass grafts) secondary to damage to the vagus nerve, or stroke (Hogue et al., 1995). A history of coronary artery bypass graft or vocal changes following cardiac surgery should alert the dysphagia clinician to potential airway protection problems. Additional complications associated with the surgical procedure and intubation include decreased base of tongue strength and elevation. This may occur secondary to the continuous pressure of the endotracheal tube resting on the base of the tongue (Logemann, 1993).

Patients with cardiopulmonary conditions are susceptible to even minor changes in the work of breathing related to an increased need for oxygen. Stress on the patient will be quickly reflected in increased cardiac or respiratory rate. Frownfelter and Dean (1996) commented that exercise, or increased energy need, "affects all steps in the oxygen transport pathway" (p. 20). This includes both cardiac output and ventilation (gas exchange). Therefore, fluctuations in pulse and respiratory rate during a dysphagia assessment or a meal must be monitored. The dysphagia clinician should know what signs and symptoms are indicative of impending cardiac–respiratory difficulties and contact other team members accordingly.

Implications of Tracheostomy and Ventilator Dependence on Impaired Pulmonary Function

Increasingly, and in a variety of health care settings, the dysphagia clinician is called on to evaluate the patient who is tracheostomized and ventilator dependent. Two of the primary indications for a tracheostomy are to provide an artificial airway, because of the inability of the patient to protect the airway, and the need for connection to mechanical ventilation. In general, if a patient has required an endotracheal tube and mechanical ventilation for 14 to 21 days and is not expected to be easily weaned from the ventilator, a tracheotomy is performed (Heffner, 1993). A tracheotomy may also be performed for individuals who cannot maintain adequate ventilation due to failure of the respiratory musculature as a result of insufficient vital capacity (Bach, 1996c). A tracheotomy, however, need not be done for ventilatory impairment alone (Bach, 1996b). Bach (1996b) described the use of noninvasive techniques to provide long-term ventilatory support. When feasible, noninvasive techniques can avoid the many complications associated with long-term tracheotomy.

Dysphagia is one complication associated with tracheotomy. Many tracheostomized or ventilator-dependent individuals will continue to eat orally, especially if there is no discrete oropharyngeal dysphagia secondary to neurologic dysfunction or structural abnormalities. However, the potential for dysphagia is heightened by the physical presence of the tube itself, as well as by the underlying condition that precipitated the need for the artificial airway (Dettelbach, Gross, Mahlmann, & Eibling, 1995). Additionally, patients who are tracheostomized and ventilator dependent are at increased risk of infections such as pneumonia due to the presence of the tracheostomy tube and their reliance on mechanical ventilation. Nosocomial pneumonia is an infection that is acquired in a health care setting, commonly in an acute care unit. Niederman, Ferranti, Ziegler, Merrill, and Reynolds (1984) noted that persistent bacterial colonization often occurs in individuals with tracheostomy and ventilator dependence and may lead to serious respiratory infections and other complications. These individuals, usually acutely ill, often have other risk factors for respiratory infection, including depressed immune systems and bacterial growth in the oropharynx (Kirsch & Sanders, 1988). When excessive aspiration of the bacterial flora from the mouth occurs, tracheostomized and ventilator-dependent individuals are less likely to successfully combat infection. They are also more likely to aspirate secondary to the mechanical and physiologic complications of the tracheostomy tube and ventilator (DeVita & Spierer-Rundback, 1990; Tolep, Getch, & Criner, 1996). Therefore, nosocomial pneumonia is a common and often fatal infection of tracheostomized and ventilator-dependent patients, and aspiration is believed to be a common route of infection. For many tracheostomized and ventilator-dependent individuals, dysphagia will contribute to the likelihood of aspiration and infection. Figure 8.2 illustrates the multiple factors that may interact and lead to dysphagic impairment in the patient in the acute care medical setting. The etiologies of the dysphagic impairment are multiple, but are often due to physiologic (airflow) or mechanical causes. For the mechanically ventilated patient, there are additional causal factors.

Airflow Issues

The reduction, or cessation, of airflow through the upper respiratory tract in individuals with tracheostomy and ventilator dependence poses the most significant disruption to normal swallowing physiology

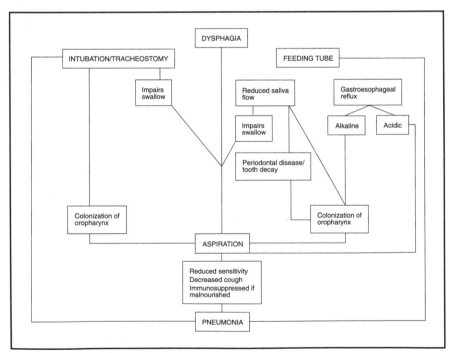

Figure 8.2. Diagnostic algorithm for the assessment of patients with dysphagia. From "Dysphagia in Neurologic Patients in the ICU Setting," by S. E. Langmore, 1996, *Seminars in Neurology, 16,* p. 335. Copyright 1996 by Thieme Medical Publishers. Reprinted with permission.

and function. A vital mechanism for bolus movement through the pharynx is the use of upper airway flow to generate pharyngeal pressures. These pressures also assist in propelling the bolus into the esophagus (McConnel, Cerenko, & Mendelsohn, 1988). The lack of adequate airway pressures can result in the accumulation of pharyngeal residue and, subsequently, aspiration after the swallow.

Eibling and Diez-Gross (1996) discussed the contribution of subglottic air pressure to swallowing, measuring airflow and pressure peaks through a tracheostomy tube at the moment of the swallow. The authors noted that individuals with open, unoccluded tracheostomy tubes experienced expiratory air leakage from the tube that prevented the achievement of a pressure peak during the pharyngeal swallow. The placement of a one-way speaking valve (Passy-Muir) restored a more normal, "closed" system and eliminated the air leakage, restoring the accumulation of positive pressure peak of an average of 10 cm H₂O. Only minimal pressures were noted with open tracheostomy tubes. The authors theorized that the loss of positive subglottic air pressures is a major contributing factor to dysphagic impairment in tracheostomized individuals. These findings were confirmed during their videofluoroscopic studies. Subjects with open tracheostomy tubes aspirated, whereas individuals wearing Passy-Muir valves failed to exhibit this phenomenon. Eibling and Diez-Gross (1996) suggested that in the tracheostomized patient, lack of sufficient subglottic air pressure to signal glottic closure and the cessation of respiration places the patient at increased risk of aspiration. It should be noted that the Passy-Muir speaking valve is currently the only one-way ventilator valve listed by the Food and Drug Administration (FDA) for purposes of improving swallowing function.

Scintigraphy has also been used to document aspiration in tracheostomized individuals. Stachler, Hamlet, Choi, and Fleming (1996) demonstrated that aspiration in tracheostomized individuals was reduced when a one-way speaking valve (Passy-Muir) was in place, as compared with an open tracheostomy tube. The authors identified the restoration of positive subglottic air pressure as one mechanism in the reduction of aspiration.

Leder, Tarro, and Burrell (1996) did not find that occlusion of the tracheostomy tube influenced the prevalence of aspiration in their short-term study of 20 subjects. The type of tracheal occlusion was not specified, but the authors did not use one-way speaking valves. They believed that the etiology of aspiration in these individuals was related to other aspects of their medical status and individual dysphagic impairment. The authors suggested that tracheal occlusion be carefully investigated in future studies of aspiration.

The loss of upper airflow in tracheostomized and ventilator-dependent individuals also affects other aspects of swallowing function. As previously discussed, swallowing is a complex physiologic process finely coordinated with respiration. Normally, swallowing interrupts expiration, but this pattern may be disrupted in individuals with restrictive pulmonary disease. An inspiration rather than an expiration may follow the swallow (Shaker et al., 1992). In their study, tracheostomized and ventilator-dependent individuals commonly had underlying lung disease, and were at risk of this discoordinated swallowing pattern and increased risk of airway protection problems even before the tracheotomy. In individuals with pulmonary disease and open tracheostomy tubes, an inspiration *during* the swallow, perhaps in the presence of increased pharyngeal residue, would increase the risk of laryngeal penetration or aspiration.

When aspiration does occur, coughing and resultant airway clearance is a normal response. Loss of airflow through the upper respiratory tract decreases the sensation of the larynx to penetrated and aspirated material (Buckwalter & Sasaki, 1984; Feldman, Deal, & Urqhart, 1966). This is especially true for patients who have had inflated tracheostomy tube cuffs for extended periods. While cuff inflation has an immediate and negative effect on the cough, airflow changes create an additional impact. Over time, possibly a period of months, the cough will become ineffective secondary to the desensitization created by the loss of airflow through the glottis. When upper airway flow is eventually restored, after cuff deflation or decannulation, the reflexive cough is often initially absent in response to airway penetration.

The productivity of the cough is also impaired in individuals with tracheostomy and ventilator dependence. If the individual with an open tracheostomy does attempt to initiate a cough, little air is available to generate the necessary clearing forces (Eibling & Diez-Gross, 1996). Clearance of the material from the airway by suctioning, mechanical insufflation–exsufflation, or assisted cough techniques is required.

Finally, airway protection may be affected at the level of the vocal folds in tracheostomized patients. The integrity of the glottic closure response has been studied with regard to subglottic air pressure (Ikari

& Sasaki, 1980; Sasaki & Buchwalter, 1984). A weakened laryngeal closure response has been demonstrated in tracheostomized individuals (Ikari & Sasaki, 1980; Sasaki, Suzuki, Horiuchi, & Kirchner, 1977) and appears related to the lack of air building up beneath the glottis. Subglottic pressure appears to be necessary for a glottic closure response to occur and provide airway protection at this level (Eibling & Diez-Gross, 1996).

Mechanical Complications of Tracheostomy

Reduced laryngeal excursion secondary to the physical restrictions of the tracheostomy tube, the cuff, or both has long been recognized as one contributing factor to dysphagia in tracheostomized individuals (Bonanno, 1971; Feldman et al., 1966). If the anterior and superior movement of the larynx is significantly limited, several aspects of the pharyngeal swallow will be impacted. The shortening of the pharynx and contact of the arytenoids with the base of the epiglottis will be diminished. In this circumstance the larynx will not move out of the path of the descending bolus, increasing the risk for penetration and aspiration. Also, the mechanical leverage, which assists in pulling the cricopharynx open, is decreased. This has been associated with decreased pharyngeal clearance and pyriform sinus pooling, and can increase risk of aspiration after the swallow. The degree of laryngeal fixation can be heightened by several factors, including the location and size of the tracheotomy incision and the presence of an inflated cuff.

To allow the tracheostomy tube to move easily with the larynx, vertical tracheotomy incisions are favored over horizontal (Nash, 1988). However, individual surgical technique and patient anatomy may affect the incision created. Additionally, scarring and granuloma around the stoma site may occur, more frequently in longer term tracheostomy. Decreased laryngeal excursion is also possible in individuals who have been orally intubated (Stauffer, Olson, & Petty, 1981). Potentially, the weight and pressure of the endotracheal tube decreases lingual excursion and strength. This may also affect the elevation and retraction of the tongue base, reducing the driving force of the tongue during the swallow.

Cuff inflation has been identified as a significant factor in dysphagia. The inflated cuff drags along the tracheal wall and can further anchor the larynx, limiting laryngeal excursion (Bonanno, 1971; Buchwalter &

Sasaki, 1984). Tracheomalacia is also a potential complication produced by the friction of the cuff on the tracheal wall. Impingement of the inflated cuff on the esophagus can create a physical barrier to the passage of a bolus, as illustrated in Figure 8.3. A typical clinical finding relating to esophageal compression by a tracheostomy tube cuff is expulsion of saliva, secretions, or food particles from the stoma site. The bolus cannot pass through the compressed esophagus, is forced into the pharynx and eventually the larynx, and is aspirated below the vocal folds.

Complications of Mechanical Ventilation

Many factors create an increased risk of dysphagia in the patient receiving invasive mechanical ventilation. These include the potential complications of intubation and tracheotomy discussed earlier, and additional factors related directly to mechanical ventilation. Tolep et al. (1996) discussed swallowing dysfunction in patients receiving mechanical ventilation. They noted that 80% of patients receiving mechanical ventilation (without concomitant neuromuscular disorders) had abnormal findings on videofluoroscopic swallowing studies. Multiple etiologies for the dysphagia were posited. DeVita and Spierer-Rundback

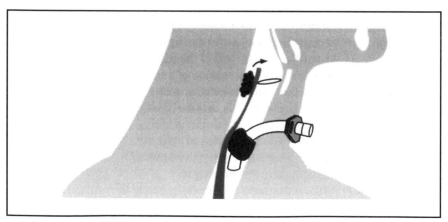

Figure 8.3. Obstruction of the esophagus by an inflated tracheostomy tube cuff. From *Communication and Swallowing Management of Tracheostomized and Ventilator-Dependent Adults* (p. 244), by K. J. Dikeman and M. S. Kazandjian, 1995, San Diego: Singular Publishing Group. Copyright 1995 by Singular Publishing Group, Inc. Reprinted with permission.

(1990) also discussed the prevalence of dysphagia in individuals who had been intubated and tracheostomized. These authors noted that dysphagia was present in individuals whose primary impairment was tracheostomy and ventilator dependence, and discussed the discoordination of respiration and swallowing as a precipitating factor.

Typically, when a patient is receiving positive-pressure, invasive mechanical ventilation, the tracheostomy tube cuff is kept inflated. The combined anchoring effect of the cuff, coupled with the weight of the ventilatory tubing, has a significant mechanical effect upon swallowing. Humidification devices may add weight and bulk, further limiting laryngeal excursion.

Although cuff deflation can often facilitate safe swallowing in the ventilator-dependent patient, crucial timing aspects of the swallow may be disrupted. Loss of the normal apneic interval occurs in individuals who have difficulty timing airway closure with a swallow and the mandatory mechanical breath supplied by the ventilator (Tippett & Siebens, 1991). Cuff deflation and placement of a one-way speaking valve, such as a Passy-Muir ventilator valve, may normalize the ability to coordinate swallowing with the ventilator breath by restoring subglottic air pressure.

Role of Pulmonary Assessment Measures in the Dysphagia Evaluation

Bedside monitoring of pulmonary function parameters will provide dysphagia clinicians with an indication of the mechanics of ventilation. Information obtained is useful in assessing the patient's ability to participate in the swallowing evaluation. Bedside monitoring most typically incorporates physical assessment coupled with objective monitoring tools, including spirometry, oximetry, and capnography.

Physical Assessment

Physical assessment is an important part of the total evaluation process. It incorporates observation of the patient's color, respiratory rate, and breathing pattern. The respiratory care practitioner or nurse also obtains vital signs (pulse rate, temperature, and blood pressure). A cyanotic or bluish discoloration of the nail bed and skin is monitored as a potential sign of hypoxia or failure of tissue oxygenation. Respiratory rate is the number of breaths per minute, normally between 12 and 20. A respiratory rate in excess of 35 per minute may be an indication of impending respiratory failure. Breathing patterns vary depending on the underlying pulmonary condition. The breathing effort should be minimal on inhalation and passive on exhalation.

The diaphragm is the primary muscle of inspiration. Significant increases in the effort of breathing, as seen in some respiratory abnormalities, may cause the accessory muscles of respiration (the scalene and the sternocleidomastoid muscles) to be active. Abnormalities in any of the physical assessment parameters will prompt the dysphagia clinician to consult with the medical team regarding possible etiologies and ongoing intervention. The dysphagia clinician often defers an evaluation when clinical parameters seem abnormal, unless the team indicates that the observed respiratory pattern represents the patient's baseline status. At times, medical support by respiratory or nursing staff can permit at least a limited dysphagia evaluation despite an abnormal physical assessment.

General Pulmonary Function Tests

In addition to the physical assessment, the respiratory care practitioner and physician obtain further diagnostic information through pulmonary function tests. Pulmonary function tests measure lung volumes and capacities and direct the respiratory care practitioner in appropriate intervention. Tidal volume, vital capacity, and peak expiratory flow are the critical measures of pulmonary function that can be obtained with a spirometer.

Tidal volume is the amount of air moved into and out of the patient's lungs with each normal breath. Normal tidal volume is estimated at 5 to 7 ml/kg of ideal body weight. The portion of tidal volume not participating in gas exchange is termed anatomical dead space. Anatomical dead space must be filled with inhaled volume before air can reach the contributing airways (i.e., alveoli). When tidal volume decreases, due to respiratory muscle fatigue or accumulation of secretions, only a small amount of tidal volume participates in gas exchange. If the tidal volume is not sufficient, hypoxia and respiratory failure can occur.

Vital capacity is the maximum amount of air that can be fully exhaled after a maximum inhalation. Forced vital capacity is the maximum amount of air that can be *forcefully* and quickly exhaled after a maximum inhalation. Measurement of vital capacity requires a patient's cooperation and effort and is an indicator of ventilatory reserve and the potential ability of the respiratory muscles to sustain ventilation. Vital capacity measurements decrease as respiratory muscle weakness increases. Normal vital capacity is estimated at 65 to 75 ml/kg of normal body weight. If a patient's vital capacity is less than 10 to 15 ml/kg of normal body weight, the patient may exhibit impairment in the ability to cough, clear, or mobilize secretions; to prevent atelectasis (collapse of the alveoli); and to sustain adequate ventilation.

Peak expiratory flow rate (PEFR) is the maximum flow rate achieved during a forced vital capacity maneuver. This requires patient coordination and is effort dependent. PEFRs are expressed in liters per minute or second. Normal PEFRs are > 600 L/min (10 L/sec). PEFR identifies the severity of airway obstruction, airway resistance to flow, and expiratory muscle strength. This relates to the patient's ability to produce a forceful cough. A more direct parameter is peak cough flow (Bach, 1996a).

Noninvasive Monitoring Tools

Noninvasive monitoring allows clinicians to monitor a patient's condition without entering the body or puncturing the skin. These methods are generally easy to use, less risky, more comfortable for the patient than are invasive techniques, and provide continuous monitoring of the patient's condition. Pulse oximetry and capnography are two of the most widely used noninvasive monitoring tools.

Pulse Oximetry. Pulse oximetry is based on the principles of light absorption and pulse detection. A light-emitting diode in the probe (usually placed on a finger or an ear lobe) transmits light of two different wavelengths through tissue and hemoglobin. Measurements can be affected by patient movement, dark skin pigmentation, dark finger nail polish, bright external light in the room, and several disease processes that affect circulation (Oakes, 1994). Pulse oximetry is used for the measurement of oxyhemoglobin saturation (expressed as S_pO_2)

and heart rate. It is an important aid in detecting clinically unsuspected hypoxemia or abnormally low oxygen in the blood. This technique can assist the dysphagia clinician by providing a baseline pulse rate and oxygen saturation level and then monitoring changes that occur when any demands (i.e., trial swallows) are introduced, or when mucus or food are aspirated. An oxygen saturation (S_pO_2) level of > 94% when a patient is receiving room air is considered normal. Values are accurate to within 2% of arterial blood gas (ABG) values.

Capnography. Capnography provides continuous, noninvasive monitoring of ventilation via the measurement of end-tidal carbon dioxide ($ETCO_2$). $ETCO_2$ is the carbon dioxide in the air at the end of expiration. Capnography provides a numeric and graphic display of the carbon dioxide level and waveforms measured at the airways. Capnography uses infrared light absorption to measure the exhaled carbon dioxide. There are two types of carbon dioxide monitoring techniques. One type, mainstream sampling, can be used only with patients who have endotracheal or tracheostomy tubes. The other type, side stream sampling, can be used for patients with or without artificial airways. $ETCO_2$ may not coincide exactly with arterial blood carbon dioxide ($PaCO_2$). Normal $ETCO_2$ levels are 35 to 45 mmHg. $ETCO_2$ provides an excellent trending tool, which can be used to continuously monitor a patient's exhaled carbon dioxide levels. Oximetry and capnography are both helpful during the dysphagia assessment process; however, the physician and respiratory care practitioner will obtain arterial blood gases for analysis whenever there is a discrepancy between the patient's clinical status and the noninvasive measurements. A dual pulse oximetry and capnography unit is pictured in Figure 8.4.

The Clinical Assessment

History Taking

The evaluation of the patient with pulmonary disease demands the same competence and similar protocols as used with any individual with dysphagia. Traditionally, the first stage of the comprehensive dysphagia assessment is the clinical or bedside swallowing evaluation. During this evaluation, the special needs of the patient with pul-

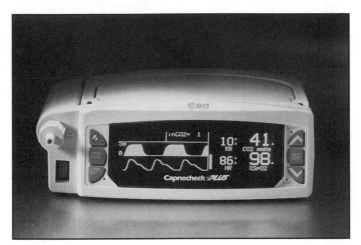

Figure 8.4. A dual oximetry and capnography unit (Capnocheck Plus, Model 9004). Photo courtesy of BCI International.

monary disease are identified. The information gained during this initial step will guide the clinician in selecting other, relevant assessment procedures. The clinician may choose to include both standard instrumental procedures, as well as those tailored to the individual with pulmonary disease.

The most important aspect of the clinical swallowing evaluation is a thorough review of the medical record and an interview with the staff, family, and, when feasible, patient. As described by Groher in Chapter 1 of this text, information gathering should include the current medical condition, relevant medical history, and medications. Other concomitant clinical factors, such as repeated pneumonia, upper respiratory infections, atelectasis, and weight loss or decreased albumin levels, are particularly relevant. The history taking will often identify symptoms of progressive pulmonary impairment and perhaps dysphagia. For example, the clinician may uncover long-standing decreased appetite and gradual weight loss that result in a hospital admission for dehydration. Closer questioning by the intuitive clinician may reveal complaints of fatigue during a meal. What is revealed is not necessarily a discrete dysphagia, but an interaction between deglutition and impaired respiratory function. In this section of the chapter, we provide specific questions to be asked during the evaluation of patients with respiratory diseases or conditions. Many of these questions are applicable to more than one disease or condition, such as the patient's overall pulmonary status including vital capacity and peak cough flow measures. Also, fatigue will play a significant role in any of these conditions. Finally, the impact of the work of breathing should be considered for all patients. By gathering this information obtained through the following questions, the clinician will be better prepared to evaluate and manage the dysphagia, whatever the particular clinical presentation.

Chronic Obstructive Pulmonary Disease. What may be particularly puzzling to the dysphagia clinician is the incidence of swallowing difficulties in the patient with a diagnosis of COPD in the absence of neurologic impairment. As previously discussed, the characteristics of this disease affect the patient's ability to coordinate respiration with deglutition. Higher energy requirements for the maintenance of adequate oxygenation may also reduce the amount of usable calories available to the body, as more calories are diverted for ventilation needs. Specific questions that will guide the initial steps in the clinician's decision-making process for these individuals include the following:

1. At what point in the disease process did the swallowing difficulties begin? That is, has the patient complained of some type of swallowing dysfunction for many years, or can the difficulty be linked to a more recent event, such as a pneumonia, exacerbation of the disease, or intubation?

2. Does the patient have difficulty completing a meal because of fatigue or shortness of breath? Fatigue may result from the physical demands of eating, or energy expenditure, which increases respiratory demands.

3. Does the patient report feeling "full" after only a few spoonsful of food or liquid? The displacement of the diaphragm by the distended stomach may impinge upon the patient's hyperinflated lungs and compromise already reduced lung volumes (Edgar, 1994).

4. Does the patient complain of a loss of appetite? Loss of appetite is a side effect of many medications. In addition, a decreased sense of smell and taste is common for tracheostomized or ventilator-dependent patients and can reduce appetite and intake.

5. Does the patient complain of thick or copious mucus, which he or she may or may not be able to expectorate? Decreased hydration can result in thicker, more viscous secretions, which prove more difficult to clear. When this is coupled with decreased vital capacity, airway obstruction, and collapse, the result is a less forceful, nonproductive cough. Clearance failure has direct implications for reduced airway protection.

6. What is the patient's forced vital capacity? Did any decline in forced vital capacity coincide with the onset of dysphagic symptoms? Forced vital capacity provides an indication of overall pulmonary status and is indicative of the ability to generate sufficient expiratory airflow for coughing.

Neurodegenerative Diseases and Conditions. Information gathering for the patient with neurologic disease includes a careful analysis of dysphagia symptom onset and progression. The clinician must determine whether dysphagic symptoms have worsened over time, and how they relate to changing pulmonary function. Pertinent questions that the dysphagia clinician may ask include the following:

1. Is the swallowing difficulty progressive, and can the clinician expect the dysphagic symptoms to change? Determining the status of the disease, whether static or degenerative, will guide the decision-making process as it relates to oral intake.

2. When was the onset of dysphagia symptoms in relation to changes in motor and pulmonary status? For progressive neurologic conditions, a decline in respiratory musculature affects endurance, as the patient must use any available energy for breathing. This type of individual is often given mechanical ventilatory assistance.

3. Does the patient complain of coughing or choking on particular consistencies? Is the patient able to successfully clear the material from the throat? Airway protection signs may be initial indicators of declining pulmonary status. This is sometimes evidenced on particular consistencies, more frequently with thin liquids.

4. Is the patient able to follow directions? This may limit the patient's ability to participate with particular assessment techniques.

Cardiopulmonary Conditions. Dysphagia clinicians in the acute care environment are frequently called to the cardiac intensive care and step-down units for clinical swallowing evaluations. In the immediate postsurgical period, extubated patients may experience dysphagic symptoms. These symptoms are often related to dysfunction of the laryngeal mechanism and reduced base of tongue strength. Questions the dysphagia clinician may ask include these:

1. Did the onset of swallowing difficulties coincide with any surgical procedures or were they more slowly progressive? A history of intubation may coincide with decreased base of tongue strength and laryngeal changes causing airway protection problems or dysphonia; cardiac aneurysms may also result in airway protection problems secondary to pressure on the vagus nerve. This is seen especially in the geriatric population.

2. Is vocal quality normal or does the patient report that his or her voice has changed? Again, a large aneurysm may press on the left recurrent laryngeal nerve and subsequently cause vocal fold dysfunction.

3. Has the patient failed in attempts to wean from mechanical ventilatory support or from tracheostomy? Microaspiration may affect pulmonary status. Additionally, a weakened pulmonary status may limit a patient's ability to take sufficient food by mouth, affecting nutritional status.

Tracheostomy and Ventilator Dependence. The presence of a tracheostomy tube with or without mechanical ventilation will require the dysphagia clinician to gather additional specific information. Questions may include the following:

1. Did the dysphagia coincide with intubation or tracheotomy? The clinician should consider the surgical procedure or the

mechanical and physiologic effects of tracheostomy or ventilator dependence as possible etiologies for the dysphagia.

2. Does the patient ever expel food or liquid from or around the tracheostomy tube while eating? If this is reported, it may be indicative of aspiration secondary to insufficient airway protection or mechanical blockage of the esophagus by the tracheostomy tube cuff.

3. Is the cuff inflated or deflated while the patient eats? An inflated cuff will limit information gathered during the clinical assessment. As discussed, inflated cuffs contribute to physiologic or mechanical dysphagia.

4. What are the type and size of the tracheostomy tube? Is it fenestrated or nonfenestrated? Larger tubes decrease airflow through the upper airway. Fenestrations may provide additional airflow when patients are not using their ventilators.

5. How frequently must the patient be suctioned? Copious or viscous secretions may indicate infection or repeated aspiration; the patient's ability to expectorate secretions provides airway protection information.

6. Does the patient receive respiratory treatments and are they frequently needed *after* a meal? Such an occurrence may be related to increased work of breathing, bronchospasm, or microaspiration during meals.

7. Does the patient require supplemental oxygen during a meal? This is often related to increased respiratory demands and subsequent increased work of breathing caused by the coordination of respiration and deglutition while eating. Gross aspiration, as identified by oxygen desaturation and the need for supplemental oxygen during each meal, should alert the clinician to the high probability of airway protection problems.

8. Does the patient receive mechanical ventilation during mealtime? Mechanical ventilation may either disrupt the timing of respiration and deglutition or, conversely, support the patient's respiratory efforts during a meal.

Oral-Peripheral Examination

The clinical evaluation continues with a thorough examination of the oral motor mechanism. Dysphagia clinicians working with patients who have pulmonary disease will concentrate on particular aspects of oral motor, pharyngeal, and laryngeal function in addition to those areas that are typically addressed during the clinical evaluation (see Chapter 2 of this text).

Observation of saliva and secretion management provides the clinician with information regarding general oral motor status, the presence of a functional pharyngeal swallow, and expectoration ability. Significant drooling is a sequela of inadequate lip and tongue control, as well as the patient's inability to trigger frequent and efficient saliva swallows. Bulbar function is more commonly impaired in the neurogenic and neurodegenerative population (Gilardeau, Kazandjian, Dikeman, Bach, & Tucker, 1995). The patient with obstructive and restrictive pulmonary conditions, but without a neurologic history, will usually present with adequate overall oral motor status. However, secretion management may vary depending upon the amount and quality produced, as well as the patient's ability to protect the airway from any penetrated or aspirated material. The tracheostomized or ventilator-dependent patient can pose a unique problem to the dysphagia clinician. The presence of the tracheostomy tube itself predisposes the patient to produce larger amounts of secretions in the airway (Bach, 1996a). Additionally, the presence of the inflated tracheostomy tube cuff eliminates the airflow needed to effectively clear secretions from the pharynx and larynx. These individuals are dependent upon the mechanical removal of secretions via oral or tracheal suctioning.

Decreased lingual function—specifically impaired base of tongue movement—is sometimes associated with oral intubation, especially prolonged intubation (Logemann, 1993). Many patients who have experienced respiratory insufficiency are intubated during their hospital course. A history of intubation may explain the presence of a mild dysphagia in a patient who does not have a history of neurologic impairment. The dysphagia clinician will use resistance techniques via tongue blade or commercially available devices to assess lingual strength. Also, Cooper and Perlman (1997) reported on electromyographic techniques that can be used to more objectively assess the patient's ability to use particular muscles during the swallow. They reported that the genioglossus muscle is active in both maintaining an open airway during respiration and functioning during oral preparation of a bolus. Impairment of this muscle may affect swallowing efficiency. Decreased base of tongue function affects the efficiency of the oral–pharyngeal swallow, including effective oral bolus control, hyoid and laryngeal elevation, and generation of adequate pharyngeal pressures.

Respiratory rate and breath patterns can easily influence safe swallowing. This may be most evident during a meal when the dysphagia clinician can observe the patient's attempt to coordinate breathing with swallowing. Observation of the patient's rate of breathing and use of accessory musculature will provide the clinician with information about the work of breathing during eating. An increase in respiratory rate associated with oral feeding is often a response to the demands of the task, which stress the patient's weakened respiratory system. In addition, if the patient is aspirating, the dysphagia clinician may observe shortness of breath and hypoxia (Teba & Omert, 1995). These symptoms may be identified both clinically and via objective monitoring.

Cervical Auscultation

Cervical auscultation, as discussed in Chapter 2 of this text, is a useful tool for the clinician working with the patient with pulmonary dysfunction. Used to detect the sounds of the swallow during deglutition, the technique can also assess the ability to achieve and maintain airway closure (Zenner, Losinski, & Mills, 1995). For the patient with pulmonary impairment, pairing laryngeal palpation with cervical auscultation provides a method of identifying discoordination between breathing and swallowing. Additionally, pharyngeal secretion management, problematic in such diagnoses as COPD, may be effectively evaluated prior to trial swallow attempts with cervical auscultation. Cued by vocal changes or audible airflow through a secretion-filled pharynx, the clinician may first use cervical auscultation to assess saliva swallows, secretion management, and candidacy to advance to trial bolus swallows. If the clinician hears secretions in the airway that cannot be cleared either by the patient or mechanically, trial swallows should be deferred. The sounds of the swallow identified via cervical auscultation may also be recorded and analyzed for more objective information (Takahashi, Groher, & Michi, 1994).

Tracheostomy Cuff Deflation Techniques

Cervical auscultation has particular relevance for the tracheostomized and ventilator-dependent patient. It assists the dysphagia clinician in identifying upper airway flow during the dysphagia assessment, especially when the patient has a cuffed tracheostomy tube. Speech–language pathologists, respiratory care practitioners, and nurses use auscultation as part of minimal occluding volume and minimal leak techniques. These techniques use a stethoscope, placed on the cervical area, to listen to airflow that travels through the upper airway. Minimal occluding volume involves inserting air into the tracheostomy tube cuff just to the point where upper airway flow ceases and measuring the volume now in the cuff. During the minimal leak technique, air is inserted into the cuff until an air seal is obtained. When air can no longer be detected via the stethoscope (or through the mouth) during delivery of a positive pressure ventilator breath, it is assumed that a seal has been obtained between the cuff and tracheal wall. A small amount of air is then removed from the cuff. The dysphagia clinician will take the minimal leak technique one step further, with physician clearance, as additional air is removed to ensure that adequate upper airway flow is accomplished.

The establishment of a partial cuff leak attempts to provide a patient with the airflow needed for generation of an effective swallow and airway protection. It is not possible to indicate a standard amount of air (e.g., 5 cc) at which partial cuff deflation will be obtained because of the variation of tracheostomy tube size relative to the size of the patient's tracheal lumen. However, the dysphagia clinician can use the patient's ability to phonate, cough, throat clear, and elevate the larynx as indicators of partial cuff deflation and adequate upper airway flow. The following provides a sample protocol for cuff deflation in the tracheostomized patient. It should be emphasized that a speech–language pathologist performs these procedures only when specifically allowed under clinical privileges in his or her facility.

1. Obtain physician order or medical clearance for cuff deflation during the dysphagia assessment.

2. Communicate with the nurse or respiratory care practitioner to determine the need for their presence at the bed-

side for preoxygenation or assistance with suctioning or bagging.

3. With the cuff inflated and according to established facility protocol, suction the patient via the tracheostomy and the mouth.

4. Reinsert the suction catheter into the tracheostomy tube. Connect a 10 ml syringe to the cuff valve and slowly begin withdrawing air as suction is applied simultaneously.

5. An alternate or adjunct method of clearing the airway of secretions during cuff deflation is to place a manual resuscitation bag (the football-shaped "ambu bag") to the tracheostomy tube and apply positive airway pressure to push the secretions upward into the mouth. There they may be expectorated or removed manually. This technique can be more easily performed with a patient who is cooperative and able to participate in the process.

6. Ensure that the cuff is fully deflated by observation of an empty pilot balloon on the outside of the tracheostomy tube.

7. Use cervical auscultation if the patient is unable to achieve voicing with tracheal occlusion and if the clinician is unsure whether airflow is actually escaping around the sides of the tracheostomy tube into the upper airway.

8. If there is a concern regarding secretion management or difficulty maintaining oxygenation in the presence of the fully deflated cuff, reinflate to partial cuff inflation. With medical approval, increase oxygen delivered from the ventilator or via the tracheostomy collar.

9. Monitor the patient for tolerance of upper airway flow. At the conclusion of the dysphagia assessment, determine whether the patient's cuff will be maintained in an inflated or deflated state. Use proper technique to reinflate the cuff, ensuring adequate cuff volume.

Cuff deflation in the ventilator-dependent patient will necessitate special considerations. The tracheostomy tube cuff is used to assist in maintaining a closed system between the patient and the ventilator. When the cuff is deflated, an air leak is created through the upper airway. Although this has positive implications for both swallowing and speech production, it may also affect the adequacy of the patient's ventilation and oxygenation. The patient's lung must receive the adequate tidal volumes to maintain normal lung ventilation. The dysphagia clinician must work closely with the respiratory care practitioner during the assessment process to ensure that appropriate levels of ventilation and oxygenation are maintained during cuff deflation. The respiratory care practitioner may change ventilator-delivered volume, rate, or even mode of ventilation (Bach & Alba, 1990). Objective monitoring tools are always used while deflating the cuff of an individual who is ventilator dependent. Baseline S_pO_2 and optimally $ETCO_2$ measurements are obtained prior to deflating the cuff and when making any modifications to the ventilator. A spirometer can be used to quantify the amount of delivered volume that is lost when the leak from cuff deflation is created. Whenever a dysphagia assessment with a patient who is ventilator dependent is performed, the assistance of the respiratory care practitioner or the nurse must be obtained.

Trial Swallows

The clinician decides whether to proceed to actual test swallows based on many factors. The decision is made more easily for the patient already receiving an oral diet. The clinician may decide to evaluate the patient during a mealtime to monitor endurance and the effect of pulmonary impairment. Some patients may not exhibit overt dysphagic symptoms at the beginning of the meal, but gradually fatigue and demonstrate increased breath rate and work of breathing, decreased food intake, and clinical signs of airway protection problems as the meal progresses.

Individuals who do not take food orally are approached more conservatively, as the clinician must rely on clinical signs such as vocal changes and reflexive coughing to judge pharyngeal stage management and airway protection abilities. Pharyngeal dysphagia can be easily overlooked during the clinical examination, especially in the patient with decreased airway protection (Splaingard, Hutchins, Sulton,

& Chaudhuri, 1988). A less sensitive larynx may not respond to penetrated or aspirated material (Sasaki et al., 1977). Additionally, the
patient with pulmonary dysfunction may be particularly intolerant to
aspiration due to previous, recurrent infections, decreased vital capacity, and inadequate airway flows. The presence of an inflated tracheostomy tube cuff further complicates airway protection abilities. Trial
swallows for this patient could consist of saliva swallows only or the
use of a few ice chips to provide lubrication and the stimulus for the
pharyngeal swallow response.

For the tracheostomized and ventilator-dependent patient, the tracheostomy tube cuff *must* be at least partially deflated in order to make
an adequate assessment of the airway. This will allow the dysphagia
clinician to briefly occlude the tracheostomy tube to determine vocal
fold status and the ability to generate airflow for vocalizing, coughing,
throat clearing, and expectorating secretions. Recall that when the cuff
is inflated, air will not reach the vocal folds and pharynx, and airflow
and air pressures for swallowing will be severely impacted. Therefore,
diagnostic information obtained when the tracheostomy tube cuff is
inflated is limited to oral phase management and the ability to trigger
a pharyngeal swallow. When medical status contraindicates even brief
cuff deflation due to copious secretions or an unstable pulmonary status, trial swallows should be deferred.

Blue Dye Test

During the clinical assessment, the clinician does have a method to
identify gross aspiration in the patient who is tracheostomized and
ventilator dependent. This technique, originally called the Evans blue
dye test, as described by Cameron, Reynolds, and Zuidema (1973), is
now commonly called the modified Evans blue dye test or simply the
blue dye test. Although this procedure does not objectively assess
swallowing safety, it will alert the dysphagia clinician to an undesirable
connection between the mouth and the trachea when the results are
positive for aspiration (Dikeman & Kazandjian, 1995). The blue dye
test initially involves placing a few drops of sterile water mixed with
food coloring on the tongue. The patient is cued to swallow and is suctioned immediately and in 15-minute intervals for 1 hour. The most
dramatic indication of inadequate airway protection and aspiration of
saliva will be seen in the immediate presence of blue dyed secretions in

the tracheal suctioning. If the results of the blue dye test are negative, the dysphagia clinician may consider trial swallows of food or liquid boluses mixed with blue dye. This decision to proceed with trial bolus swallows is made in the same manner as with the nontracheostomized patient, and carries the same risks and limitations.

During the actual administration of trial bolus swallows, the clinician should use only one consistency at a time (i.e., either semisolids or liquids). Mixing consistencies will confound the results of this subjective evaluation, as the clinician will see only the presence of some type of blue dyed material in the tracheostomy tube. The patient should be suctioned several times, at intervals, after the administration of one bolus type. When viscosity of the bolus increases, the potential of pharyngeal retention also increases. The presence of blue dye in suctioned secretion hours after the test may be a sequela of this retention and eventual aspiration. The clinician will have no idea of the presence, location, or extent of pharyngeal residue, and therefore it is vital that other staff are aware that the test has been performed and that they use a standard format to report a positive result (Dikeman & Kazandjian, 1995). In some facilities, a positive blue dye test is used to determine the need for an instrumental dysphagia assessment (Tippett & Siebens, 1995).

The importance of cuff deflation is clearly demonstrated during the blue dye test. If a test is performed with the tracheostomy tube cuff inflated, and the patient aspirates, most of the aspirated material will at least briefly collect in the trachea above the cuff (see Figure 8.5). The clinician must deflate the cuff with the suction catheter in place to obtain accurate results. While one clinician deflates the cuff, a second is ready to suction the material that would otherwise drop into the trachea. However, recall that the presence of the cuff itself may affect safe swallowing, so that the results of a blue dye test performed with an inflated cuff are confounded. When the test is performed with the cuff deflated, the clinician can use clinical indicators such as coughing, throat clearing, and vocal changes as potential signs of poor airway protection. The procedure for performing a blue dye test is detailed in Table 8.1. Patients who are tube fed only, but are suspected aspirators due to reflux, may also benefit from a version of the blue dye test. The dysphagia clinician may suggest that blue dye be added to enteral feedings in order to document aspiration of formula.

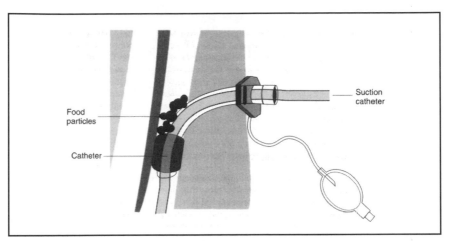

Figure 8.5. Food particles pooled on top of an inflated tracheostomy tube cuff. From *Communication and Swallowing Management of Tracheostomized and Ventilator-Dependent Adults* (p. 248), by K. J. Dikeman and M. S. Kazandjian, 1995, San Diego: Singular Publishing Group. Copyright 1995 by Singular Publishing Group, Inc. Reprinted with permission.

Glucose Oxidase Testing

A helpful addition to the blue dye test is the use of glucose oxidase test strips, which are placed in secretions obtained from the tracheostomy tube or from around the stoma. These test strips measure the glucose level in a substance and are sensitive to the presence of aspirated food or formula in secretions. Standard directions provide the user with guidelines for interpretation. Glucose oxidase test strips have been reported as more sensitive than blue dye visualization in detecting refluxed enteral formula (as glucose) in pulmonary secretions (Potts, Zaroukian, Guerrero, & Baker, 1993).

Instrumental Examination Techniques

Fiberoptic Assessment of Swallowing

The use of nasopharyngolaryngoscopy is one of the objective evaluation techniques at the disposal of the dysphagia clinician that is particularly relevant to the patient with pulmonary impairment. As described

Table 8.1

Protocol for Testing Swallows Using Blue Dye
During a Clinical Swallowing Evaluation

For *tracheostomized* patients who normally maintain inflated cuffs, the optimal procedure for test swallows is:

1. Deflate cuff fully or partially (follow suctioning protocol)
2. Occlude tracheostomy tube
3. Dry test swallow
4. Check vocal quality; encourage cough/throat clear
5. Bolus test swallow
6. Check vocal quality; encourage cough/throat clear
7. Suction (cuff deflated)
8. Rest interval (+5 minutes; reinflate cuff partially if risk of aspiration is high)
9. Resuction
10. **Negative:** continue with larger amounts or different consistencies; **positive:** terminate test; try different bolus types.

For *ventilator-dependent* patients with inflated cuffs, the test swallow procedure is:

1. Deflate cuff fully or partially (follow suctioning protocol)
2. Institute ventilator modifications as tolerated; allow patient time to adjust to settings
3. Dry test swallow
4. Check vocal quality; encourage cough/throat clear utilizing ventilator flow if possible
5. Bolus test swallow
6. Check vocal quality; encourage cough/throat clear
7. Suction (cuff deflated)
8. Rest interval (+5 minutes; partially reinflate cuff if needed between suctioning intervals)
9. Resuction
10. **Negative:** continue with different consistencies; larger amounts; **positive:** terminate test.

Note. From *Communication and Swallowing Management of Tracheostomized and Ventilator-Dependent Adults* (p. 323), by K. J. Dikeman and M. S. Kazandjian, 1995, San Diego, CA: Singular Publishing Group. Copyright 1995 by Singular Publishing Group, Inc. Reprinted with permission.

by Langmore, Schatz, and Olsen (1988) and in Chapter 5 of this text, the Fiberoptic Endoscopic Evaluation of Swallowing (FEES®) not only provides a method of assessing management of various bolus consistencies, but also allows the dysphagia clinician to visualize the impact of respiratory patterns upon deglutition. Secretion management can be assessed in the presence of direct fiberoptics. Any pooling of secretions in the pharyngeal area and any entry of secretions into the larynx can be noted prior to administering food boluses. The clinician can document pooling and retention of food boluses that are not immediately detected with a blue dye procedure. The patient's frequency of swallowing and the ability to close the airway at the appropriate time during the swallow, maintain airway closure, and manage secretions can also be documented (Murray, Langmore, Ginsberg, & Dostie, 1996). A modification of the FEES, the Fiberoptic Endoscopic Evaluation of Swallowing with Sensory Testing (FEESST®), incorporates endoscopic sensory testing of the pharynx and larynx into the procedure (Aviv, Martin, Keen, Debell, & Blitzer, 1993). In addition to saliva and bolus swallows, measured air pulses are delivered to assess the sensitivity of the laryngeal closure mechanism. This relatively new procedure is a helpful addition to the instrumental dysphagia evaluation. Pulmonary disease inherently places patients at risk of compromised airway protection. The FEESST procedure can provide valuable information regarding potential aspiration risk due to decreased laryngeal sensitivity (Aviv et al., 1996).

When used with the tracheostomized and ventilator-dependent patient, the fiberoptic endoscopic technique will be far more useful when at least partial cuff deflation is accomplished prior to endoscopic assessment. This will allow the patient to first adapt to the change in airflow before a new procedure is introduced. Some patients may need time to adjust to the sensation of airflow passing through the upper airway and react to the initial cuff deflation with prolonged coughing. The clinician should leave ample time between procedures to transition the patient through any of these difficulties. The portability of FEES and FEESST procedures allows ventilator-dependent patients, even those who are bedridden or in the ICU, to receive an objective dysphagia assessment.

Videofluoroscopy

The videofluoroscopic swallowing examination, or the modified barium swallow, is a dynamic radiologic study of the oral, pharyngeal, and esophageal phases of swallowing which integrates both evaluation of structure and function with a review of the effectiveness of treatment procedures (see Chapter 4 in this text). This procedure objectively documents the etiology of airway protection problems. The clinician may document whether aspiration occurs secondary to incomplete airway closure or is due to poorly timed airway closure.

Additionally, the ability to move the bolus through the pharynx is dependent on generation of adequate airway pressures. Difficulty with pharyngeal transit can be noted during videofluoroscopy in individuals with unoccluded tracheostomy tubes and inflated tracheostomy tube cuffs.

The environmental constraints of transporting the patient who receives oxygen, or who is tracheostomized and ventilator dependent, to radiology for the videofluoroscopic study must be considered prior to performing the study. In acute care facilities the respiratory care practitioner usually assists in transporting ventilator-dependent patients to radiology. There must be support in the fluoroscopy suite to assist with placing the patient on portable mechanical ventilation and with positioning the patient and the ventilator for the videofluoroscopy. Personnel trained to perform suctioning must be available during the study. Optimally, the tracheostomy tube cuff should be deflated and, if applicable, a one-way speaking valve placed in line. However, as with the endoscopic evaluation, the dysphagia clinician should not perform the *initial* cuff deflation or one-way valve placement during the videofluoroscopy. There are also more specific procedures that can be used with the tracheostomized and ventilator-dependent patient during the modified barium swallow (Dikeman & Kazandjian, 1995). These would require the presence and active participation of a respiratory care practitioner and the use of objective monitoring tools such as oximetry and capnography. Patients who receive oxygen only are less problematic, but the logistics and extra time required for transportation and setup should be factored into the clinician's schedule.

Special Considerations During Objective Assessments

Patients with pulmonary disease often cannot tolerate the multiple compensatory strategies and postural modifications normally performed during the diagnostic assessment. Although it is important to objectively document the success of the treatment techniques, the clinician should consider the increased work of breathing that, for example, an "effortful" swallow may create. The patient may accomplish the strategy for one or two swallows, but it may not be functional to ensure safe swallowing during an entire meal. Martin (1994) and O'Connor (1994) observed changes in baseline cardiac and respiratory rate and oxygen saturation levels when physiologic demands, in the form of the consumption of a meal, were placed on a compromised respiratory system. Modifications of food and liquid viscosity and simple postural changes are often more feasible for these individuals. Tracheostomized and ventilator-dependent individuals cannot perform supraglottic swallows or Mendelsohn maneuvers unless the tracheostomy tube cuff is deflated and finger occlusion, a one-way valve (Passy-Muir), or a tracheostomy button closes the tracheostomy tube.

Related Pulmonary Assessment Instruments

Specialized pulmonary assessment techniques have a role in the dysphagia assessment process. The oxygen saturation (S_pO_2) levels obtained with pulse oximetry monitor the patient's arterial oxygen levels during a dysphagia assessment procedure. A downward trend from baseline levels observed during the dysphagia assessment can alert the clinician to fatigue, increased work of breathing, and possibly aspiration. If this occurs during a meal, the patient may require smaller meals or a change in food consistency (e.g., a mechanical soft diet changed to puree), which lowers the mechanical demands on the patient. Oxygen desaturation during trial swallows, or during an actual meal, has been used to identify individuals at risk for aspiration (Rogers, Msall, & Shucard, 1993; Zaidi et al., 1995). As material penetrates and enters the airway, airflow through the trachea is reduced due to bronchospasm or the partial airway obstruction caused by the aspirated bolus. This results in a consequent decrease in oxygen levels available to the patient. Zaidi et al. (1995) found that the degree of oxygen desaturation in acute stroke patients while swallowing 10 ml of water was greater than for normal and nonneurologic controls. These individuals were also identified during clinical swallowing assessments by speech pathologists as "likely to aspirate." It was not clear, however, if the desaturation in oxygen was actually identifying aspiration below the level of the vocal cords. The use of oximetry continues to be investigated in conjunction with videofluoroscopy to determine its reliability as an indicator of laryngeal penetration or aspiration, and to provide values, that a clinician can use to monitor aspiration risk.

Pulse oximetry instrumentation that measures oxygen saturation simultaneously monitors pulse rate. An ongoing measurement of the patient's heart rate is very sensitive in detecting increased demands placed on the patient during oral intake, even before oxygen saturation begins to decrease. For example, the dysphagia clinician may note that a patient has to expend more effort during a meal to maintain consistent levels of S_pO_2 and $ETCO_2$. This is evidenced by rapid breathing, more use of accessory respiratory musculature, and increased pulse rate. Edgar (1994) noted that postmeal measures of maximum inspirations for individuals with COPD decreased when compared to premeal measures, suggesting that fatigue of inspiratory musculature may play a role in this difference. A patient with this pattern may eventually fatigue to the point that adequate arterial blood saturation and carbon dioxide levels cannot be maintained.

Capnography is a useful pulmonary assessment instrument, especially when paired with oximetry during the dysphagia evaluation. When monitoring a patient with pulmonary impairment, the dysphagia clinician may observe changing trends in $ETCO_2$ during oral intake. When work of breathing increases either because of aspiration or respiratory muscle inadequacy, elevated CO_2 levels may be observed, reflecting a decrease in the patient's ability to adequately ventilate the lungs. For individuals who are ventilator dependent, the respiratory care practitioner can compensate by increasing the support provided by the ventilator during meals. This may mean that a patient who is being weaned, a process that demands considerable patient effort, will be changed to a higher level of support (i.e., assist control) during meals (Chua et al., 1997).

Pulmonary function tests provide the dysphagia clinician with additional information regarding vital capacity, peak cough flow, and the ability to generate a forceful and effective cough. Individuals who exhibit a vital capacity lower than 65 ml/kg of ideal body weight may be at risk for insufficient peak cough flows and, consequently, inadequate airflow to clear penetrated/aspirated material and productively expectorate secretions. Siebens, Tippett, Kirby, and French (1993) discussed the importance of airflow as a clearing mechanism for the larynx, and measured peak airflow velocities reaching 7 liters per second in normal subjects. Individuals who are unable to generate the expiratory airflow needed for an effective cough appear at increased risk of aspiration. Bach (1996b) stated that a patient will have difficulty clearing secretions when spontaneous or assisted peak cough flows cannot exceed 5 liters per second. Tracheostomized and ventilator-dependent individuals are at even greater risk when they are unable to use the vocal folds for their normal protective function of modulating upper airway flow (Muz, Mathog, Nelson, & Jones, 1989; Siebens et al., 1993). Cuff deflation and one-way speaking valve use may assist the restoration of upper airway flow and allow patients access to normal clearing mechanisms (Tippett & Siebens, 1991). Recommendations for oral feeding should be made cautiously in the face of poor airway protection, decreased vital capacity, and an ineffective cough.

Summary

The dysphagia evaluation of the patient with pulmonary disease demands that the dysphagia clinician have a multifactorial understanding of the potential causes of dysphagia in these individuals. Joint consultations between the speech pathologist, physician, respiratory care practitioner, dictician, nurse, and other team members will guide the clinician through the decision-making process and assist in referrals for other diagnostic assessments and, eventually, in treatment planning. The dysphagia clinician is an essential member of the team who addresses the multiple medical issues involving these complex patients.

References

Ardran, G. M., & Kemp, F. H. (1967). The mechanism of the larynx: II. The epiglottis and closure of the larynx. *British Journal of Radiology, 40,* 372–389.

Aviv, J. E., Martin, J. H., Keen, M. S., Debell, M., & Blitzer, A. (1993). Air pulse quantification of supraglottic and pharyngeal sensation: A new technique. *Annals of Otology, Rhinology and Laryngology, 102*(10), 777–780.

Aviv, J. E., Martin, J. H., Sacco, R. L., Zagar, D., Diamond, B., Keen, M. S., & Blitzer, A. (1996). Supraglottic and pharyngeal sensory abnormalities in stroke patients with dysphagia. *Annals of Otology, Rhinology and Larynology, 105*(2), 92–97.

Bach, J. R. (1996a). Conventional approaches to managing neuromuscular ventilatory failure. In J. R. Bach (Ed.), *Pulmonary rehabilitation: The obstructive and paralytic conditions* (pp. 285–301). Philadelphia: Hanley & Belfus.

Bach, J. R. (1996b). Pathophysiology of paralytic-restrictive pulmonary syndromes. In J. R. Bach (Ed.) *Pulmonary rehabilitation: The obstructive and paralytic conditions* (pp. 275–283). Philadelphia: Hanley & Belfus.

Bach, J. R. (1996c). Prevention of morbidity and mortality with the use of physical medicine aids. In J. R. Bach (Ed.), *Pulmonary rehabilitation: The obstructive and paralytic conditions* (pp. 303–330). Philadelphia: Hanley & Belfus.

Bach, J. R., & Alba, A. (1990). Tracheostomy ventilation: A study of efficacy with deflated cuffs and cuffless tubes. *Chest, 97,* 679–683.

Bonanno, P. C. (1971). Swallowing dysfunction after tracheotomy. *Annals of Surgery, 174,* 29–33.

Buckwalter, J. A., & Sasaki, C. T. (1984). Effect of tracheotomy on laryngeal function. *Otolaryngologic Clinics of North America, 17,* 41–48.

Cameron, J. L., Reynolds, J., & Zuidema, G. D. (1973). Aspiration in patients with tracheostomies. *Surgical Gynecological Obstetrics, 136,* 68–70.

Chua, R., Kazandjian, M., Chan, R., Dikeman, K., Ferreras, B., Fleming, R., Perez, F., & Zamora, A. (1997, June). *Evaluation, monitoring and management of ventilator dependent patients while using one-way speaking valves.* Paper presented at The 6th Congress of Asia Pacific Association for Respiratory Care, Manilla, Phillipines.

Cooper, D. S., & Perlman, A. L. (1997). Electromyography in the functional and diagnostic testing of deglutition. In A. Perlman & K. Schulze-Delrieu (Eds.). *Deglutition and its disorders: Anatomy, physiology, clinical diagnosis and management* (pp. 255–284). San Diego: Singular.

Dettelbach, M. A., Gross, R. D., Mahlmann, J., & Eibling, D. (1995). Effect of the Passy-Muir on aspiration in patients with tracheostomy. *Journal of Sciences and Specialties of the Head and Neck, 17*(4), 297–300.

DeVita, M. A., & Spierer-Rundback, L. (1990). Swallowing disorders in patients with prolonged orotracheal intubation or tracheostomy tubes. *Critical Care Medicine, 18,* 1328–1330.

Dikeman, K. J., & Kazandjian, M. S. (1995). *Communication and swallowing management of tracheostomized and ventilator dependent adults.* San Diego: Singular.

Edgar, J. D. (1994). *Meal related patterns of respiration and deglutition in patients with COPD.* Unpublished doctoral dissertation, University of Minnesota, Minneapolis.

Eibling, D. E., & Diez-Gross, R. D. (1996). Subglottic air pressure: A key component of swallowing efficiency. *Annals of Otology, Rhinology, and Laryngology, 105*(4).

Eubanks, D. H., & Bone, R. C. (1990). *Comprehensive respiratory care.* St. Louis: Mosby.

Feldman, S. A., Deal, C. W., & Urqhart, W. (1966). Disturbance of swallowing after tracheotomy. *Lancet, 1,* 954–955.

Frownfelter, D., & Dean, E. (1996). *Principles and practices of cardiopulmonary physical therapy.* St. Louis: Mosby.

Gilardeau, C., Kazandjian, M., Dikeman, K., Bach, J., & Tucker, L. (1995). The evaluation and management of dysphagia in Duchenne muscular dystrophy. *Seminars in Neurology, 15*(1), 46–51.

Heffner, J. E. (1993). Timing of tracheostomy in mechanically ventilated patients. *American Review of Respiratory Disease, 147,* 768–771.

Hogue, C. W., Lappas, G. D., Creswell, L. L., Ferguson, T. B., Sample, M., Pugh, D., Balfe, D., Cox, J. L., & Lappas, G. (1995). Swallowing dysfunction after cardiac operations: Associated adverse outcomes and risk factors including intraoperative transesophageal echocardiography. *Journal of Thoracic and Cardiovascular Surgery, 104,* 1510–1517.

Hoo, G. W. S., Dhanani, S., & Santiago, S. (1995). Restrictive lung disease and swallowing disorders. *Seminars in Respiratory and Critical Care Medicine, 16,* 490–502.

Ikari, T., & Sasaki, C. T. (1980). Glottic closure reflex: Control mechanisms. *Annals of Otology, Rhinology and Laryngology, 89,* 220–224.

Kirsch, C. M., & Sanders, A. (1988). Aspiration pneumonia: Medical management. *Otolaryngologic Clinics of North America, 21*(4), 677–689.

Langmore, S., Schatz, K., & Olsen, N. (1988). A fiberoptic endoscopic examination of swallowing safety: A new procedure. *Dysphagia, 2,* 216–219.

Langmore, S. E. (1996). Dysphagia in neurologic patients in the ICU setting. *Seminars in Neurology, 16*(4), 329–340.

Leder, S. B., Tarro, J. M., & Burrell, M. I. (1996). Effect of occlusion of a tracheostomy tube on aspiration. *Dysphagia, 11,* 254–258.

Logemann, J. A. (1993, April). *Management of tracheostomy tubes, intubation, ventilators during swallowing assessment and treatment.* Paper presented at Special Consultations in Dysphagia, Northern Speech Services, Chicago.

Martin, B. J. W. (1994, October). *Biomechanical and temporal characteristics of laryngeal closure in patients with pulmonary disease.* Paper presented at The Third Annual Dysphagia Research Society Meeting, McClean, VA.

Martin, B. J. W., Logemann, J. A., Shaker, R., & Dodds, W. J. (1994). Coordination between respiration and swallowing. Respiratory phase relationships and temporal integration. *Journal of Applied Physiology, 76,* 714–723.

Martin, B. J. W., & Robbins, J. (1995). Physiology of swallowing: Protection of the airway. *Seminars in Respiratory and Critical Care Medicine, 16*(6), 448–458.

McConnel, F. M. S., Cerenko, D., & Mendelsohn, M. S. (1988). Manofluorographic analysis of swallowing. *Otolaryngologic Clinics of North America, 21,* 625–637.

Murray, J., Langmore, S. E., Ginsberg, S., & Dostie, A. (1996). The significance of accumulated oropharyngeal secretions and swallowing frequency in predicting aspiration. *Dysphagia, 11,* 99–103.

Muz, J., Mathog, R. H., Nelson, R., & Jones, L. A. (1989). Aspiration in patients with head and neck cancer and tracheostomy. *American Journal of Otolaryngology, 10,* 282–286.

Nash, M. (1988). Swallowing problems in the tracheostomized patient. *Otolaryngologic Clinics of North America, 21*(4), 701–709.

Niederman, M., Ferranti, R. D., Ziegler, A., Merrill, W. W., & Reynolds, H. Y. (1984). Respiratory infection complicating long term tracheostomy: The implication of persistent gram-negative tracheobronchial colonization. *Chest, 85*(1), 39–44.

Nishino, T., Yonezawa, T., & Honda, Y. (1995). Effects of swallowing on the pattern of continous respiration in human adults. *American Review of Respiratory Disease, 132,* 1219–1222.

Oakes, D. F. (1994). *Clinical practitioner's pocket guide to respiratory care.* Old Town, ME: Health Educators Publications.

O'Conner, A. (1994, October). *Influence of eating and drinking on cardiopulmonary function in adults.* Paper presented at The Third Annual Dysphagia Research Society Meeting, McClean, VA.

Potts, R. G., Zaroukian, M. D., Guerrero, P. A., & Baker, C. D. (1993). Comparison of blue dye visualization and glucose oxidase test strip methods for detecting pulmonary aspiration of enteral feeding in intubated adults. *Chest, 103*(1), 117–121.

Rogers, B., Msall, M., & Shucard, D. (1993). Hypoxemia during oral feedings in adults with dysphagia and severe neurological disabilities. *Dysphagia, 8,* 43–48.

Sasaki, C. T., & Buchwalter, J. (1984). Laryngeal function. *American Journal of Otolaryngology, 5,* 281–291.

Sasaki, C. T., Suzuki, M., Horiuchi, M., & Kirchner, J. A. (1977). The effect of tracheostomy on the laryngeal closure reflex. *Laryngoscope, 87,* 1428–1433.

Shaker, R., Li, Q., Ren, J., Townsend, W. F., Dodds, W. J., Martin, B. J., Kern, M. K., & Rynders, A. (1992). Coordination of deglutition and phases of respiration: Effects of aging, tachypnea, bolus volume and chronic obstructive pulmonary disease. *American Journal of Physiology, 263,* 750–755.

Siebens, A. A., Tippett, D. C., Kirby, N., & French, J. (1993). Dysphagia and expiratory airflow. *Dysphagia, 8,* 266–269.

Smith, J., Wolkove, N., Colacone, A., & Kreisman, H. (1989). Coordination of eating, drinking and breathing in adults. *Chest, 96,* 578–582.

Splaingard, M. L., Hutchins, B., Sulton, L. D., & Chaudhuri, G. (1988). Aspiration in rehabilitation patients: Videofluoroscopy vs. bedside clinical assessment. *Archives of Physical Medicine and Rehabilitation, 69,* 637–640.

Stachler, R. J., Hamlet, S. L., Choi, J., & Fleming, S. (1996). Scintigraphic quantification of aspiration reduction with the Passy-Muir valve. *Laryngoscope, 106,* 231–234.

Stauffer, J. L., Olson, D. E., & Petty, T. L. (1981) Complications and consequences of endotracheal intubation and tracheostomy. *American Journal of Medicine, 70,* 65–75.

Takahashi, K., Groher, M. E., & Michi, K. (1994). Symmetry and reproducibility of swallowing sounds. *Dysphagia, 9,* 168–173.

Teba, L., & Omert, L. A. (1995). Postoperative respiratory insufficiency. *American Family Physician, 51,* 1473–1480.

Tippett, D., & Siebens, A. (1991). Speaking and swallowing on a ventilator. *Dysphagia, 6,* 94–99.

Tippett, D., & Siebens, A. (1995, November). *Validating the modified Evans blue dye test.* Seminar presented at the American Speech-Language-Hearing Association Annual Convention, Tampa, FL.

Tolep, K., Getch, C. L., & Criner, G. J. (1996). Swallowing dysfunction in patients receiving prolonged mechanical ventilation. *Chest, 109,* 167–172.

West, J. B. (1990). *Respiratory physiology.* Baltimore: Williams and Wilkins.

Zaidi, N. H., Smith, H. A., King, S. C., Park, C., O'Neill, P. A., Connolly, M. J. (1995). Oxygen desaturation on swallowing as a potential marker of aspiration in acute stroke. *Age and Aging, 24,* 267–270.

Zenner, P. M., Losinski, D. S., & Mills, R. H. (1995). Using cervical auscultation in the clinical dysphagia examination in long-term care. *Dysphagia, 10,* 27–31.

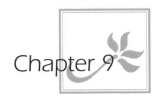

Chapter 9

The Use of Scintigraphy in the Evaluation of Dysphagia

Sue Fleming

Fleming provides the reader with an orientation to the use of scintigraphy in the evaluation of dysphagia. Although scintigraphy is not a commonly employed technique, it offers unique advantages in the evaluation of dysphagia.

1. *Most dysphagia clinicians rely on the videofluoroscopy and fiberoptic endoscopy to detect the presence of aspiration. Scintigraphy can also detect the presence of aspiration. What else can scintigraphy do that these other techniques cannot?*

2. *Why is it not possible to study more than one test material type during a single scintigraphic test?*

3. *What distinction does Fleming make between glottal and pulmonary aspiration?*

4. *Why is the distinction between glottal and pulmonary aspiration important for dysphagia clinicians to appreciate?*

❦   ❦   ❦

Scintigraphy is a diagnostic process that uses radioisotopes to yield information regarding specific anatomic areas of interest. As it is applied to swallowing disorders, the patient ingests food or liquid that has been mixed with a radioisotope. The patient is positioned in front of a gamma camera that determines the quantity of the isotope at various locations within the body. Scintigraphy can be used to quantify oral, pharyngeal, and esophageal transit, and, more important, pulmonary aspirate. Prior to a discussion of the technique, a historical perspective will illustrate why this method is beneficial in the evaluation of dysphagia.

Historical Perspective

Prior to the 1970s dysphagia was generally assumed to have an esophageal or gastric origin. As a consequence, the literature of the time was primarily devoted to discussions of achalasias, gastroesophageal reflux, Schatake's rings, esophageal webs, and hiatal hernias. Because of this limited view of dysphagia, primarily physicians were concerned with dysphagia. Those physicians who were involved were most often specialists such as gastroenterologists and radiologists. Because the esophagus and stomach were the principal areas of interest, there was little opportunity for nonphysicians to contribute to the study of dysphagia.

Insofar as the deglutition process is concerned, the initial application for scintigraphy was the assessment of gastric function. Gastric emptying, for example, used scintigraphy to study volume flow. Volume flow studies provide information on how rapidly specific amounts of test material pass or clear anatomic areas of interest. In the late 1960s and the 1970s, clinicians began to expand the use of scintigraphy in the assessment of esophageal function. The scintigraphic assessment of the esophagus evaluated volume flow through the upper, middle, and lower esophageal segments. The technique also provided information regarding the presence and severity of gastroesophageal reflux. In many cases these data were correlated with endoscopic, pH monitoring, and manometric findings.

In the 1970s a growing awareness developed that dysphagia was hardly limited to the esophagus. It was apparent to me, as well as other health care professionals, that a variety of patients, of all ages and with a multitude of medical problems, experienced dysphagia. There were major considerations of oral and pharyngeal origin that directly impacted swallowing. It was then that the potential role of scintigraphy in the evaluation and management of oropharyngeal dysphagia was first posed. Although scintigraphy has its benefits in the evaluation and management of dysphagia in both children and adults, the focus of this chapter is its use as an evaluation tool in adult dysphagia.

Fundamentals and Rationale

Scintigraphy depends on a technology that is foreign to most dysphagia clinicians. Fundamentally, it is a technique in which a test material that has been laced with a radioactive tracer is swallowed. The patient's body is then scanned with a gamma camera that is sensitive to the radiation emitted by the isotope. In this way it can be determined where the isotope went (i.e., the stomach vs. the lungs). The radioactive substances commonly used in scintigraphy are technetium 99, thallium, iodine 123, and gallium. When the isotope is detected by the camera, it is processed by the system's computer and displayed as a map of sparkling emissions that can be recorded on videotape or on a film plate as a static image. The intensity or brightness of the image captured correlates directly with the amount of the radioactive substance in a particular part of the body. In this way scintigraphy can quantify pulmonary aspiration (Hamlet et al., 1996; Hamlet, Muz, Farris, Kumpuris, & Jones, 1992; Hamlet, Muz, Patterson, & Jones, 1989; Humphreys et al., 1987). This is a very powerful feature of the technology.

The ability of scintigraphy to quantify aspiration has important implications in dysphagia management. Equally important is the fact that a comparison of scans taken immediately following a swallow with those completed later can determine the extent to which the pulmonary protective functions have cleared the aspirate (Klein & Steigbigel, 1983). Scintigraphy's ability to document the natural defenses to aspiration may be its most important application. The availability of scintigraphic analysis has empowered physicians and others to optimize the management of patients with dysphagia in important ways. It can provide three-phase (oral, pharyngeal, and esophageal) information regarding bolus flow, as well as information about presence or absence of aspiration and its clearance. It is also a management tool, allowing the dysphagia clinician to quantify and document the level of safety associated with a particular bolus type or avenue of nutritional intake.

Dysphagia clinicians encounter a substantial number of patients who have been placed on nothing per oral (NPO) status. For these patients nutrition and hydration are supported by a nasogastric feeding tube or perhaps a surgically placed percutaneous endoscopic gastrostomy (PEG) tube (Griggs, 1997). Once the alternate feeding route has been selected and a PEG has been placed, the patient must be monitored to determine whether there is a continuing need for the alternate avenue of intake. In a number of the etiologies commonly seen by the dysphagia management team, improvement over time can be anticipated and, therefore, the need for an alternate avenue of feeding is temporary. Unless these patients are periodically reviewed, a risk remains that some patients will continue to be fed in this manner when it is no longer needed. Considering the substantial risks associated with tube feeding, it must be discontinued as soon as the patient is able to advance to an oral diet. Some states have mandates that require interim (e.g., quarterly) reassessment of the maintenance of a feeding tube.

The monitoring is most frequently done by use of clinical and videofluoroscopic evaluations of swallowing. Often the determination of when a patient can advance to an oral diet rests heavily on a determination of whether the patient continues to evidence significant aspiration of per oral (PO) delivered foods and liquids. It is clear from the literature that this determination cannot be reliably made for many patients based on the clinical examination. For the most part, repeat videofluoroscopic evaluations of swallowing are used to detect change. Although viable, videofluoroscopic examination lacks the ability to quantify the degree of immediate aspiration. Further, it does not allow the clinician to appreciate the amount of aspirate that the patient is able to remove from the lungs over time. For these reasons, scintigraphy offers a distinct advantage. It can offer quantification of aspiration and clearance across points in time. These are significant pieces of data needed by the dysphagia clinician who is considering a recommendation to remove a patient from tube feeding.

The clinician needs to consider certain factors about glottal and pulmonary aspiration. Glottal aspiration occurs when a foreign substance passes the level of the glottis. Pulmonary aspiration occurs only when the foreign material passes to the level of the lower bronchus and below. In some professions, such as speech pathology, glottal aspiration is estimated based on judgment at the time of videofluoroscopy. In my opinion these values tend to be high relative to the amounts that actually reach the lungs. Also, they are only estimates of the true amount aspirated. Pulmonary aspiration amounts aspirated tend to be significantly lower than the values estimated with glottal aspiration. The beauty of scintigraphy is that pulmonary aspiration is quantified. Based on experience with the technology, I have found that clinically pulmonary aspiration of greater than 3% is significant. The clinician needs to understand that glottal aspiration does not obligate one to have pulmonary aspiration, much less to develop aspiration pneumonia.

In the examination the clinician chooses one medium that is administered to the patient. The nuclear medicine technician mixes the isotope with the texture. The clinician drapes and positions the patient and presents the material.

Radiation Safety Issues

Radiation physicists indicate that the amount of radiation exposure to the patient in scintigraphy is less than in most videofluoroscopic studies. Thus, in the event of a repeat scintigraphic evaluation (choosing a different texture), radiation exposure is not a limiting issue. Because scintigraphy involves the use of ionizing radiation by health care workers, oversight is provided by the Nuclear Regulatory Commission (NRC) and the Occupational Safety and Health Administration (OSHA). Each has specific requirements for personnel monitoring; laboratory monitoring; isotope storage, handling, and accountability; and decontamination. For an overview of these considerations, the reader is referred to Early (1995).

In the interest of routine safety, the patient and the clinician must wear disposable gloves. Whenever dealing with isotopes the clinician must be careful never to touch the material. It is also important that it not be allowed to spill on either the patient's or the clinician's clothing. It is helpful to tape a disposable absorbent blue pad on the patient to serve as a bib. As a safety measure, as in the event of coughing and spraying the gamma camera, the camera is also covered with disposable blue pads. If spillage does occur the blue pads are later removed, and the radioactive spillage is measured and then disposed of safely and in accordance with the Nuclear Regulatory Commission standards. Any other contaminated items are disposed of in a similar manner.

Choice of Test Materials

One of the limitations of scintigraphy is that only one food texture should be tested at a sitting. Dysphagic symptoms often depend on food texture and viscosity. The choice of test materials depends primarily on the clinical questions the clinician is attempting to answer. If the clinician wishes to know whether safe oral gratification is possible, then perhaps a thickened liquid or pureed food might be selected for testing. If the clinician wishes to know whether the patient can consume thin liquids without aspiration, then water might be selected as the medium in which to suspend the isotope.

Patient Selection Criteria

Scintigraphy is a practical technique when it is desirable to move patients from an NPO or extremely limited oral intake status to a status that significantly increases their oral intake. Cost-benefits are not maximized when scintigraphy is routinely applied to those patients who have little hope for improvement. The best candidates for scintigraphic swallowing assessment are patients who have been NPO for a period of longer than 3 months, give no clinical signs of pulmonary aspiration, and are able to sit up or otherwise alter trunk position. Other viable candidates for scintigraphic swallowing assessment are those patients, frequently hospitalized, whose dysphagia management considerations would reduce length of stay, reduce intensive care stays, or reduce the use of other procedures that may be costly. Patient selection for scintigraphic swallowing assessment should consider the issues often found in weighing the benefits of other tests. The most important issue is that of aspiration. If glottal aspiration is known or strongly suspected, it is valuable to know how much material is actually reaching the lungs.

Typically, scintigraphic swallowing assessment is not immediately recommended for patients who (a) are known heavy aspirators, (b) are suspected of having a temporary condition resulting in dysphagia for 2 months or less, or (c) have a progressively deteriorating condition such as amyotrophic lateral sclerosis. There are exceptions to these guidelines, however. Quality of life issues, such as finding even one safely tolerable texture, cannot be dismissed. In such cases scintigraphic swallowing assessment can be helpful.

Types of Scintigraphic Studies

Over time, I have worked with Sandra Hamlet on scintigraphic investigations for clinical and research purposes. Among the scintigraphic protocols we have generated are those for transit and static scintigraphic studies. A transit study evaluates 10 seconds of isotope flow through the patient's system and is used primarily for research purposes to assess volume flow. This type of study allows the identification of areas (oral, pharyngeal, or esophageal) that may contribute to subsequent aspiration. The static study occurs at the completion of transit or when the majority of the bolus is in the gastric or pulmonary regions. In this type of study, the amounts of the isotope in specific body locations are measured. Because the static study is the type more often used for *clinical* purposes, I discuss in this chapter its use as a means of detecting and quantifying pulmonary aspiration. I do not discuss the transit study protocol in further detail.

Protocol for Static Scintigraphic Images

Scintigraphic swallowing assessment takes place in a hospital's nuclear medicine section. Communication and good interpersonal professional interactions with the nuclear medicine staff are essential. To perform the examination a scintigraphy system with gamma camera and computer is needed. In addition, three external cobalt markers are needed for placement on the patient's body at specific anatomic points. Because the scintigraphic images are devoid of anatomic structures, the markers help to orient the clinician during data analysis. A cobalt marker should be taped (a) just over the anterior cricoid cartilage, (b) at the sternal notch, and (c) on the mastoid just behind the right ear. These markers are particularly useful for transit studies, but also are helpful for static scan studies as described in this protocol.

The scintigraphic study will use a radioactive isotope, typically a dose of 5 millicurie of technetium sulfur colloid (Tc 99m). The clinician will also need 120 ml (4 oz) of the one texture that will be ingested by the patient. The radioisotope is a controlled substance and must be dispensed by nuclear pharmacy and by order of the nuclear medicine radiologist. It is carefully mixed with the 120 ml of fluid or food that has been selected for the patient to consume. The technology will allow the testing of only a single texture during each scintigraphic study.

Patient Positioning and Test Material Delivery

In preparation for the study, the patient is seated and draped as previously described or standing and draped as illustrated in Figure 9.1.

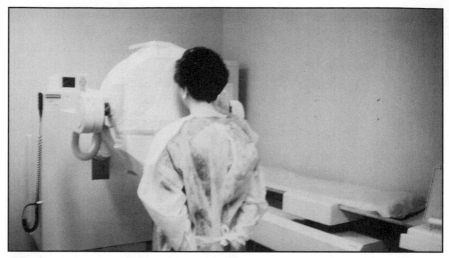

Figure 9.1. *The patient is standing in anticipation of the anterior static view. Once the scintigraphic acquisitions actually begin, the patient will need to be positioned even closer to the gamma camera. Note that both the patient and the gamma camera are draped.*

Immediately before the initiation of the study, the 5 mCi of the isotope is carefully mixed with 120 ml of the selected food or liquid. The patient is encouraged to drink or eat the test material in a manner that is customary for meals. The rate of ingestion, as well as the use of any learned compensatory swallowing strategies, should reflect what the patient will normally do while eating or drinking. It is important to note the start time of ingestion as well as the start time of each of the static scans that follows so that radioactive decay may be factored into the counts. The patient should not be given anything else to eat or drink once the 120 ml of test material has been ingested.

Data Acquisition: The Static Scan

The static scans of the patient's body are made after the patient ingests the test material. It is important for the clinician to note the time that the patient finished ingesting the test material. Although static scans may be obtained immediately after ingestion, I typically wait 30 minutes before taking the first static scan. For accurate counts the patient must be placed very close to the gamma camera for data acquisition. This is usually accomplished with the patient in a standing position. Minimally, a right anterior oblique (RAO) view and an anterior (ANT) view should be obtained. Both of these views, RAO and ANT, tend to be most reliable if the patient is able to stand. If standing is not possible, then sitting in a wheelchair, provided the gamma camera can be positioned for such, or lying in a supine position is a good alternative. Figure 9.2 shows a right anterior oblique 2-minute static scintigraphic acquisition. During data acquisition the gamma camera counts the radioactivity whenever the scintilation occurs internally. Each time a static scan is done, the data acquisition period takes 2 minutes.

When patients retain the food in oral or pharyngeal recesses, showing retention due to poor peristalsis or glottally aspirated material, it takes time for the food to resolve its course. It is often necessary to perform delayed interim static RAO and ANT static scans. In other words, it is not uncommon to do 30-minute static scans, 60-minute scans, and

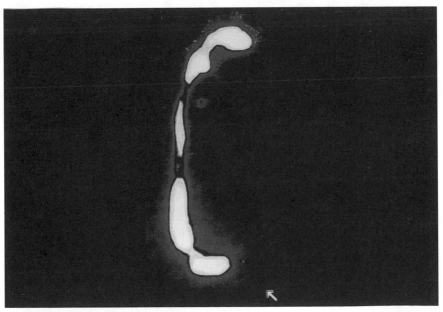

Figure 9.2. A right anterior oblique (RAO) 2-minute static scintigraphic acquisition. The arrow is pointing to the gastric area.

even 120-minute scans. Note that during the entire static scan series, the patient ingests nothing else. Once the patient has consumed the initial 120 ml with the radioactive material mixed in, that is all that the patient may ingest.

Data Analysis

Outlining Anatomic Areas. The data analysis process begins as the clinician selects and encircles regions of interest on the computer screen. This is accomplished through the computer system by use of a mouse. Normally the clinician outlines oral, pharyngeal, upper and lower esophageal, and gastric areas. The regions of the left and right lungs are also marked. Because the human eye is not adept at detecting counts as displayed on the computer screen, the clinician should be certain to use wide margins to demonstrate the aforementioned regions. In other words, all scintillation should be in a region and accounted for in establishing the outline. If high concentrations of activity are in the image, then it is possible for the clinician to be unable to see an adjacent area of trace activity. The outlining process that is done directs the computer to provide a count of the radiation emitting from each of these areas.

Specifics of Anatomic Areas of Interest. In performing the outlining process, the clinician will be dealing with representations of anatomic structures that may be foreign to his or her training and experience. When studying the image the clinician will see that the oropharyngeal boundary occurs where the overall image starts downward from oral horizontal to vertical pharyngeal. The boundary will result in approximately a 45-degree line. The pharyngeal–esophageal boundary will be just above the cricoid marker. The esophageal gastric boundary will be at the narrowest point of inferior vertical imaging. As the gastric area fills, on subsequent static films the esophageal–gastric area may be difficult to ascertain secondary to high gastric scintillation activity. The aforementioned outlining technique may be used to better determine that boundary, but from a practical standpoint the exact placement of the esophageal–gastric boundary is not critical for the purposes of this particular study.

Once the regions of radioactive activity have been outlined, the clinician should look for any activity inferior to the oral and anterior to the pharyngeal regions. Activity in this area would indicate subglottic aspiration. Such activity should also be outlined. More significantly, the clinician should look for any scintigraphic activity, albeit trace, lateral to the esophagus and superior to the previously outlined gastric area. This activity would represent pulmonary aspiration. The separate regions that are drawn should include all areas of scintillation activity. Figure 9.3 shows an example of right bronchus aspiration quantified at 0.5%. It is very important to make sure that high scintillation activity, particularly in the gastric region, does not mask trace activity in the lungs' lower lobes. The clinician needs to bear in mind that, due to diaphragm excursion during respiration, the lower lobes will show an excursion range of approximately 5 cm in an adult.

Collecting the Counts. Once the areas have been circled, the computer is directed to perform a 2-minute scan of the patient. It will do so and report its counts in each circled area. As each is completed the clinician records them. The sum of counts by each of the regions yields total count. The total count will serve as a reference for determining the percentage of aspiration in either of the lung fields.

Once the total count and regional counts have been obtained for the RAO view, the same process occurs for the ANT view. The RAO view is used in measuring transit and clearance of regions such as the oral or pharyngeal cavities. The ANT view is better used for establishing regions of potential pulmonary aspiration.

Factors Influencing Radioactivity Counts

The amount of radioactivity that is detected by the system depends on two factors: isotope half-life and the patient's tissue density. These must be accounted for to achieve accurate counts.

Isotope Half-life. Radioisotopes decay exponentially, and the term half-life is used to designate this phenomenon. Half-life refers to the amount of time necessary for a radionuclide to be reduced to half of its initial existing activity. One should know the half-life of the radionuclide being used. The half-life of Tc 99m, which is used for the majority of nuclear medicine studies, is about 6 hours. From the time the Tc 99m is mixed, its decay, begins. This decay will, of course, influence the counts in progressive static scans. There are at least two methods for

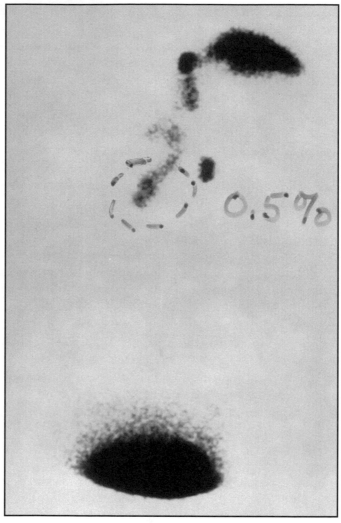

Figure 9.3. Right bronchus aspiration quantified at 0.5%. Additional follow-up 2-minute static scintigraphic acquisitions will show either resolution or pulmonary aspiration that will be quantifiable.

accounting for decay. First, a total count can be made as soon as the patient finishes the 120 ml of test texture. That number serves as reference and can be adjusted for decay. Alternatively, one can get a later total area scan. An anterior abdominal static scan should be obtained to encompass all of the regions that the test material reached. Getting accurate total area counts is important because the total count is used as the reference for determining percentage of aspiration.

Should the clinician opt to repeat the scintigraphic swallowing study for another food texture with a patient, then he or she should wait at least 72 hours if Tc 99m has been used. This waiting period is associated with the half-life of Tc 99m.

Patient Tissue Composition. Body tissue and composition will influence the accuracy of region counts. Hamlet, Choi, Kumpuris, Holliday, and Stachler (1994) have developed a method for converting for tissue attenuation. If tissue attenuation correction is not done, the counts from the proximal trachea will overestimate the amount of aspirate, and counts from the bronchi will underestimate the amount of aspirate. When in doubt, a radiation physicist should be consulted because accurate results are essential to correct interpretation.

Interpretation of Results

The percentage of pulmonary aspirate that is considered to be safe is an unresolved issue. Researchers have not yet determined what percentage of pulmonary aspirate should be evidenced on scintigraphy for an NPO recommendation to be made. Such a recommendation cannot be made without considering a number of elements that reflect the patient's overall health status and history. As other chapters in this text indicate, factors such as pulmonary immune system, dental status, and overall medical status need to be considered. Other factors such as feeding dependency and oral health status are also important. Based on experience in correlating clinical findings with scintigraphic data, I can provide two benchmarks. It appears that a reasonably healthy but dysphagic person can often handle up to 1% pulmonary aspiration without developing adverse health consequences. This value represents a combined count from both lungs. However, that same person might be physically challenged if that pulmonary aspiration were to exceed 3%. As the body of knowledge grows, clinicians will correlate scintigraphic swallowing results with arterial blood gases, pulmonary function tests, duration of intubation, presence of aerobic infection, albumin levels, and so on. The outcome will be the development of profiles for the low-tolerance aspirator. The detection of this patient profile will mandate more cautious clinical management.

Case Study

As mentioned earlier, the inception for scintigraphic application came about through clinical observation. Over 10 years ago I had the opportunity to observe four patients who had had feeding tubes. Three of these patients had had percutaneous endoscopic gastrostomies (PEGs), and one patient had had a Dobhoff nasogastric feeding tube. These four patients had received tube feedings for periods from 6 months to a little over 2 years. All patients had three factors in common: (1) they had all returned to work or to a normal lifestyle; (2) during the interval none demonstrated confirmed or clinically symptomatic signs of pulmonary aspiration; and (3) when they underwent interim videofluoroscopic assessments, they all showed pharyngeal swallowing problems including penetration into the laryngeal vestibule and, in two cases, glottic aspiration. In short, their videofluoroscopic results suggested to me that development of pneumonia was probable. Yet in reality, no pneumonia occurred in any of these four patients.

It occurred to me that, given these patients' progress and status, perhaps they had developed strategies to eliminate or significantly reduce pulmonary aspiration in spite of their videofluoroscopically demonstrated pharyngeal problems. I presented the four patients and their physicians with a proposal designed to assess their swallowing status. I proposed that each patient be given 4 oz (120 ml) of each of three different textures (solid, puree, liquid) during scintigraphic study. The multiple-texture design was proposed so that a more complete assessment of the patients' normal intake could be made. The volume of 120 ml was selected because it is a volume that would likely be consumed in the normal PO diet. The study was designed to assess bolus volume transit rates and, most important, quantify any pulmonary aspiration. The patients and their physicians agreed to the proposal.

The results of the scintigraphic assessment of the swallowing of these four patients were pleasantly surprising. None of the four patients demonstrated any pulmonary aspiration on the solid texture. When the puree texture was presented, one patient demonstrated .76% pulmonary aspiration. The remaining three patients demonstrated no pulmonary aspiration. Upon presentation of the liquid texture, the patient who aspirated .76% on the puree showed a greater level of aspiration, .882%. None of the remaining three patients showed any pulmonary aspiration on the liquid texture.

Following the scintigraphic assessments, each of the four patients and their respective physicians were contacted. The results proved very significant in determining the feeding recommendations for these patients. The three patients who failed to demonstrate pulmonary aspiration on any of the textures had their tube feedings replaced by oral feedings. The patients were asked to continue to use any swallowing strategies they had been taught. The patient who demonstrated pulmonary aspiration of less than 1% kept his PEG for hydration and was told to take solids orally and maintain the swallowing strategies he had been taught.

In follow-up completed 2 years later, none of the four subjects had developed a clinical episode of pulmonary aspiration. The implications of these outcomes are significant in terms of health care costs and quality of life. The use of scintigraphy played a pivotal role in moving these patients from tube feeding to oral diets. Without the scintigraphic data that quantified the extent of aspiration, the physicians would not have been willing to support this change. It truly produced positive outcomes for all four patients.

Summary

Because it quantifies pulmonary aspiration, scintigraphy is a powerful tool in the management of the patient with dysphagia. However, the scintigraphic swallowing assessment should not supplant other assessment mechanisms. Each of the evaluation technologies that have evolved has its strengths and weaknesses. The scintigraphic swallowing assessment is proving to be indispensable in the management of the patient with dysphagia. Clinicians can optimize the management of dysphagia by incorporating scintigraphic swallowing assessment into their assessment protocols.

References

Early, P. J. (1995). Radiation safety. In P. J. Early & D. B. Sodee (Eds.), *Principles and practice of nuclear medicine* (pp. 323–336). St. Louis: Mosby.

Griggs, B. A. (1997). Nursing management of swallowing disorders. In
M. Groher (Ed.), *Dysphagia diagnosis and management* (pp. 316–336).
Boston: Butterworth–Heinemann.

Hamlet, S. L., Choi, J., Kumpuris, T., Holliday, J., & Stachler, R. J.
(1994). Quantifying aspiration in scintigraphic deglutition testing: Tissue attenuation effects. *Journal of Nuclear Medicine, 35,*
1007–1013.

Hamlet, S. L., Choi, J., Zorrneier, M. Shamsa, F., Stachler, R., Muz, J., &
Jones, L. (1996). Normal adult swallowing of liquid and viscous
material: Scintigraphic data on bolus transit and oropharyngeal
residues. *Dysphagia, 11,* 41–47.

Hamlet, S. L., Muz, J., Farris, R., Kumpuris, T., & Jones, L. (1992).
Scintigraphic quantification of pharyngeal retention following
deglutition. *Dysphagia, 7,* 12–16.

Hamlet, S. L., Muz, J., Patterson, R. L., & Jones, L. (1989). Pharyngeal
transit time: Assessment with videofluoroscopic and scintigraphic
techniques. *Dysphagia, 4,* 4–7.

Humphreys, B., Mathog, R. H., Rosen, R., Miller, P., Muz, J., & Nelson,
R. (1987). Videofluoroscopic and scintigraphic analysis of dysphagia in the head and neck cancer patient. *Laryngoscope, 97,* 25–32.

Klein, R. S., & Steigbigel, N. H. (1983). Aspiration pneumonia. In
L. Weinstein & B. N. Fields (Eds.), *Seminars in infectious disease:
Volume V. Pneumonias.* New York: Thieme-Stratton.

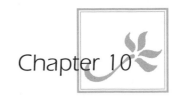

Chapter 10

Infection Control for the Dysphagia Clinician

Russell H. Mills and Brian Kobylik

Mills and Kobylik discuss a variety of diseases that can be transmitted while dysphagia services are provided. They make the point that disease transmission is multidirectional and that effective protection depends on the dysphagia clinician's appreciation of the avenues of transmission.

1. *During the clinical interaction the dysphagia clinician and patient may both be at risk for disease transmission. Who else in the clinician's environment might then receive the disease?*

2. *According to the authors, what is the single most effective thing the dysphagia clinician can do to prevent the transmission of disease?*

3. *While tuberculosis is spread primarily via an airborne route, hepatitis and HIV are spread by what route?*

4. *Although most dysphagia clinicians do not use needles in their practice, how might they be exposed to the risk of needle stick injury?*

5. *What vaccinations are available to the dysphagia clinician to protect him or her from disease?*

✢   ✢   ✢

Over the centuries health care has advanced across a broad front. Many of the concepts and technologies used today are so ingrained that it seems that they have always existed. But at some point in time, each was a revelation, a breakthrough. Many

299

dysphagia clinicians provide their services from within the framework of a modern medical center. However, there was a time when hospitals did not exist. In the Middle Ages monasteries provided way stations called "hospitalia" for sick and needy travelers. Brieger (1978), in his historical review, stated that hospitals did not appear until the 18th century and did not become commonplace until after 1900. To a significant extent it was war that prompted the necessary collection of the injured into common facilities that would allow their treatment. In 1752 John Pringle assessed medical care in the military and noted that over-crowded conditions in hospitals, barracks, and transport vessels led to "pent-up air" and illness among the soldiers. Early medical facilities were crowded, dank, and lacking in sanitation and ventilation. Hospital deaths due to what we now know to be infections was so common in England that a prominent physician of the day, Benjamin Rush, argued in 1810 that the United States of America should avoid England's error and not embrace the hospital concept (Brieger, 1978). He believed that for many patients the mortality risk was much reduced if the patient was cared for at home.

At about this time in England, a correlation was found between the number of beds in a hospital and the risk of death for patients who had undergone limb amputation. The greater the number of beds, the greater the risk of death. Although there was only a limited understanding of the cause of these high death rates, in fact many were due to the development of infection, passed from one patient to another or from the staff to the patients. Florence Nightingale served the wounded as a nurse from 1854 to 1855 during the Crimean war. She expounded on the terrible conditions that existed in hospitals of that day and argued for buildings that were designed as separate pavilions to provide adequate ventilation and for a decrease in the number of patients per bed (Centers for Disease Control and Prevention [CDC], 1987a).

Much was learned from the work of Louis Pasteur and others in the mid-1800s about the existence of microorganisms. Joseph Lister applied Pasteur's findings in 1867 to the antiseptic surgical treatment of patients. Lister proposed the use of carbolic acid dressings and other means of reducing infection. He became a diligent investigator and a prolific writer who defended his theory over the next two decades. His methods were applied in the Glasgow Royal Infirmary in England and reduced death rates from 45% to 14% for patients who had undergone amputation. By the end of the 1880s, there was growing understanding of infection and the adoption of Lister's infection control techniques became widespread.

Although much has been gained in the 130 years since the introduction of antiseptic practices, modern hospitals continue to be populated by infectious organisms. Often these organisms produce nosocomial infections, those contracted by a patient that arise from within a medical facility. We expand that definition to include the transmission of infections to health care workers from within the work site. The risk of a patient developing a nosocomial infection has varied among studies, but 5% is commonly accepted as a median value (Fahlberg & Groschel, 1978). Although antiseptic technique is the standard of practice, universal precautions have been adopted, and more powerful antibiotics have been introduced, the incidence of institutionally acquired infections has remained essentially unchanged. The dysphagia clinician must take protective measures while working in this environment of infectious organisms and persistent nosocomial infections to avoid increasing the extent to which his or her patients are placed at risk.

Controlling the risk of infection is particularly important for the dysphagia clinician who services an elderly population. In this population the potential receiver of an infection, the host, is often compromised in a variety of ways. Favero (1978) evaluated the effects of metabolic and nutritional status on the risk for development of postsurgical infection. The author showed that when there were no compromising metabolic or nutritional factors, the risk was 7.1%. When diabetes mellitus was present, as it is in many adult dysphagic patients, then the risk factor rose to 10.4%. The highest level found was when surgery occurred in the presence of severe malnutrition. In this case the risk factor jumped to 22.4%. Thus, if through ineffective infection control procedures, the dysphagia clinician causes the transmission of an organism to patients, then many will likely develop infection. Mills (1998) reported that many of the elderly dysphagic patients studied exhibited suppressed immune system function. Thus, the transmitted infection may have severe consequences.

Scores of organisms can result in nosocomial infections. In this chapter we can focus on only a few that pose significant risks to patients and health care workers in the medical center environment. For a complete review of the variety of infectious diseases, the reader is referred to Benenson (1995). We also discuss the routes of transmission (i.e., airborne, contact, vehicle, and vector). With the routes of transmission known, the clinician will be better prepared to understand and employ infection control measures to prevent the transmission of the disease.

The Multidirectional Nature of the Infection Process

A review of the literature reveals an extensive discussion of infectious diseases in the hospital environment. One portion of the literature discusses the risks posed to patients by infectious organisms. Although important, this literature does not reveal the complete picture. Another segment of the literature discusses the risk of infection to health care workers. This, too, is important but also incomplete. Only when both portions of the literature are considered together can an important concept be appreciated. Combined, the literature reveals that infectious disease does not respect directionality. Figure 10.1 shows that four groups of people—the clinician, the patient, other staff, and family members—can serve as sources for disease transmission. When

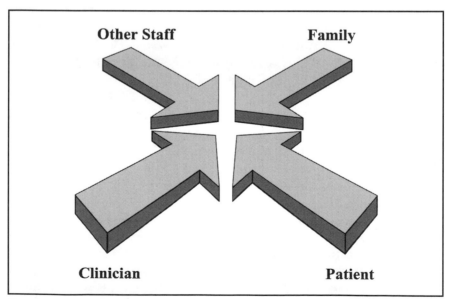

Figure 10.1. A multidirectional model of infectious disease transmission.

members of these groups interact, each has the potential for transmitting disease to members of any of the other three groups. In this way disease transmission is multidirectional. All possible interactions must be considered as infection control measures are applied.

The model also illustrates that care workers and patients can receive infections from each other. Transmission in either direction presents the possibility that the newly acquired infection can then be passed to others who were not a part of the episode of care that originally transmitted the infection. For the newly infected patient, it raises the potential for infecting other providers, patients, or visiting family members. When the worker has been infected, then passing the infection to coworkers, friends, and family members becomes possible or probable depending on the organism and its route of transmission.

Routes of Infectious Disease Transmission

Infectious disease can be transmitted in any of four primary ways: by an airborne route, by contact (direct and indirect), by an intermediate vehicle such as food or water, or by vector such as mosquito (Garner & Simmons, 1983). Some microorganisms may be transmitted by more than one route. When transmission is by an airborne route, the organism may be released in the expired air from the airway of one who is infected. The organism is then available for inhalation by the host. While the airborne route of transmission is common for tuberculosis, some droplets may not actually be inhaled into the lungs of the person receiving the organism, but merely come to rest in the oral and nasal mucosa. Consequently, some authors consider transmission in this case to be by droplet contact rather than inhalation. Organisms such as those responsible for the production of methicillin-resistant staph aureus (MRSA), vancomycin-resistant enterococci (VRE), hepatitis B (HBV), and human immunodeficiency virus (HIV) are best transmitted by direct contact between two persons. This is the most common form of transmission for nosocomial infections. MRSA and VRE are transmitted from one patient to another or to staff members by touching infected tissue or fluids (direct contact) or by touching a contaminated environmental object (indirect contact). In the case of HBV and HIV, transmission is best accomplished when there is direct blood-to-blood contact. Outside of the medical center, sexual contact is most often responsible for transmission of HBV and HIV. In the hospital, transmission of these infections is most often accomplished through a needle stick or a sharps injury. Because infectious diseases transmitted by food and water and vectorborne organisms are not professional practice issues for the dysphagia clinician, they are not addressed in this chapter.

Tuberculosis

Tuberculosis (TB) is a bacterial infection with acute and chronic phases that is caused by the organism *Mycobacterium tuberculosis* (*M. tuberculosis*). It infects the lungs and often the larynx, although other organs of the body are sometimes involved. It is estimated that one third of the world's population has been infected, although most do not develop active tuberculosis. When the immune system of the host is compromised, *M. tuberculosis* may overcome the organism's defenses and active TB may develop. Worldwide, 8.8 million cases of active TB and 3 million deaths per year are seen. More deaths occur worldwide from TB than any other infectious disease (Bloom & Murray, 1992).

For years TB was on the decline in developed nations. However, it has reemerged in the United States as a significant public health problem. Between the years 1985 and 1993, there was a 14% increase in cases reported to the CDC. Of particular concern is the significant increase in the numbers of drug-resistant and multi–drug-resistant (MDR-TB) cases of TB. In 1995 New York State reported that 13% of all positive TB cultures were resistant to at least one antibiotic. With a complete 6- to 12-month multidrug treatment course, most TB can be cured. The death rate for untreated TB is 40% to 60%. The mortality rate for those with MDR-TB who are treated is 50% to 80% (Dooley, Jarvis, Martone, & Snyder, 1992). Thus, multiple-drug resistance adds significantly to the mortality risk.

Transmission of Tuberculosis

M. tuberculosis is contained in tiny infectious droplet nuclei that are approximately 1 to 5 microns in diameter. The primary transmission of

M. tuberculosis is via an airborne route, although some may actually be transmitted through mucosal contact. As the infected person coughs, sneezes, speaks, sings, or spits, microscopic droplets are expelled from the oral and nasal cavities. The droplets may contain bacilli that can be inhaled by another individual within the same air space. The droplets are sufficiently small that room air currents can keep them suspended and circulate them to other parts of a building for an extended period of time. The expelled droplets usually contain few bacilli. Consequently, transmission of the disease is more likely with prolonged contact with an infected individual. For this reason, family members and residential caregivers are at greatest risk.

Evolution of the Tuberculosis Infection

When droplets containing *M. tuberculosis* are inhaled, it is common for the bacteria to settle in the air sacs (alveoli) of the lungs. When the body detects the presence of these "invaders," it summons macrophages to combat them. Macrophages attack the bacterium by ingesting them. Although many bacterium will die, others may survive and multiply within the alveoli. During the initial 2 to 8 weeks of the infection, T-lymphocytes become aware of the presence of the bacterium and respond with a hypersensitivity reaction. It is this reaction that will cause the tuberculin skin test (Mantoux) to become significant. A significant response to the skin test does not mean that the individual has developed tuberculosis disease, but that at some time he or she has been infected with the organism.

The T-lymphocytes' response to the infection may cause infected macrophages to be "walled off" to form hard capsules known as tubercles. In this way *M. tuberculosis* is confined. The only evidence of the disease may be a continuing response to the skin test. It is common for those who are infected to have the disease lie dormant for months, years, or even decades. In approximately 10% of cases—that is, in about 15 million persons in the United States—the disease is reactivated by exogenous or endogenous factors and develops into active TB. Development of active disease is more likely when the patient's immune system is compromised, as in the elderly, the malnourished, or those with HIV. Then the disease may break out of the tubercules and become active.

Making the Tuberculosis Diagnosis

The diagnosis of TB depends on the medical history, physical examination, skin test, chest X-ray, and microscopic examination and culture of sputum samples. Other diagnostic tests such as bronchoscope may be ordered. The primary screening test is the tuberculin skin test or Mantoux test, which is based on putrefied protein derivative (PPD) that is injected just under the skin. It is also known as the PPD skin test. Two to 3 days following injection, it is "read." An induration with a diameter of 10 to 15 mm at the injection site is evidence that the individual has been infected with *M. tuberculosis*, not necessarily evidence that the individual has developed TB.

Tuberculosis Risk to Health Care Workers

Health care workers have been identified as having a heightened exposure to TB (Meredith, Watson, & Citron, 1996). Elpern and Girzadas (1993) identified health care occupations in general, and nursing specifically, as high risk for TB infection. A recent study of 1,303 health care workers in a New York City hospital revealed that physicians and nurses, along with housekeepers, laundry workers, and security personnel, were in the highest tuberculin conversion group (Louther et al., 1997). McKenna, Hutton, Cauthen, and Onorato (1996) found that inhalation therapists showed elevated rates, whereas Esposito (1992) observed increased TB infection rates among nursing home workers. Concern for the welfare of the health care worker has increased with the development of an increased number of drug-resistant strains (Baker, 1995).

Risks and Prevention for the Dysphagia Clinician

The level of TB risk to health care workers is tied to a number of factors, including the nature of the patient population and especially the amount and type of involvement the worker has with such patients. Esposito (1992) reported that 13% of hospitals had received reports of nosocomial TB transmission to health care workers, and concluded that the application of sound prevention and control measures could reduce the occupational transmission of the disease (Louther et al., 1997). The CDC (1994b) issued guidelines for health care facilities to follow to reduce the likelihood of TB transmission in health care settings. Although the CDC did not specifically address the activities of the dysphagia clinician, the following sections describe elements that apply to the dysphagia clinician's practice.

Medical Surveillance Programs. The medical center must provide a medical surveillance program for employees who are at risk. Dysphagia clinicians should be in that surveillance program. A central part of that program is TB skin testing and appropriate follow-up of employees who are considered to be at risk. Follow-up to a new PPD test conversion is to include a physical examination, laboratory tests, chest X-ray, and other tests as indicated. Although the institution is mandated by OSHA to monitor PPD test results, the prudent clinician will be aware of his or her testing schedule and results and take appropriate action to ensure that follow-up is provided when needed.

Delays in Diagnosis and Treatment. Schwartzman, Loo, Pasztor, and Menzies (1996) reported that when diagnostic delays occur, there is increased risk of TB infection for health care workers. Patients with active TB appear at medical centers, where other patients have come for the alleviation of their symptoms. They may experience persistent cough, bloody sputum, night sweats, weight loss, and fever, all of which are commonly associated with TB. Unfortunately, these symptoms are not fully diagnostic because they are shared with other disease entities. A variety of tests may be needed to make the differential diagnosis. Consequently, during the initial days of hospitalization, the patient may be highly mobile, traveling to a variety of locations for diagnostic testing. If symptoms of dysphagia coexist, then such a patient might appear for a dysphagia evaluation before being diagnosed and isolated.

Appropriate Signage. Signs must be provided to alert health care workers of the presence of TB risk and proper precautions to be taken. That signage will be located at the entry door to the patient's isolation room and may state "AFB Isolation" (acid-fast bacilli). The sign will specify those elements of protection that are required. It is the clinician's responsibility to know the proper precautions to be taken and to follow the institution's policies.

Locations for the Delivery of Dysphagia Services. When active TB is suspected or diagnosed, the CDC recommends that the patient be placed in a negative pressure isolation room. The room is maintained with an air pressure slightly less than the rest of the hospital. Thus, air flows into the room but room air is exhausted outside of the building to prevent the spread of *M. tuberculosis.* CDC also recommends that when a patient is known to have active TB, services should be provided, as much as possible, in the patient's negative pressure isolation environment.

For a patient with TB and dysphagia, CDC's recommendations seem to suggest that performing a clinical examination, a Fiberoptic Endoscopic Evaluation of Swallowing (FEES), or fluoroscopy with a C-arm system brought to the isolation room would be appropriate ways to evaluate while reducing risk of infection to others in the medical center. There is increased risk of disease transmission when services are provided to patients in non–negative pressure environments, such as small treatment rooms or rooms with poor ventilation. If it is necessary to transport the patient to the radiology department to complete a fluoroscopy examination, then the patient should wear a surgical mask to reduce the spread of infected droplets. In some cases it may be warranted to delay the dysphagia evaluation until the patient is no longer infective, which may require several weeks. Whether such a delay is appropriate will depend on factors specific to the individual case.

Cough-Inducing Procedures and TB Transmission. CDC makes special mention of procedures that stimulate the cough. This is especially important when the clinician is in close proximity to the patient's oral cavity. A cough or sneeze when the clinician is in this location will encourage the direct transmission of *M. tuberculosis* into the clinician's lungs. Per oral aspiration followed by a spontaneous cough is a common occurrence in dysphagia evaluations. When clinical and FEES examinations are performed, the clinician's face is often close to the oral cavity, increasing the likelihood of inhaling droplets into his or her airway. The dysphagia clinician must be aware of the risk factors and be prepared to employ adequate precautions.

The Use of Protective Barriers to Reduce the Risk of TB. Although the TB organism is transmitted through the airborne route, gloves are still recommended for clinical procedures as a commonsense part of universal precautions. Respirators (see Figure 10.2) were created to protect the wearer from inhaling organisms or contaminants that are present in the air. This is also a function ascribed to surgical masks, although they were not designed to perform this function. They were designed to prevent the respiratory secretions of the wearer from reaching the environment. With this function in mind, it would make sense for the patient with active TB to wear a surgical mask when outside of the negative pressure isolation environment. It would not be appropriate for a dysphagia clinician to wear a surgical mask as a means of protection from *M. tuberculosis*.

Each medical center has an infection control committee that determines which employee groups will be provided with particulate respirators. Each respirator is individually fitted to provide an airtight seal between the mask and the wearer's face. The respirator must meet 42 CFR, Part 84 standards adopted by CDC and OSHA (CDC, 1994a). When properly fitted, the respirator will filter particles as small as 1 micrometer with at least 95% efficiency.

Clinicians must wear respirators when entering rooms housing individuals with suspected or confirmed infectious TB. They must also be worn when performing high-hazard procedures with these

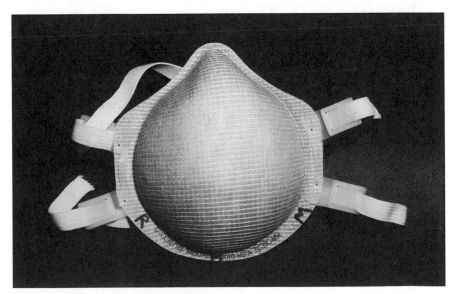

Figure 10.2. A particulate respirator for protection from airborne pathogens.

patients. High-hazard procedures should include those that are likely to produce coughing and those performed with the clinician in close proximity to the oral cavity. Although dysphagia clinicians are not considered at great risk, the procedures they provide must be considered hazardous. Careful considerations must be given to the implementation of protective measures, including the use of a respirator.

Viral Hepatitis

Hepatitis is an inflammatory disease of the liver. It may be caused by a variety of toxins, medications, or infectious agents. Most infectious hepatitis is caused by viruses. There are several forms of the hepatitis virus (HV): hepatitis virus A, B, C, Delta, and E. They share the fact that they all have similar clinical presentations and produce damaging effects in the liver. Although they are grouped together, they differ in important ways, including route of transmission, degree of risk posed for the health care worker, and the protective measures that are appropriate.

Hepatitis Virus A (HAV)

HAV has a fecal–oral route of transmission (direct contact). The prevalence of exposure in developing countries is extremely high. In Cameroon 94% of children entering primary school were found to have the anti-HAV antigen that indicates previous exposure to HAV (Stroffolini et al., 1991). In developed countries it is most commonly found in day care centers where contamination through diaper changing spreads the disease. It is also found in school-age populations. Widespread outbreaks that occurred in the United States in 1961, 1971, and 1989 were associated with contaminated food and water (vehicle route). It has also been associated with raw or undercooked shellfish harvested from contaminated waters and contaminated produce such as lettuce and strawberries (vehicle route). A vaccine now exists for HAV, but it is not universally mandated (Kane, 1992).

Commonly, the individual infected with HAV experiences fever, anorexia, nausea, abdominal discomfort, and jaundice, symptoms that are similar to those of other forms of viral hepatitis. The patient usually remains infectious for approximately 7 days following the onset of jaundice. The illness lasts a few weeks, or in rare cases several months. Complete recovery without lasting effects is the rule for HAV. Overall, the case fatality rate is low at 1 per 1,000 cases. Among persons greater than 50 years of age, however, the mortality rate rises to 27 per 1,000 (Benenson, 1995).

The Use of Protective Barriers To Reduce the Risk of HAV. Because of the fecal–oral route of transmission, the most effective means of limiting its spread is religious hand washing. In day care centers it is important that hands are washed between each diaper change and that soiled diapers are disposed of properly. To interrupt the cycle it is necessary that day care workers, food processors, and food handlers all take the same precautions. The risks may be greater for dysphagia clinicians who provide services to the pediatric population than those who service the elderly. If commonsense infection control practices are employed, risks should be minimal.

Because the transmission of HAV is not airborne, masks are not required. Gowns are indicated only if soiling is likely. Gloves should be worn if infected material will be touched. In that it is unknown what portions of the patient's skin or clothing may have had contact with fecal material, gloves are recommended for all procedures that the dysphagia clinician performs. The greatest single thing the dysphagia clinician can do to protect against the transmission of HAV is to wash his or her hands after and between procedures. The importance of this recommendation cannot be overstated.

Hepatitis E (HEV)

HEV was formally called Enteric Non-A Non-B. The disease is most often associated with contaminated water (vehicle route) and, like HAV, probably has a fecal–oral route of transmission. HEV is most common in countries with poor environmental sanitation and is associated with waterborne epidemics. The only cases seen in the United States are in people who have traveled to countries where the disease is endemic. It is the one form of viral hepatitis that has only an acute phase. Most clinicians will never encounter this virus in the patients they treat, unless the patient has traveled to areas where HEV is endemic.

The Use of Protective Barriers To Reduce the Risk of HEV. As with other diseases that are spread by contact, wearing gloves and hand washing are the best protections during professional practice.

Hepatitis Virus B (HBV)

HBV was formerly called serum hepatitis. Like the other forms of the hepatitis virus, HBV targets the liver. HBV is found in virtually all of the infected patient's body secretions and excretions. It is estimated that between 10% and 25% of those who contract hepatitis B may develop chronic active hepatitis that can lead to cirrhosis and death (CDC, 1982). CDC estimates that 300,000 new HBV infections occur each year in the United States and 0.3% of the population is composed of chronic carriers of the disease (CDC, 1987b). Although the incidence of HBV among health care workers has decreased due to the availability of an effective vaccine and improved infection control measures, the prevalence of patients who are HBV positive has increased (Lanphear, 1997). Thus, there is a significant opportunity for the dysphagia clinician to encounter patients who are positive for HBV.

Blood, serum, saliva, semen, and vaginal fluids have shown the ability to transmit the virus by percutaneous and permucosal routes (direct contact). In the social environment, HBV transmission is most frequently linked to sexual contact. Transmission has also been demonstrated in the transfusion of blood and blood products, needle sharing, hemodialysis, acupuncture, tattooing, and needle sticks. In the health care setting a common method of transmission is via a sharps injury, usually a needle stick injury. Although HBV is stable on environmental surfaces (indirect contact) for as long as 7 days, transmission by contact with environmental surfaces is far less likely than any of the above methods. Unlike HAV, transmission by the fecal–oral route has not been demonstrated. In approximately 35% of cases, the mode of transmission has not been determined.

HBV is the most common form of viral hepatitis to be found in the health care worker population (Lanphear, 1997). A screening study of health care workers in Japan found that 1.1% showed evidence of the HBV surface antigen, indicating exposure to the disease (Miyajima et al., 1997). In 1983 it was estimated that 500 to 600 health care workers whose jobs entail exposure to blood and body fluids are hospitalized annually, with over 200 deaths due to fulminant hepatitis, cirrhosis, and liver cancer (Palmer, Barash, King, & Neil, 1983). Employees in a medical center who are not exposed to blood and other body fluids are at no greater risk than the general public. It has been estimated that over the long term there is a 15% to 30% chance for health care workers in high-risk categories to develop an HBV infection (Chin, 1982). It is important for clinicians to recognize that the risk of contracting the disease for those who are exposed to HBV greatly exceeds the risk for those exposed to HIV (Vlahov & Polk, 1987). The risk of acquiring HBV from a needle stick injury by a contaminated needle ranges from 6% to 30%, which is substantially greater than the 0.3% risk associated with a similar event when the needle is contaminated with HIV (CDC, 1985; Vlahov, 1987).

Reducing the Risk of HBV Transmission. High-risk employment categories include those that will expose the worker primarily to blood or blood-containing body fluids or that have the potential for sharps injury. Included in this list are pathologists, surgeons, internists, dentists, dental technicians, emergency room staff, dialysis workers, IV therapy teams, ICU nurses, hematologists, blood bank personnel, and others. Although dysphagia clinicians may be exposed to saliva and vomitus that contain blood, they are not normally exposed directly to a patient's undiluted blood. Thus, while their risk may be greater than for some health care occupations, they likely do not fall into the high-risk category.

Health care workers tend to underestimate the occupational risk imposed by blood-borne pathogens, and consequently show low compliance in infection control measures (Ippolito et al., 1995). The dysphagia clinician must appreciate the risk imposed by HBV and the health consequences associated with infection. Actions that the dysphagia clinician can take to effectively reduce the risk are not based on the disease, but reflect the route of HBV transmission. Consequently, they are appropriate whenever there is the risk that the clinician will be contaminated by contact with blood or body fluids. In practice these are universal precautions for blood-borne pathogens.

One of us (Kobylik), an infection control nurse, always reminds clinicians, "If it's wet, protect." This comment reflects the CDC's (1987a) recommendations that work practices should be based on the assumption that all body fluids and tissues are infectious. Thus, the protective measures that are applied are independent of whether the diagnosis is known, posted on the wall, or recorded in the medical chart. Assuming the infectious nature of blood, tissue, and fluids allows the clinician to be properly protected with all cases. Thus, if it is possible that the clinician will contact blood or body fluids ("If it's wet"), then he or she should respond with protection.

Vaccination To Protect Against HBV Infection. Since 1982 a vaccine has been available to protect workers from HBV exposure. Initially, vaccines were prepared using inactivated hepatitis B surface antigen particles obtained from the blood of donors infected with HBV. Now they are genetically engineered using yeast cells. The vaccine is given in three injections, with the second and third given 1 and 6 months following the first. The vaccine is 90% effective in preventing an HBV infection. However, not all persons have an equal likelihood of being protected by the vaccine (Occupational Safety and Health Administration, 1983). Some data have shown that obesity and smoking can reduce the likelihood of receiving protection from vaccination. The CDC evaluated the safety of the vaccine in a series of 200,000 cases and found only 62 episodes of illness that might have been vaccine related. Only 6 of these were considered serious. Thus the CDC has concluded that the vaccine is quite safe.

If the vaccine protects 90% of the employees who receive it, then 10% remain unprotected following inoculation. Approximately 6 weeks following the completion of the HBV vaccination series, the dysphagia clinician should ask that a titer be run to determine whether he or she has developed antibodies to HBV. A sample of blood is then taken and evaluated for the presence of antibodies. If the clinician is reactive, then resistance to the disease has developed. If not, then a booster is provided. Later, the clinician should again ask that a titer be run to determine whether the booster has imparted resistance to HBV.

Infectious HBV Signage. The CDC recommends that hospitals adopt a method of signage to inform health care workers and visitors of the presence of certain infections. Often a pink card is posted on the door or near the bed stating "Blood/Body Fluid Precautions" or "Hepatitis B." The card informs the clinician of the type of precautions that are required upon entering the room. The dysphagia clinician is obligated to be aware of the signs and apply appropriate protection.

The Use of Protective Barriers To Reduce the Risk of HBV. Because HBV is not transmitted via an airborne route, masks are not indicated as a means of protecting the clinician from infection. Gloves are indicated where the clinician may contact blood, body fluids, or saliva. Saliva may be encountered during feeding or when performing an oromotor examination, a clinical examination for swallowing, or a FEES examination. When a tracheostomy is present, the risk of such contact is elevated. As a practice, dysphagia clinicians should not engage in any of these clinical activities with any patient without first donning disposable gloves. Once gloves have been donned, they should be checked for splits and tears. As shown in Figure 10.3, defects are possible and can compromise protection.

Gowns should be worn when blood, body fluid, or saliva may contaminate clothing. A face shield should be worn when there is risk that food contents or saliva may be spit or ejected into the clinician's face. When serving the adult population, this should be an unusual occurrence. For each case, the dysphagia clinician should evaluate the procedure to be performed and the behavioral characteristic of the patient to determine when a gown or face shield may be prudent.

Reusable Equipment. CDC has provided specific recommendations that require reusable equipment to be sterilized or decontaminated. It

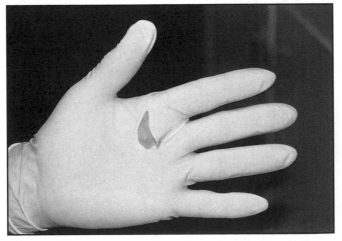

Figure 10.3. Infection protection breached by a glove tear.

is recommended that, where possible, only disposable items be used in dysphagia evaluation and management.

Protection from Needle Stick Injuries. The greatest risk for the transmission of HBV in the hospital is infection via a needle stick injury. Henry and Campbell (1995) stated that 800,000 needle sticks are reported each year but that many others are not reported. Although dysphagia clinicians do not routinely use syringes coupled to needles, they do use syringes without needles. Syringes may be used in feeding, bolus presentation in the dysphagia examination, and tracheostomy cuff inflation. Although these uses seem harmless enough, a risk exists. All syringes, with or without needles, are considered to be hazardous waste and must be discarded in a sharps container, usually placed in strategic locations on the ward or in examination rooms. Such a container is shown in Figure 10.4. These boxes are designed with a protective cover that prevents one from reaching in while disposing of an item. Because the boxes are not always emptied before they become full, it is possible to reach toward the container to dispose of a syringe, only to find needles protruding from the top. While not a common occurrence, this situation places the dysphagia clinician at risk for a

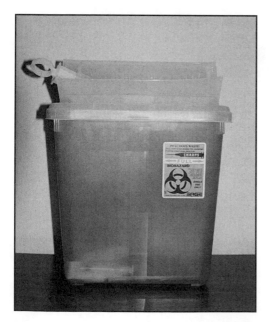

Figure 10.4. A sharps container for the disposal of syringes and needles.

needle stick injury. Clinicians should always be careful when making these disposals.

Hand Washing. The single most effective thing the clinician can do to limit the transmission of disease is to wash his or her hands. Even when gloves are worn during a procedure, hands should be washed as soon as the gloves are removed. If patients are to be seen in succession, hand washing should take place before the next set of gloves is donned. To complicate matters, frequent hand washing and the use of disposable gloves can produce skin damage that may make percutaneous transmission of disease more likely (Larson, Friedman, Cohran, Treston-Aurand, & Green, 1997). Latex allergies also complicate the situation for some people. Consequently, dysphagia clinicians must be vigilant for the presence of skin lesions and scaling, and change to a different type of soap or gloves when necessary.

Actions Necessary Following HBV Exposure. If the clinician's eyes, mouth, or broken skin becomes exposed to blood or saliva, or if a sharps injury occurs, it is important to immediately notify the infection control nurse or employee health physician, who can provide advice regarding any actions that should be taken. In some cases the infection control physician might recommend Hepatitis B immune globulin (HBIG), which can modify an HBV infection (CDC, 1981). To ensure the highest probability of effectiveness, the HBIG must be given within 48 to 72 hours of the injury.

Hepatitis D (Hepatitis Delta or HDV)

Hepatitis Delta is very similar to HBV in its signs and symptoms. The most important feature of HDV is that it always coexists with HBV. It appears that in the past, 25% to 50% of the fulminant cases thought to be due to HBV were actually due to the effects of HDV. The disease may be self-limiting or progress to chronic hepatitis.

The Use of Protective Barriers To Reduce the Risk of HDV. Methods of protection for this virus should follow those outlined for HBV since they share common routes of transmission. It is important to note that vaccination against HBV also protects the individual from contracting HDV.

Hepatitis C (HCV)

Hepatitis C was formerly called Hepatitis non-A non-B. It has an insidious onset with an incubation period of 6 to 9 weeks. Symptoms of the disease, similar to other forms of viral hepatitis, include anorexia, abdominal discomfort, nausea, and vomiting. A smaller percentage of HCV patients progress to jaundice than do patients with HBV. The disease is transmitted through percutaneous exposure to blood and plasma derivatives. The most common form of transmission in the health care environment is needle stick injury. In over 40% of cases the risk factors that lead to infection cannot be determined. A diagnostic test for anti-HCV antibodies has been developed, but a vaccine is not available at this time.

In 75% of cases the acute illness from HCV is only mild. Fulminating and fatal cases are rare. Of concern is that more than 80% of patients with HCV will show evidence of chronic liver disease. Of these, 30% to 60% may develop chronic active hepatitis and up to 20% will develop cirrhosis of the liver. Studies indicate that approximately 2.5% of health care workers are reactive in HCV testing, indicating previous exposure to the virus (Goetz, Ndimbie, Wagener, & Muder, 1995; Miyajima et al., 1997).

The Use of Protective Barriers To Reduce the Risk of HCV. Because the known route of transmission is percutaneous, the prevention measures recommended for HBV are appropriate for HCV. Based on the absence of identified risk factors in a significant number of HCV cases, these protections may be incomplete.

Human Immunodeficiency Virus

The human immunodeficiency virus (HIV) produces a progressive disease that damages the immune system, as well as other organ systems. In later stages the disease is labeled acquired immunodeficiency syndrome (AIDS). AIDS was first recognized in 1981. A serologic test for the detection of HIV became available in 1985. In 1995 the World Health Organization estimated that there were approximately 4.5 million cases of AIDS worldwide. Although the largest groups affected in the United

States are homosexual men and injecting drug users, the largest recent increases have been among women and minority populations. Women constituted 7% of AIDS cases in 1981 and 23% in 1998 (CDC, 1998).

Evolution of the Disease

Within the first weeks or months following exposure, many of those infected with HIV will develop a short-term mononucleosis-like illness with a 1- to 2-week duration. Most will produce antibodies within the first 1 to 3 months that can be detected by laboratory tests. The initial illness is often followed by a period of months or years during which the individual is free from symptoms. When this period ends, it is with the onset of clinical illness that is marked by a variety of opportunistic infections and clinical symptoms, including lymphadenopathy, anorexia, chronic diarrhea, weight loss, fever, and fatigue (Benenson, 1995). This late stage of the disease is termed AIDS. The degree to which the body is invaded by a host of opportunistic infections is characteristic of the degree of damage to the immune system.

Mode of HIV Transmission

Casual or social contact with HIV-infected persons carries no risk of disease transmission. The routes of transmission are the same as those for HBV. Outside of the hospital the predominant means of transmission is through sexual contact. The sharing of needles and syringes by drug users has also been a significant source of infection. Although HIV has been found in tears, pulmonary secretions, urine, and saliva, transmission after contact with these fluids has not been documented (Benenson, 1995). Within the medical center environment, HIV has been transmitted to patients through the transfusion of blood and blood products. The greatest occupational risk is associated with needle stick or sharps injury. Seroconversion rates following needle stick injuries with HIV-infected needles have been reported at approximately 0.3%. For the needle contaminated by HBV, 25% is a reasonable estimate. To put this difference into perspective, for each 1,000 employees experiencing a needle stick injury, 3 employees will be positive for HIV whereas 250 will be infected by HBV. Clearly, HBV presents a much greater risk from needle stick.

The Use of Protective Barriers
To Reduce the Risk of HIV

HIV, like HBV, is a blood-borne pathogen. As such, HIV requires the same methods of protection. Although masks are not required, facial protection should be worn if there is the potential for spattering. Gloves should be worn if the clinician may be touching infected tissue, blood, or fluids. Gowns are required if blood or fluids may soil the clinician's clothing.

Methicillin-Resistant
Staphylococcus Aureus

Staphylococcus aureus (*S. aureus*) represents a group of pathogens that are commonly found on the skin. They do not always produce disease, but *S. aureus* has been associated with the infection of decubitus ulcers (bedsores) and surgical wounds and pneumonia, meningitis, endocarditis, and sepsis (Benenson, 1995). Over 60% of the strains of *S. aureus* have demonstrated resistance to antibiotics and the number is growing (Ibelings & Bruining, 1998). These resistant forms have been labeled methecillin-resistant *Staphylococcus aureus* (MRSA). MRSA represents a major nosocomial problem in hospitals. Not only is MRSA a common cause of infection, but when contracted by a compromised host, it may be extremely difficult to eliminate. The resistance that has been developed by MSRA has produced significant increases of morbidity and mortality in medical centers. A study of 10,038 hospitalized patients in Europe found that 21% of ICU patients had acquired MRSA (Ibelings & Bruining, 1998). At Frankfurt University hospital a strong correlation was found between the severity of MRSA and the length of stay with a 28.6% mortality rate among those patients who had acquired MRSA (Wichelhaus, Westphal, Kessler, Schafer, & Brade, 1998).

Method of Transmission

Health care workers can serve the nosocomial transmission process in different ways. First, the worker may be a carrier of an MRSA strain. Second, the worker may transport the organism directly from one patient to another through direct contact. Finally, he or she may transmit the organism to an environmental object. At a later time, another health care worker or patient may contact the environmental object and transfer the organism to another patient. Boyce, Potter-Bynoe, Chenevert, and King (1997) found environmental contamination in the rooms of 73% of the patients infected with MRSA. Contaminated items included floors, bed linens, the patient's gown, tables, and blood pressure cuffs. In the course of their duties, 42% of health care workers who had no direct contact with infected patients contacted environmental objects and transferred the organism to their gloves. Data also indicate that there may be other environmental factors, as evidenced by an outbreak of the EMRAS-15 strain that was directly linked to contamination of a ventilation system (Kumari et al., 1998). Medical centers and health care workers must employ diligent infection control measures with respect to MRSA.

The Use of Protective Barriers To Reduce the Risk of MRSA

Because contact with the patient tissue, particularly wound sites, is a major factor in transmission, the clinician should wear gloves when providing any procedure that may involve touching the patient's tissues. The clinician also needs to be aware of environmental surfaces that he or she may touch, as these may be a source of contamination for future staff and patients. A gown is recommended if a patient's body part or fluid might contact the clinician's clothes. Due to the potential for nares acquisition, a mask should be worn when care is provided to the skin or a wound. Wearing the mask may prevent colonization of the health care worker. As always, hand washing is the most important way to prevent the spread of these resistant organisms.

Vancomycin-Resistant Enterococci

Under normal conditions enterococci are organisms that inhabit the stomach and intestines. They are very durable organisms and can live in a wide range of temperatures, pH conditions, and oxygen saturation levels. Only two forms of enterococci infect the human, *E. faecium* and *E. faecalis,* and they are responsible each year for 176,000 cases of bacteremia, urinary tract infections, wound infection, and endocarditis in the United States. Risk factors to consider include prolonged hospital-ization, multiple antibiotics, high severity of illness score, intraabdom-inal surgery, renal insufficiency, enteral tube feedings, and exposure to specific hospital units, nurses, or contaminated objects in patient care areas. Reports began to appear in the 1980s that described increased resistance of enterococci to penicillin. Vancomycin-resistant enterococci (VRE) is now a well-established infectious disease problem in medical centers. Between 1989 and 1993 VRE increased more than 20-fold in this country (Huycke, Sahm, & Gilmore, 1998). Of particular concern is the laboratory-based finding that *Staphylococcus aureus* has been ren-dered vancomycin resistant through transfer of resistance from the VRE organism (Noble, Virani, & Cree, 1992). This means that one bacterium that was antibiotic resistant passed that trait to another bacterium. The consequences of such a transfer occurring in the human body could be disastrous.

Transmission of VRE

As an enterococcus, VRE is found in the gut and human feces of those who are infected. Thus, the best opportunity for the spread of VRE is by the hands of health care workers or by contact with medical devices. Lack of hand washing and the soiling of environmental objects such as bed rails, sinks, faucets, and doorknobs enhance the likelihood of a transmission. It is important that efforts to avoid environmental con-tamination be rigorous, including appropriate cleaning.

The Use of Protective Barriers
To Reduce the Risk of VRE

Because VRE is transmitted by contact, precautions of the type that are appropriate for HBV, HIV, and MRSA are appropriate. Although a mask is not needed, gloves should be worn and gowns donned should it be likely that blood or body fluids will soil the clinician's clothing.

Summary

The spread of nosocomial infections is a major problem facing medical centers. The risk for transmission of infectious diseases applies not only to patients, but also to dysphagia clinicians. Although risks exist, so do effective measures to prevent and control the spread of disease. To operate safely the clinician must be aware of the routes by which infections are transmitted. With this information the clinician can apply appropriate precautions to ensure the safety of the parties involved. Above all, the single most effective action the clinician can take is the religious washing of hands after each and every procedure.

References

Baker, S. A. (1995). Airborne transmission of respiratory diseases. *Journal of Clinical Engineering, 20*(5), 401–406.

Benenson, A. S. (1995). *Control of communicable diseases manual.* (16th ed.). Washington, DC: American Public Health Association.

Bloom, B. R., & Murray, C. J. L. (1992). Tuberculosis: Commentary on a reemergent killer. *Science, 257,* 1055–1064.

Boyce, J. M., Potter-Bynoe, G., Chenevert, C., & King, T. (1997). Environmental contamination due to methicillin-resistant Staphylococcus aureus: Possible infection control implications. *Infection Control and Hospital Epidemiology, 18*(9), 622–627.

Brieger, G. H. (1978). Hospital infections: A brief historical appraisal. In W. J. Fahlberg & D. Groschel (Eds.), *Occurrence, diagnosis, and sources of hospital associated infections* (pp. 95–125). New York: Marcel Dekker.

Centers for Disease Control and Prevention. (1981). Immune globulin for protection against viral hepatitis. *Morbidity and Mortality Weekly Report, 30,* 423–435.

Centers for Disease Control and Prevention. (1982). Inactivated hepatitis B virus vaccine: Recommendations of the Immunization Practices Advisory Committee. *Annals of Internal Medicine, 97,* 379–383.

Centers for Disease Control and Prevention. (1985, November). Recommendations for preventing transmission of infection with human T-lymphotrophic virus type III/Lymphadenopathy-associated virus in the workplace. *Morbidity and Mortality Weekly Report, 34,* 681–686, 691–695.

Centers for Disease Control and Prevention. (1987a). *Guidelines for protecting the safety and health of health care workers: joint advisory notice.* Washington DC: Centers for Disease Control and Prevention.

Centers for Disease Control and Prevention. (1987b). Update on hepatitis B prevention. *Morbidity and Mortality Weekly Report, 36,* 353–360.

Centers for Disease Control and Prevention. (1994a). 42 CFR Part 84: Respiratory protective devices, proposed rule. *Federal Register, 59,* 26849–26889.

Centers for Disease Control and Prevention. (1994b). Guidelines for preventing the transmission of mycobacterium tuberculosis in health care facilities. *Morbidity and Mortality Weekly Report, 43,* 1–132.

Centers for Disease Control and Prevention. (1998). *HIV/AIDS Surveillance Report, 10*(2), 1–44.

Chin, J. (1982). The use of hepatitis B virus vaccine. *New England Journal of Medicine, 307,* 678–679.

Dooley, S. W., Jarvis, W. R., Martone, W. J., & Snyder, D. E., Jr. (1992). Multi-drug resistant tuberculosis [editorial]. *Annals of Internal Medicine, 117,* 257–258.

Elpern, E. H., & Girzadas, A. M. (1993). Tuberculosis update: New challenges of an old disease. *Medical–Surgical Nursing, 2*(3), 176–183.

Esposito, A. L. (1992). Pulmonary infections acquired in the workplace: A review of occupation-associated pneumonia. *Clinical Chest Medicine 13*(2), 355–365.

Fahlberg, W. J., & Groschel, D. (1978). *Occurrence, diagnosis and sources of hospital-associated infections.* New York: Marcel Dekker.

Favero, M. S. (1978). Sources of hospital-associated microorganisms. In W. J. Fahlberg & D. Groschel (Eds.), *Occurrence, diagnosis, and sources of hospital-associated infections* (pp. 95–125). New York: Marcel Dekker.

Garner, J. S., & Simmons, B. P. (1983). *CDC guideline for isolation precautions in hospitals.* Washington, DC: Centers for Disease Control and Prevention.

Goetz, A. M., Ndimbie, O. K., Wagener, M. M., & Muder, R. R. (1995). Prevalence of hepatitis C infection in health care workers affiliated with a liver transplant center. *Transplantation, 59*(7), 990–994.

Huycke, M. M., Sahm, D. F., & Gilmore, M. S. (1998). Multiple-drug resistant enterococci: The nature of the problem and an agenda for the future. *Emerging Infectious Diseases, 4*(2), 239–249.

Ibelings, M. M., & Bruining, H. A. (1998). Methicillin-resistant Staphylococcus aureus: Acquisition and risk of death in patients in the intensive care unit. *European Journal of Surgery, 162*(6), 411–418.

Ippolito, G., Sagliocca, L., D'Ubaldo, C., Ruggiero, A., Fabozzi, O. C., De Masi, S., & Petrosillo, N. (1995). The knowledge, attitudes and practice in regard to the risk for occupational HIV infection in a group of gynecologists from three Italian regions. *Epidemiolgie Prevenzione, 19*(64), 276–281.

Kane, M. A. (1992). Perspectives on the control of hepatitis A by vaccination. *Vaccine, 10*(Suppl. 1), S93–S96.

Kumari, D. N., Hiji, T. C., Keer, V., Hawkey, P. M., Duncanson, V., & Flower, E. (1998). Staphylococcus aureus causing an outbreak in an orthopaedic ward at a district general hospital. *Journal of Hospital Infections, 39*(2), 127–133.

Lanphear, B. P. (1997). Transmission and control of bloodborne viral hepatitis in health care workers. *Occupational Medicine, 12*(4), 717–730.

Larson, E., Friedman, C., Cohran, J., Treston-Aurand, J., & Green, S. (1997). Issues in infection control: Prevalence and correlates of skin damage on the hands of nurses. *Heart and Lung: Journal of Acute and Critical Care, 26*(5), 404–412.

Louther, J., Rivera, P., Feldman, J., Villa, N., DeHovitz, J., & Sepkowitz, K. A. (1997). Risk of tuberculin conversion according to occupation among health care workers at a New York City hospital. *American Journal of Respiratory and Critical Care Medicine, 156*(1), 201–205.

McKenna, M. T., Hutton, M., Cauthen, G. & Onorato, I. M. (1996). The association between occupation and tuberculosis: A population-based survey. *American Journal of Respiratory and Critical Care Medicine, 154*(3, Pt. 1), 587–593.

Meredith, S., Watson, J. M., & Citron, K. M. (1996). Are healthcare workers in England and Wales at increased risk of tuberculosis? *British Medical Journal, 313*(7056), 522–525.

Mills, R. H. (1998, November). *The use of serum based laboratory values in the management of dysphagia.* A paper presented to the annual convention of the American Speech-Language-Hearing Association, San Antonio.

Miyajima, I., Sata, M., Murashima, S., Suzuki, H., Kondo, S., Ito, Y., Kawano, H., & Tanikawa, K. (1997). Prevalence of hepatitis C antibodies in health care personnel. *Kansenshogaku-Zasshi, 71*(2), 103–107.

Noble, W. C., Virani, Z., & Cree, R. G. A. (1992). Co-transfer of vancomycin and other resistance genes from Entercoccus faecalis NCT 12201 to Staphylococcus aureus. *FEMS Microbiology Letters, 93,* 195–198.

Occupational Safety and Health Administration. (1983, November). *Hepatitis risks in the health care system* (OSHA Instruction CPL 2–2.36). Washington, DC: Author.

Palmer, D. L., Barash, M., King, R., & Neil, F. (1983). Hepatitis among hospital employees. *Western Journal of Medicine, 138,* 519–523.

Schwartzman, K., Loo, V., Pasztor, J., & Menzies, D. (1996). Tuberculosis infection among health care workers in Montreal. *American Journal of Respiratory and Critical Care Medicine, 154*(4, Pt. 1), 1006–1012.

Stroffolini, T., Chiaramonte, M., Ngatchu, T., Rapicetta, M., Sarrecchia, B., Chionne, P., Lantum, D., & Naccarato, R. (1991). A high degree of exposure to hepatitis A virus infection in urban children in Cameroon. *Microbiologica, 14*(3), 199–203.

Vlahov, D., & Polk, B. F. (1987). Transmission of human immunodeficiency virus within the health care setting. *Occupational Medicine: State of the Art Reviews, 2,* 429–450.

Wichelhaus, T. A., Westphal, K., Kessler, P., Schafer, V., & Brade, V. (1998). Methicillin-resistant Staphylococcus aureus: Risk factors for infection-colonization and clonal heterogeneity in intensive care units. *Anasthesiologie Intensivemedizen Notfallmedizen Schmerzther, 33*(8), 497–500.

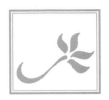

Author Index

Subject Index

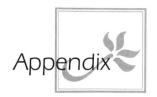

Appendix

Color Photos for Chapter 5: Endoscopic Views During the Fiberoptic Endoscopic Examination of Swallowing (FEES)

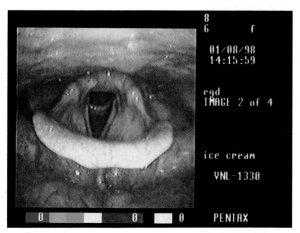

Figure A.1. View of the larynx when the endoscope is positioned just above the tip of the epiglottis.

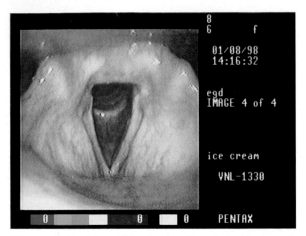

Figure A.2. View of the larynx when the endoscope is positioned over the laryngeal surface of the epiglottis.

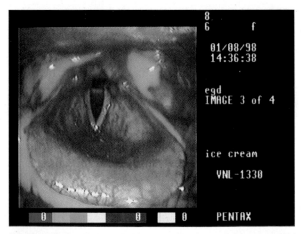

Figure A.3. Spillage of liquid (milk) around the laryngeal vestibule to the pyriform sinuses. Note that airway is open.